Materials and Components

of Interior Architecture

- -

Seventh Edition

J. Rosemary Riggs

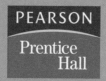

PEARSON

Prentice
Hall

Upper Saddle River, New Jersey 07458

Library of Congress Cataloging-in-Publication Data

Riggs, J. Rosemary.
  Materials and components of interior architecture / J. Rosemary Riggs. – 6th ed.
    p. cm.
  Includes bibliographical references and index.
  ISBN 978-0-13-158704-5 (alk. paper)
  1. Building materials. 2. Household appliances. 3. Plumbing–Equipment and supplies.
    4. Interior decoration. I. Title.
  TA403.R525 2007
  698–dc22

                                                        2007015968

Editor-in-Chief: Vernon R. Anthony
Acqusitions Editor: Jill Jones-Renger
Production Editor: Val Heffernan, Carlisle Publishing Services
Production Liaison: Janice Stangel
Manufacturing Manager: Ilene Sanford
Manufacturing Buyer: Cathleen Petersen
Managing Editor: Mary Carnis
Senior Marketing Manager: Leigh Ann Sims
Senior Marketing Coordinator: Alicia Dysert
Marketing Assistant: Les Roberts
Senior Design Coordinator: Miguel Ortiz
Cover Designer: Wanda Espana
Cover image: Richard Perry © 2004
Printer: RR Donnelley/Willard
Cover Printer: Coral Graphics

This book was set in New Aster by Carlisle Publishing Services. and was printed and bound by RR Donnelley Williard Company. The cover was printed by Coral Graphics

Pearson Education Ltd.
Pearson Education Singapore, Pte. Ltd.
Pearson Education Canada, Ltd.
Pearson Education—Japan
Pearson Education Australia PTY, Limited

Pearson Education North Asia Ltd.
Pearson Educación de Mexico, S.A. de C.V.
Pearson Education Malaysia, Pte. Ltd.
Pearson Education, Upper Saddle River, New Jersey

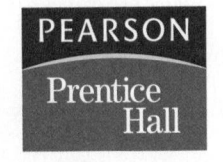

10 9 8 7 6 5 4 3 2 1
ISBN-13: 978-0-13-158704-5
ISBN-10: 0-13-158704-8

Contents

Foreword

What constitutes good design? This age-old question, when considered from a purely aesthetic viewpoint, can generate as many subjective responses as the number of individuals who answer it. When considered from a more objective perspective, however, a respondent might argue that a designed environment is good only when it delivers value by satisfying its end users' requirements. In other words, good design is what satisfies the needs of the people for whom the design is intended— whether it's the design of a product, a single room or an entire home, a conference room or a corporate headquarters, a trade show exhibit, even a university curriculum or a book's contents. It doesn't make a lot of difference how exceptional a design might appear; if it doesn't perform well, then it just isn't good design.

The Environment Group's Cary Johnson, FIIDA, argues that today's public expects, demands, and appreciates good design. "All one has to do is open the colorful advertising flyer for Target department stores to realize that our society has been exposed to and grabbed on to the notion of good design for everyone," he says. Indeed, gone are the days when cookie-cutter design ideas satisfy; design clients today want out-of-the-box thinking and innovative solutions that are custom-tailored to their own particular styles of working and living. More and more, they are also demanding solutions that are environmentally responsible, especially as the long-term, tangible benefits of sustainable design and building practices are more fully realized. Designers and architects, in particular, have a great potential to protect the earth's natural environment, as they are the ones responsible for the majority of the world's built environments.

A plethora of products and materials, many of which are explored in this latest edition of *Materials and Components of Interior Architecture*, comprise the tools with which designers create stellar interiors. A comprehensive understanding of the information presented here is essential for any practitioner to achieve success. For it is the functionality of the individual elements within an environment that impacts the performance of the space as a whole—elements that must be carefully researched and specified, as well as properly installed, in order to achieve the desired results.

The well-known sustainable design architect William A. McDonough, FAIA, has often said, "Design is the first signal of human intention." If it is your intent to bring to every project the full scope of your abilities and passion for your work, then this book is an invaluable resource to take with you on your journey. Just as creative thinking is the hallmark of the architecture and design field, knowledge and research are the foundations upon which creativity proves its worth.

Katie Sosnowchik
Co-author Sustainable Commercial Interiors

Preface

While teaching an introductory course in interior design, I noticed that the students usually chose paint or wallpaper for the walls and always used carpet on the floor, as though these were the only suitable treatments for walls and floors. I felt a need to break the cycle by exposing students to the fascinating world of materials—and so this book started to take shape.

I was unable to find a book that fully covered the exciting nonstructural materials available to the interior designer. Some authors concentrated on historical aspects of the home, both in architecture and furniture. Some emphasized upholstered furniture, draperies, and carpets; others stressed the principles and elements of design and color and the aesthetic values that make up a home. No one, however, concentrated on the "nuts and bolts" of interior design. Some books purporting to cover all types of flooring did not even mention wood floors, whereas others had only one or two paragraphs on the subject. In the fourth edition of this text, a chapter on environmental design was added, and the seventh edition has increased information on products that are environmentally sustainable. Throughout this edition, for those particularly interested in environmental concerns, products and manufacturers are mentioned that are participating in some way in the recycling process. (See Chapter 1, "Environmental Concerns.") Chapter 1 should be of prime interest to those designers (most of us) who believe that the environment is precious and worth saving. Environmental responsibility and recycling are also ways to help cope with the growing landfill problems. In researching material for the "Environmental Concerns" chapter, a representative from a very environmentally conscious company said that because she spends each day working on this problem, it has become a habit in her personal life and in the lives of other coworkers. This, of course, is the aim of the chapter. Listed at the end of the chapter are some of the companies that are helping our environment, sometimes to their financial betterment, but not always.

In the past, the interior design profession dealt mainly with the more decorative aspects of design. Today it has become increasingly necessary for interior designers to be knowledgeable not only about the finishing materials used in the design field, but also about some structural materials as well. Many interior designers are working, for or with architects, so it is important that they understand the properties and uses of all materials—thus, the *raison d'être* of this textbook. Together with the properties of materials, I also feel that students should know the historical background of the materials, as in the case of marble and the construction of wallcoverings. In the latter case, there is a considerable cost difference between various wallcoverings, and much of that difference is due to the methods of printing and the backing used. Knowledge of quality construction will help to convince clients to use the more expensive (better-made) product. The section on wallcoverings includes background information on this subject supplied by the Wallcovering Organization.

In the case of decorative laminate, I found some interesting historical background and also current uses. For example, the old "Woodie" stationwagon used laminate for the imitation wood on its sides, and today most bowling alleys are surfaced with decorative laminate. The interiors of pleasure boats are often manufactured with laminate because of the product's durability, ease of maintenance, and resistance to salt. Also included is some background on the beginnings of Jacuzzi and Moen.

Most sales representatives realize that the interior design student of today is the customer of tomorrow, but some still do not understand the scope of the interior design field. Many interior designers are women, and I have found that the ability to talk knowledgeably about materials earns the respect of both men and women in the profession.

Installation methods are discussed in this book because some contractors (luckily only a few) will use the cheapest method of installation, one that may not be the best for that particular job. Installation methods have been taken from information provided by manufacturers, associations, and institutions involved with that product. Knowledge of the correct installation procedures ensures a properly installed project. The Instructor's Manual provides many real-world examples of problems with products that have been improperly installed, and some installation problems are mentioned in this seventh edition. Your instructor will probably describe some of his or her own experiences. In researching material for this edition, I read in technical journals of various problems, such as yellowing in carpet, moisture in concrete slabs, and discoloration in vinyl flooring. Awareness of a potential problem before it occurs can prevent headaches in the future.

Maintenance information on many materials has also been included, because the cost of maintenance should be one of the deciding factors in product selection. What may be an inexpensive material at first may be the most expensive over time because of high maintenance costs.

Most of the world uses the metric system, and because the U.S. government has stressed the importance of a transition to the metric system, designers will find increasing use of millimeters, meters, grams, and kilograms as measurements for length and weight. The wallcovering industry has already converted to metric or European measurements. Some manufacturers, particularly those who sell to Canada and other foreign countries, now list their products in two systems, inches and metric. Handy conversion tables of most of the measurements used in interior design are provided at the end of the book.

In doing my research and talking to many manufacturers, I have found a growing awareness of customers' needs and wishes. Dependability is one thing the consumer requires, whether for a private home or a large commercial installation. Thus, many manufacturers offer warranties (e.g., one manufacturer offers a lifetime structural guarantee on its wood floor).

All disciplines have their own jargon. To communicate properly with contractors and architects, a designer must understand their jargon. Designers or prospective builders who have read and studied *Materials and Components of Interior Architecture* will be able to talk knowledgeably with architects and contractors about the uses of materials and their methods of installation. This understanding will also enable designers to decide for themselves which materials and methods are best for a given installation and avoid being influenced by the bias of salespeople.

One note about the spelling of *moulding:* The Architectural Woodwork Institute uses this spelling, and the term is spelled this way in Canada, where this textbook is also used. The dictionary I consulted has both spellings. To be consistent I have used *moulding* throughout this book, as some companies even have that spelling in their corporate name.

The growth of the Internet between the writing of the sixth and seventh editions is phenomenal, to such a degree that I have eliminated the two appendices from this current edition. Any question that a student has about products can easily be answered by using the Internet, and the information found will be up to date. There are so many changes in the names and ownership of companies that it is impossible nowadays to keep pace.

In selecting products to mention, I have selected those that advertise in *Interior Design Magazine* and *Interiors & Sources,* especially in the *I & S Buyer's Guides.* I am also on the e-mail list of many companies who send me information about their latest products as soon as they appear on the market. Products that have received awards are also a good source of new and well-designed materials.

This book can serve as a reference for designers who are already practicing, because it brings to their attention new materials on the market and improvements in current products, many of which have won awards in 2006. Wherever possible, generic information has been used; however, when a product is unique to one manufacturer, that manufacturer's product has been used. A contractor who read this book told me that contractors would also benefit from using it as a reference tool.

In arranging the subject matter, I placed the chapter on environmental concerns first, because all chapters on materials stress environmental concerns. The chapter on paint follows because all types of surfaces—floors, walls, and ceilings—may be painted. In this seventh edition I have also included wallcoverings in the paint chapter, as they are generally sold in paint stores. Then, starting from the bottom, the logical progression is a chapter on carpets, Chapter 3 (carpet is the most common floor covering). Chapter 4 deals with all the other types of materials available for floors.

One comment on ceramic tile is needed here. Spain is the largest producer of ceramic tile, with Italy and Brazil also being large producers. However, I have not mentioned manufacturers of imported tile because the scope of imported tile is too large. Students should be aware that many companies carrying ceramic tile also display imported tile, which can be ordered. Delivery may not be quite as easy as for domestically produced tile.

Many of the same materials used for flooring are also discussed in Chapter 5, but this time they are used on walls; the installation, finish, and maintenance vary, of course. Chapter 6 covers ceilings, areas that are usually either painted or ignored. Chapter 7 discusses all the other components that make up a well-designed room, including mouldings, doors, hardware, and hinges.

Chapter 8 explains the construction, structure, and design of fine cabinetry and could not have been written without the assistance of the Architectural Woodwork Institute. I am not suggesting that students are going to construct cabinets themselves, but they should be able to distinguish between good and bad construction and know what to look for. (The information presented in Chapter 8 also will come in handy for inspecting ready-made furniture because cabinets and furniture are constructed similarly.) Study of Chapter 8 will enable designers to provide rough drawings of cabinetry that is as economical as possible to construct. *Architectural Woodwork Quality Standards*, 8th edition, version 2.0 (2006) should be consulted for precise drawings.

Chapter 9 discusses kitchens. With the background of the previous chapter, Chapter 9 enables a designer to make an intelligent selection of the appropriate cabinetry. Chapter 9 also covers the various appliances and the newest innovations in kitchen design. Chapter 10 describes bathrooms, both residential and institutional. One comment about glass shower doors. The author was building a new home and ordered a glass shower door. The salesman asked, "Where do you live?" which points to how building codes may differ even within one county. Chapters 9 and 10 were included because designers will be called on frequently to assist in the renovation of homes—including the very expensive areas of kitchens and bathrooms. These remodeling jobs will probably cost about 10 to 15 percent of the house value. A full bath added to an older three-bedroom, one-bath house will not only guarantee recouping the cost of the improvements but will also increase resale value.

A glossary of words boldfaced in the text appears at the end of each chapter. It can be used as an aid for students studying for exams. While compiling the index for this book, I realized that it can also be an aid in preparing for comprehensive exams, such as a final or the National Council for Interior Design Qualification (NCIDQ) exam. Thus in the index, I have listed, in parentheses, all the words in the chapter glossaries. I have done this for two reasons: First, the page number enables users to find the word (the usual purpose of an index); second, students can test themselves on whether they are familiar with the word and its meaning.

If one manufacturer seems to be given more emphasis than another, it is not necessarily because its product is better than others on the market, but because the manufacturer has been extremely helpful (e.g., providing information and brochures, checking sections for accuracy, and, most important, providing photographs with which to illustrate the various sections). The photographs should not be glossed over as merely interesting illustrations but should be examined in detail as to how and where the material is used and what ambience it creates.

On the subject of photographs, this is the first edition printed all in color, thanks to a persistent editor.

I am indebted to the many manufacturers and trade organizations that have so willingly sent me technical information, from which I have compiled up-to-date data. There are several associations that I wish to mention here who have allowed me to copy drawings and descriptions verbatim. Sherwin-Williams permitted me to use its training manual, which had easier-to-comprehend definitions than the ones in previous editions. Sherwin-Williams also proofread the paint section. Thank you. The Wallcovering Association provided definitions for the various types of wallcovering. The Carpet and Rug Institute provided extensive information and granted permission to quote from its informative book, *Specifier's Handbook*. This handbook has been the basis for much of the information contained in Chapter 3. The National Oak Flooring Manufacturers Association (NOFMA) provides industry-wide standards for wood flooring installation. The Marble Institute of America reviewed the section on marble floors and walls, while the Tile Council of North America, the authority for all types of hard materials for floors and walls, provided the installation information for those materials. The Architectural Woodwork Institute supplied the information for Chapter 5, "Walls," and also for Chapter 8, "Cabinet Construction." Each of these associations is the recognized authority in its field. Thank you all for your help.

This textbook is a compilation of facts gathered with the help of high-speed Internet. I have tried to keep personal bias down to a minimum, but some may have crept in due to personal contact when building several houses for our own use. Many professionals also helped me ensure the accuracy and relevance of information presented in this text. Robert Hanks of Bridgepoint Corporation realized that proper maintenance is vital to the durability of carpet, and Zach James of Sherwin-Williams was a great help in making sure that the information in Chapter 2 was current. (There have been many technical changes in that field due to environmental controls.)

Most of all, I would like to thank my husband, sculptor Frank Riggs, for serving as a house husband and for offering his support and encouragement. He also helped with some of the line drawings in the text. I am also grateful to him for not complaining about meals served at odd times during the writing of this edition (he is getting to be a better cook with each edition). Once I get on the computer, time is irrelevant.

J. Rosemary Riggs

Introduction

For too many years, the fields of architecture and interior design have been treated as two separate disciplines involved in creating a pleasant living environment. The architect planned the exterior and interior of the home, often with little attention to where the furniture was to be placed. The interior designer had to contend with such things as walls that were not long enough to allow for placement of furniture, or heating vents placed directly under the bed or some other piece of furniture. On the other hand, designers would ruin the architect's designs by using the incorrect style of furniture, thereby spoiling the concept of the building.

Today, these problems are being resolved with many architects having interior designers on their staff, as is the case with the author of the Foreword. The result is that both disciplines cooperate from the very beginning of the project.

From the interior designer's point of view, this cooperation involves learning and appreciating the language and problems associated with architecture. The American Institute of Architects (AIA) is the professional organization for architects; the American Society of Interior Designers (ASID) and the International Interior Design Association (IIDA) are the professional organizations for interior designers. It is because of the professionalism of these organizations that the fields of architecture and interior design have gradually become aware of the need for closer cooperation. This book is dedicated to fostering that cooperation.

Trademarks

180 Walls is a trademark of Milliken & Company

3M is a trademark of the 3M Co.

A Lifetime of Pleasure is a registered trademark of Sussman Lifestyle Group

Accupro is a trademark of Jacuzzi

Add-a-Space is a trademark of Whirlpool

Advantium is a registered trademark of GE Corp.

Aged Woods is the registered trademark of Yesteryear Floorworks Co.

Allegro is a trademark of the Sussman Lifestyle Group

AlphaSorb™

Alpha base is a trademark of Roppe Corporation USA

Alumide is a registered trademark of Harris Tarkett

Anaglypta is the registered trademark of Crown Corp. N.A.

Antron is a registered trademark of EI du Pont de Nemours and Company

Anystream is a registered trademark of Speakman Company

AnyWare is a trademark of Whirlpool

Approach is the trademark of AD-AS

AquaSurge is a trademark of Frigidaire

Aquatower is a registered trademark of GROHE America

ARGUS is a registered trademark of Pittsburg Corning

Armor is a trademark of Scuffmaster Inc.

Assurance is a trademark of Mannington Mill Corp.

Assure is a trademark of Kohler

Avonite is a registered trademark of Avonite Surfaces

Avonite Surfaces is a trademark of the product group of Aristech Acrylics LLC

BioSpec is a trademark of Mannington Commercial

Brilliance is a registered trademark of Delta Faucets

Butcher Mainstay Sundance is a registered trademark of Johnson Diversey Inc.

Butcher Sundance is a registered trademark of Johnson Diversey Inc.

Chemsurf is a registered trademark of Wilsonart International

ChroMatix is a trademark of Solutia, Inc.

Clean Sweep is a registered trademark of Armstrong

Clorox is a registered trademark of The Clorox Company

Colonial Williamsburg is a registered trademark of Colonial Williamsburg Foundation

Comfort Height is a trademark of Kohler Co.

Congoleum is a registered trademark of Congoleum Corp.

Contact is a trademark of Wilsonart International

Cool Carpet is the trademark of Bentley Prince Street

Corian is a registered trademark of of EI du Pont de Nemours and Company

Cross-Grip is a trademark of Crossville, Inc.

CurvGrid is a trademark of Chicago Metallic Corporation

cXc is a trademark of Milliken Carpet

DensArmor is a registered trademark of Georgia Pacific

Designer Series is a registered trademark of Pella Corporation

DishDrawer is a registered trademark of Fisher & Paykel

Distressed by Mother Nature, Aged by Father Time is a trademark of Yesteryear Floorworks Co.

Dual-Max is a trademark of toto USA, Inc.
Duracolor is a registered trademark of Lees Carpet, a division of Mohawk Industries Inc.

Durapalm is a registered trademark of Smith & Fong

Durasan is a registered trademark of the National Gypsum Co.

DuraTech is a registered trademark of EI du Pont de Nemours and Company

DyeNamix is a trademark of Solutia, Inc.

E-ven Heat is a trademark of Maytag Corp.

Early Warning Effect is a registered trademark of RJF International

Easy Reach Plus is a trademark of Amana

ECO surfaces is a registered trademark of Dodge-Regupol

Elkay is a registered trademark of Elkay Manufacturing Company

Elumicolor is a trademark of Lees Carpet

Energy Star is a registered trademark of EPA

ErgoAire is a registered trademark of Lees Carpet

Essentials is a registered trademark of Mannington Commercial

Etch Sealer is a trademark of Skyline Design

Europlus II is a registered trademark of Grohe America

Everest is a registered trademark of Schlage

Excelon is a registered trademark of Armstrong Floors

FAULUX is a trademark of Triarch Industries, Inc.

Fill 'n Glaze is a trademark of the 3M Company

FirstStep is a registered trademark of Lees Carpets, a division of Mohawk Industries Inc.

Flexible Whiteboard is a trademark of OMNOVA Solutions Inc.

FLUSHMATE is a registered trademark of the Sloan Valve Company

Focal Point is a registered trademark of Focal Point Architectural Products Inc.

Formula 409 is a registered trademark of Clorox

FosilGlas is a trademark of Skyline Design

Frank Lloyd Wright Collection is a trademark of Frank Lloyd Wright Foundation Taliesin West

French Curve is a trademark of Kohler Co.

French Door Bottom-Freezer is a trademark of Maytag Corp.

Fresh Start QD-30® Stain Blocking Primer 202 is a registered trademark of Benjamin Moore Inc.

Frigidaire is a registered trademark of Frigidaire

GE Profile is a trademark of GE Corp.

GE Monogram Collection is a trademark of GE Corp.

Gibraltar is a registered trademark of Wilsonart International

Glass Plus is a registered trademark of Johnson Diversey

Gold Bond is a registered trademark of National Gypsum Properties, LLC

Green Building Rating System is a registered trademark of the U.S. Building Council

GREENGUARD Environmental Institute is the trademark of the Environmental Institute

GREENGUARD INDOOR AIR QUALITY CERTIFICATION is the registered trademark of the Environmental Institute

Gridset is the registered trademark of Interface Inc.

Handmold is a registered trademark of Seneca Tiles, Inc.

Hatbox is a trademark of Kohler Co.

Hi-Impact™ Gold Bond is a trademark of National Gypsum Co.

High Flex is a registered trademark of National Gypsum Co.

High Flex® Brand Wallboard is a registened trademark of National Gypsum

HiRise is a trademark of Kohler

Historic is a trademark of Kohler

Honeywell is a registered trademark of Honeywell International (formerly BASF)

i-ceilings is a registered trademark of Armstrong World Industries

IceScapes is a registered trademark of Pittsburg Corning

iCore is a registered trademark of Mannington

In-Door-Ice is a registered trademark of Whirlpool

In Sink Erator is a registered trademark of InSinkErator, a division of Emerson

Infinity is a registered trademark of Honeywell

Ingenium is a trademark of Kohler Co.

Inspirations is a trademark of Mannington Commercial

Intersept is the registered trademark of InterfaceFLOR, LLC

Jacuzzi is a registered trademark of Jacuzzi Whirlpool

Jenn-Air is a registered trademark of the Maytag Corp.

Johnsonite is a registered trademark of Johnsonite Inc.

Kal-Kore is a registered trademark of National Gypsum Properties, LLC

Kal-Kore Hi-Impact is a registered trademark of National Gypsum Properties, LLC

KoroKlear is a registered trademark of RJF International

Koroseal is the registered trademark of RJF International

Lees Squared is a registered trademark of Lees Carpets, a division of Mohawk Industries Inc.

LifeShine is a registered trademark of Moen

Lifetime is a registered trademark of Baldwin Hardware Co.

Lincrusta is the registered trademark of Crown Corp. N.A.

LiTraCon is a trademark of LiTraCon

LoadLogic is a trademark of Whirlpool

Londeck is a registered trademark of Lonseal, Inc.

Lonseal is a registered trademark of Lonseal, Inc.

MacLock is a registered trademark of MacLock, Inc.

Marmoleum is a registered trademark of Pergo

Masonite is a registered trademark of Masonite International Corp.

MasterShower is a registered trademark of Kohler Co.

Maximum-Security Accessories is a trademark of Bobrick Washroom

MemErase is a registered trademark of OMNOVA Solutions Inc.

Metalaminates is a trademark of Wilsonart International

METALWORKS is a trademark of Armstrong World Industries

Micore is a registered trademark of U.S. Gypsum

Microban is a registered trademark of Microban International, Ltd.

Millitron is a registered trademark of Milliken Carpet

Minerali is a trademark of Oceanside Glass Tile Co.

Mold & Mildew proof is a trademark of W. Zinsser & Co. Inc.

Monarch is a trademark of Chicago Metallic

Morphosis is a registered trademark of Jacuzzi Whirlpool

Moxie is a trademark of Kohler Co.

Mr. Clean is a registered trademark of Procter & Gamble

MrSauna is a trademark of the Sussman Lifestyle Group

Natural CORK is a trademark of Natural Cork, LLC

Natural Cork Floating Floor is a trademark of Natural Cork, LLC

OPTIMA is a registered trademark of Sloan Valve

Oxygen is a registered trademark of Milliken Carpet

Parallam is a registered trademark of Trus Joist MacMillan

Parallam PSL is a registered trademark of Trus Joist Macmillan

Peacekeeper is a trademark of Kohler Co.

Peachtree is a registered trademark of Peachtree Door and Windows

Pella is the registered trademark of Pella Corporation

Pergo is a registered trademark of Pergo

Perma White is a registered trademark of ZINSSER Co., Inc.

Perma-Edge is a registered trademark of Wilsonart International

Permalight is the registered trademark of American Permalight Inc.

Pforever Warranty is a registered trademark of Price Pfister

Pinecrest is a registered trademark of Pinecrest, Inc.

Plyboo is a registered trademark of Plyboo America Inc.

PolyFox is a registered trademark of Aerojet-General Corporation

Portersept is the registered trademark of Porter Paints

Power Lite is a trademark of Kohler Co.

Powerbolt is a registered trademark of Weiser Lock Products

PreFixx is the registered trademark of OMNOVA Solutions Inc.

Premier is a trademark of Premier Bathtubs

Primus is a registered trademark of Schlage

Pro-Style is a registered trademark of the Maytag Corp.

Pro-Style is a registered trademark of the Maytag Corp.

Profile is a registered trademark of GE Corp

Proform is a registered trademark of National Gypsum Co.

ProVantage is a trademark of Pittsburg Corning

Pure Air is a registered trademark of Jacuzzi

Purist is a registered trademark of Kohler Co.

QuarryCast is a registered trademark of FormGlas

Questech is a registered trademark of Crossville Inc.

Quiet System is a trademark of Asko

Quiet-Close is a trademark of Kohler Co.

Radarange is a registered trademark of Amana

Re-Bath is a registered trademark of Re-Bath LLC

Restoration Glass is a registered trademark of Bendheim Corp.

Robern is a registered trademark of Robern

SAFE-T-FIRST is a trademark of Johnsonite

SAFESEAL is a trademark of Robern

SafeTcork Slip-Resistant Tile & Tread is a trademark of Roppe Corporation USA

SafeWalks is a trademark of Mannington Floors

Schlage is a registered trademark of Ingesoll-Rand Co

Scotch-Brite is a registered trademark of the 3M Company

Scotchgard is a registered trademark of the 3M Company

Self Lock is a registered trademark of Lees Carpets, a division of Mohawk Industries Inc.

Sheetrock is a registered trademark of the U.S. Gypsum Company

Sherwin-Williams is the registered trademark of The Sherwin-Williams Co.

Sloan is a registered trademark of Sloan Valve

SmartDispense is a trademark of GE Corp.

Solitaire is a registered trademark of Broan

Soss is a registered trademark of Universal Industrial Products

Spacemaker is a registered trademark of GE Appliances

SpeedClean is a trademark of Frigidaire

SPYRA is a registered trademark of Pittsburg Corning

Sta-Smooth is a registered trademark of National Gypsum

Steam & Sauna Connection is a registered trademark of Sussman Lifestyle Group

Step Master is a registered trademark of Armstrong

Stone Panels is a registered trademark of Stone Panels Inc.

Street Shoe XL is a registered trademark of Basic Coatings

Stride is a registered trademark of Johnson-Diversey Inc.

Swanstone is a registered trademark of the Swan Corporation

Syndecrete is the registered trademark of Syndesis Inc.

Tableau is a trademark of Kohler Co.

TacFast is a registered trademark of TacFast International Inc.

Tap-N-Lock is a trademark of Wilsonart International

Tedlar is the registered trademark EI du Pont de Nemous and Company

Teflon is a registered trademark of EI du Pont de Nemours and Company

Teragren is a trademark of Teragren LLC

Texturglas is a registered trademark of Roos International

Therapro is a trademark of Jacuzzi

Thibaut is a registered trademark of Thibaut Wallcoverings

Thinline is a trademark of Pittsburg Corning

Topshield is a trademark of Forbo Industries

TOPsiders is the registered trademark of TOPsiders Inc.

Toto is a registered trademark of toto USA, Inc.

Trivection is a registered trademark of GE Corp.

Twirl is a trademark of Kohler Co.

TyKote is a registered trademark of Basic Coatings

Ultra Silent is a registered trademark of Broan

UltraGlas is a registered trademark of Ultra Glas Inc.

Ultron is the registered trademark of Solutia, Inc.

Uni-Kal is a registered trademark of National Gypsum Properties, LLC

VariSimmer is a trademark of Viking Range

Vectra is a trademark of Johnson Diversey

Vicrtex is the registered trademark of RJF International

VISTABRIK is the registered trademark of Pittsburg Corning

VKC is a trademark of Custom Laminations, Inc.

VKC-FP is a trademark of Custom Laminations, Inc.

VSH is a trademark of Viking Range Corp.

VUE is a registered trademark of Pittsburg Corning

WarmaTowel is a registered trademark of Sussman Lifestyle Group

WaterSentry is a registered trademark of Elkay

We Preserve the Past by Giving It a Future is a registered trademark of Yesteryear Floorworks Co.

WEAR-DATED is a registered trademark of Honeywell

Whirlpool Gold Kitchen is a registered trademark of Whirlpool

Wide-by-Side is a registered trademark of the Maytag Corp.

Wilsonart is a registered trademark of Wilsonart International

Zeftron is the registered trademark of Honeywell Nylon Inc.

Zodiaq is a registered trademark of Du Pont

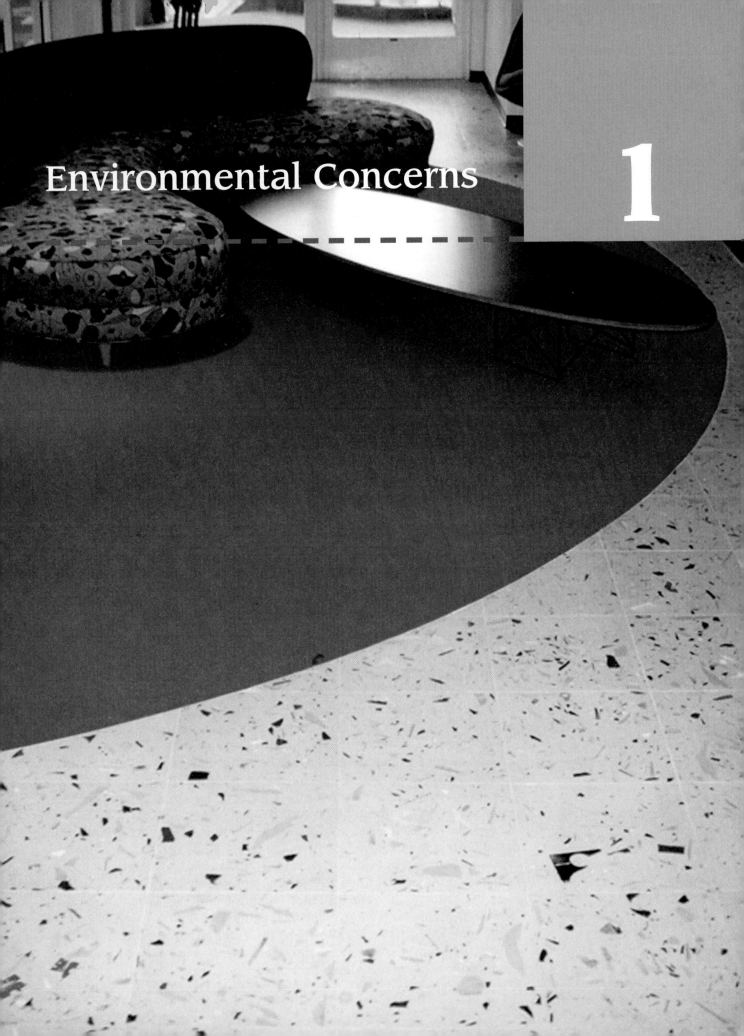

Environmental Concerns

1

The Center for Environmental Study states,

> We stand at a crossroads. For the first time in history, we face the prospect of irreversible changes in our planet's life support systems. The growing human population and the by-products of our industrial and technological society threaten our planet's air, water, climate and biodiversity. These threats present a challenge to our society—to learn to live in harmony with our planet.

The World Resources Institute defines *sustainable development* as "growth that meets economic, social, and environmental needs without compromising the future of any one of them."

Members of the design community and the manufacturers they work with can, if they wish to, lead the way in helping to save this country from overburdened landfills. This can be achieved in both the manufacturing process itself and in the disposal of products after they are no longer needed. An example would be using linoleum instead of vinyl flooring. Linoleum is a product manufactured from natural materials and will, at the end of its use, gradually biodegrade.

The Federal Trade Commission (FTC) defines "recycled content" as materials recovered or diverted from the solid waste stream, either during the manufacturing process (preconsumer) or after use (postconsumer). Scrap produced from manufacturing processes in which the end product is not for consumer use is commonly referred to as *postindustrial.*

AIR QUALITY ISSUES

The increasing awareness of indoor air quality (**IAQ**) issues and the growing incidence of sick building syndrome (**SBS**) affecting worker comfort, well-being, and productivity highlight the vital need for improved workplace air quality worldwide.

Probably the best-known examples of environmental concerns are the precautions taken when dealing with any form of asbestos. Before the mid-1980s, one of the ingredients used in the resilient flooring industry and in acoustical ceiling tiles was asbestos. This mineral has been proven injurious to health; therefore, the Resilient Floor Covering Institute (RFCI), a trade association of resilient flooring manufacturers, has developed a set of recommended work practices for the removal of resilient flooring, regardless of whether or not it contains asbestos. Following the RFCI's recommendations will ensure that the removal of an older resilient floor complies with Environmental Protection Agency (**EPA**) and Occupational Safety and Health Administration (**OSHA**) regulations regarding the handling of asbestos-containing materials, should it be determined that removal is necessary.

Asbestos is hazardous to health when it becomes "friable," or freefloating and airborne, as in a dust form. However, asbestos used in resilient flooring manufactured prior to the mid-1980s is firmly encapsulated in the product because of the manufacturing process. The EPA has determined that encapsulated, or nonfriable, asbestos-containing products are not subject to extensive regulatory requirements as long as they remain in that state. Resilient flooring, either vinyl composition tile or sheet vinyl, is nonfriable provided that it is not sanded, sawed, or reduced to a powder by hand pressure.

To ensure that any asbestos present in resilient flooring does not become dislodged and friable, the RFCI has recommended work practices that specifically prohibit sanding, dry scraping, mechanically pulverizing, or beadblasting the resilient flooring or felt backing. In other words, workers should refrain from any procedure that produces dust.

The Envirosense® Consortium, Inc. is a nonprofit membership organization that promotes a proactive approach to indoor air quality issues. Members of the Consortium include interior product manufacturers, architectural and design firms, energy and utility companies, and research and development firms and laboratories.

Members of the Consortium promote a three-part "total systems approach" to indoor air quality: building systems, product systems, and maintenance systems. In addition, members of the Consortium meet twice yearly to present case studies, updates, and research results to one another so they can assure the most up-to-date answers for customers who call for assistance.

Following is a list of those manufacturers of products covered in this textbook that are members of Envirosense Consortium, Inc.:

Bentley Prince Street—carpet
The Center for Health Design—health care
Interface Flooring Systems, Inc.—carpet
Interface Research Corporation—technical help
Re: Source—service network
Rocky Mountain Institute—energy research and consulting
Trane—air conditioning

Through its comprehensive website, Envirosense offers online newsletters, product updates, IAQ discussion areas, IAQ product profiles, e-mail directories, and access to the latest technical papers and case studies. A wealth of information is available on control of microbial sources and volatile organic compound emissions. Twelve Consortium members lend their knowledge to provide a site where interested parties can "one-stop shop" on the Internet.

Other Approaches to Environmental Issues

Many contemporary buildings are sealed environments in order to increase **HVAC** (heating, ventilating, and air conditioning) efficiency. This means that pollutants derived from such manufactured materials as synthetic fabrics, plywood, carpets, and paints are not cleared from the building. A study funded by the National Aeronautics and Space Administration (NASA) directed by Dr. B. C. Wolverton, a 20-year veteran in horticultural research, proved that the plants commonly used in interior plantscaping cleanse the air of many harmful pollutants, such as formaldehyde, benzene, and trichloroethylene. Golden pothos, philodendron, corn plants, and bamboo palms are particularly effective in cleansing the air of formaldehyde. Spathifhyllum (peace lily), dracena warneckei, and dracena "Janet Craig" remove quantities of benzene, such as is found in tobacco smoke. Marginata, warneckei, and spathiphyllum work well in removing trichloroethylene. The Plants for Clean Air Council recommends one potted plant for each 100 square foot of floor space.

"People worry so much about outdoor air, but indoor air may be a far more serious problem," said Dr. Wolverton. "This study demonstrates that plants are a natural solution to indoor air pollution—not just in future NASA space ships but in the offices and homes of today." When the air is too dry, people are susceptible to colds and flu. When the humidity is too high, people can develop other ailments. Through their natural processes of transpiration and evaporation, office plants add moisture to the dry, overheated air often found in sealed office environments. At the same time, studies show that plants do not add moisture in significant amounts when the air is already moist. A study conducted at Washington State suggested that plants help regulate humidity. When plants were added to an office environment, the relative humidity stabilized within the recommended "healthy" range of 30 to 60 percent. By using a professional plantscaping service, offices will have design uniformity throughout the workplace, plants in peak condition, and plants for correct light levels and HVAC conditions found in a particular workplace. TOPsiders® Panel Mount Planters are aesthetically correct, 6" × 6" × 24" or 30" (this size provides proper scale and proportion for open plan systems), and are easily installed and taken down. TOPsiders® have brackets for mounting on tops, sides, and corners of partitions and are available in metal or marble finishes and 13 colors. (See Figure 1.1.) Matching ROUNDZ are also available.

Companies may need to alter their HVAC systems, according to Joseph Milam of Environmental Design International, Ltd.:

FIGURE 1.1
TOPsiders® Panel Mount Planters provide scale and proportion for open plan systems and are easily installed and taken down. The TOPsiders® shown fit on top of the partitions. (Photo courtesy of TOPsiders®)

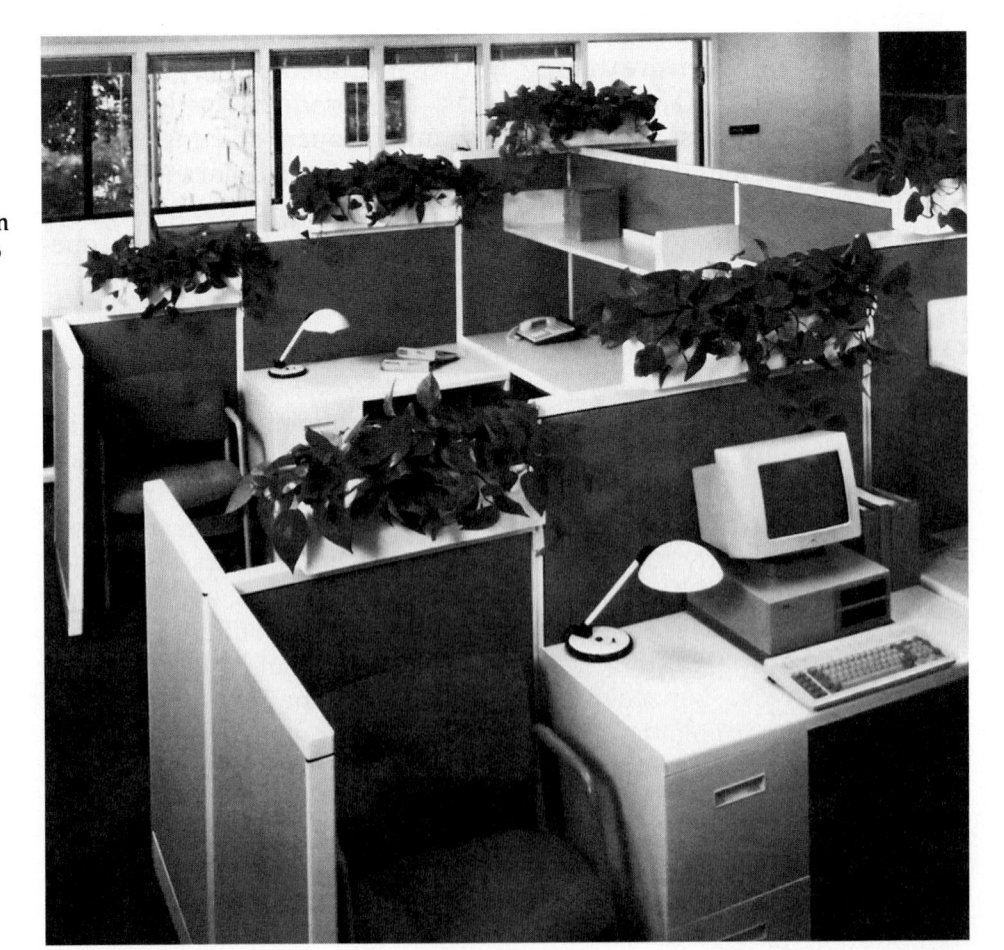

New cost cutting concepts of hoteling, telecommuting, and teaming are driving businesses to change how they configure their office space. In many cases these changes result in fitting the same number of people into less space. Older HVAC systems were designed for one person per 150 to 200 usable square feet, and a PC on every third or fourth desk. In a modern office with higher-occupant densities, the HVAC system needs to accommodate personal computers on every desk as well as more people in less space. Most mechanical systems that are seven or more years old generally provide five to 7½ cubic feet per minute (cfm) of outside air per person. Today's standards ASHRAE 62-1989 require 20 cfm per person.[1]

It is important to clarify and identify the different types of carpet recycling, so you can select a carpet that provides the most environmental benefits without sacrificing any performance requirements. *Carpet recycling* is often used as a generic term encompassing all types of recycling and reclamation of various carpet parts, including fibers and backing.

The following definitions are supplied by Honeywell Inc. at www.hfri.nist.gov:

Carpet reclamation—Typically refers to cleaning and repairing of carpet for reinstallation. The carpet is not reprocessed or remanufactured in any way; rather, it is cleaned and repaired using heavy-duty, commercial techniques.

Downcycling—A form of recycling in which carpet fibers are separated and remelted for use in low-value, noncritical, nonaesthetic plastics applications. This is the standard practice for recycling carpet fibers of nylon type 6,6. Eventually, the nylon quality is degraded to the point where it can no longer be recycled and is disposed of. Recycling PET soda bottles into carpet fibers is also a form of downcycling, since the resulting fibers are disposed of at the end of the carpet life.

Closed-loop recycling—The most sophisticated form of recycling, where carpet fibers are chemically renewed in a depolymerization process and manufactured into first-quality carpet fibers again. A true closed-loop process allows sustainable renewal of fibers over and over again without loss of any properties and without the use of a landfill. This allows maximum-value recovery of the original materials. Nylon type 6 is renewable in a true closed-loop process using new, breakthrough technology.[2]

According to the Carpet and Rug Institute,

Carpet manufacturers are striving to minimize the quantities of natural and energy resources used in day-to-day operations. They are reducing waste, reusing and recycling raw materials, packaging materials, waste, and by-products. Individual companies are pursuing environmental efforts at different points in the manufacturing process. . . . Advanced monitoring systems and processes in the mills help conserve water, electricity and other fuels. As an example, new developments in dyeing techniques require less water. Dye materials are removed from waste water; the waste water is monitored, reprocessed, and then reintroduced into the manufacturing system. New systems recycle thermal-energy, capturing, condensing, and then re-heating the water for use in the finishing of carpet. Oil waste is sold to recycling companies or is used as a boiler fuel. . . . Although more efficient manufacturing is reducing excess carpet waste, such as selvedges, trimmings, and shearings, the industry has found creative uses for carpet by-products, to avoid the use of local landfills. Individual companies are engaged in recycling efforts, including the following.

Fiber and yarn that cannot be reused in manufacturing are often sent to yarn vendors that sell them for crafts and other end uses. Excess carpet is cut into mats and sold.[3]

Similarly, "DuPont offers the Carpet Reclamation program as a service to ensure that the old carpet you remove does not go into a landfill. DuPont will take anything back regardless of origin when you purchase a new carpet of DuPont Antron®." Because of the importance of this issue, reclamation guidelines are in place.[4]

In the public interest, the Carpet and Rug Institute (CRI) has developed three IAQ testing programs that will minimize the potential of emissions from new carpet installations. The programs cover carpet, carpet cushion, and floor covering adhesive products. The goal for the programs is to help consumers with their buying decisions by identifying products that have been tested and meet stringent IAQ requirements.

In the testing programs for carpet, separate carpet cushion, and floor covering adhesives for carpet installations, samples are collected from the manufacturer's production process. Each sample is tested individually for chemical emissions by an independent laboratory, using highly sophisticated, dynamic, environmental chamber technology.

The test procedure follows an approved methodology recognized by the Environmental Protection Agency (EPA) and the American Society for Testing and Materials (ASTM D-5116). The **VOC** emissions are identified and quantified as though the products were in a real building situation. Products are retested on an on-going basis to ensure that the required emission levels are not exceeded.

The products that meet the emission criteria are allowed to display the [CRI] label [See Figure 1.2.] If the products exceed the emission criteria, the manufacturer is so advised and is requested to make process or formulation changes in order to reduce the emissions. After the appropriate product modification, the manufacturer may resubmit the product for additional testing. Products that do not meet the test criteria will not thereafter be allowed to affix the label until they meet the test program criteria . . .

In each of these programs the authorized label displayed on the product contains an identification number assigned specifically to the individual manufacturer for each product that meets the criteria.

It is also important to know that with most products, adequate ventilation can lower concentrations and minimize the impact on indoor air quality. Regular and effective cleaning also adds to good air quality.[5]

The CRI serves the industry and consumers with practical, technical, educational, and issue-related information. The CRI only deals with three

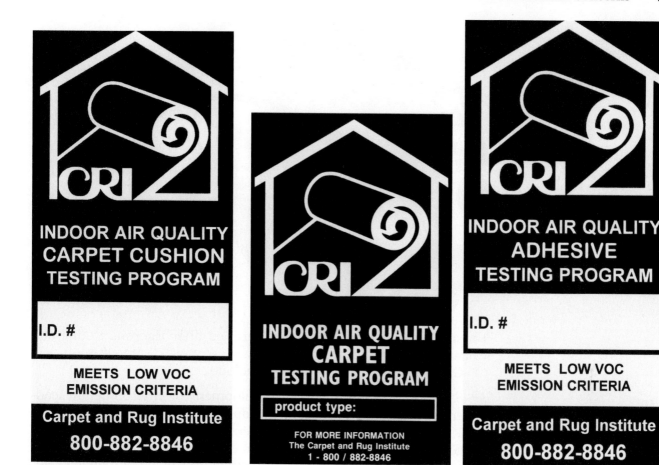

FIGURE 1.2

The three labels of the CRI Indoor Air Quality Testing Program. (Labels courtesy of the Carpet and Rug Institute, Dalton, GA)

carpet installation products. See the CRI's website (www.carpetrug.com) for more detailed information.

The carpet industry has taken many steps to ensure carpet's positive role in the indoor environment. The CRI's Indoor Air Quality Testing and Labeling Program mentioned earlier is one step. The following information, not previously covered, is condensed from *Covering the Future,* a CRI brochure. Installation guidelines for consumers and installers have been developed to maintain good indoor air quality during the installation of new carpet. With adequate air ventilation, the minimal emissions from carpet will dissipate within the first 48 to 72 hours of installation. Formaldehyde is *not* used in the manufacturing of carpet, contrary to popular belief. The industry emphasizes consistent guidelines for preventive, daily, and restorative carpet maintenance to ensure good indoor air quality.

Green Seal

Green Seal works with manufacturers, industry sectors, purchasing groups, and governments at all levels to "green" the production and purchasing chain. They utilize a life-cycle approach, which means we evaluate a product or service beginning with material extraction, continuing with manufacturing and use, and ending with recycling and disposal.

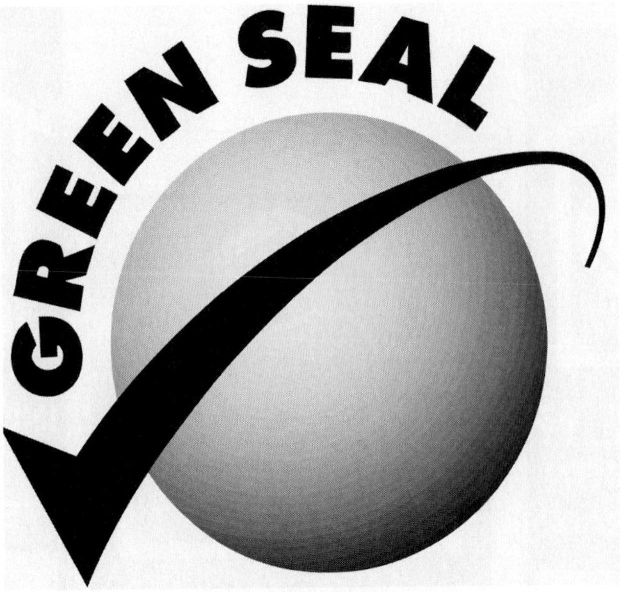

FIGURE 1.3
Green Seal emblem.
(Emblem courtesy
of Green Seal)

Products only become Green Seal certified after rigorous testing and evaluation, and including on-site visits.

Green Seal's specific programs include:

- *Standard and Certification*—development of environmental leadership standards for specific products categories and certification of products and services that meet them.
- *Greening Your Government*—technical assistance to all levels of government in their purchasing, operations, and facilities management.
- *Choose Green Reports*—technical reports on products in a variety of categories, giving specific brand recommendations of those that meet screening criteria.
- *Greening the Lodging Industry*—long-term project with hotels and motels to green their operations and purchasing, including certification of specific properties.
- *Policy*—leadership in green procurement policy (products recommendations), internations policy for ecolabeling, etc.[6]

LEED

The Leadership in Energy and Environmental Design (LEED) Green Building Rating System™ is the nationally accepted benchmark for the design, construction, and operation of high-performance green buildings. LEED gives building owners and operators the tools they need to have an immediate and measurable impact on their buildings' performance. LEED promotes a whole-building approach to sustainability by recognizing performance in five key areas of human and environmental health: sustainable site development, water savings, energy efficiency, materials selection, and indoor environmental quality.[7]

Designers will find the LEED endorsement occurring frequently when looking at materials that are environmentally friendly.

The following information is from *Interiors & Sources* magazine:

An environmentally friendly paint developed by polymer science researchers at the University of Southern Mississippi, Hattiesburg,

MS, serves the dual purpose of reducing pollutants in the atmosphere and increasing market opportunities for farmers. . . .

Within the next year, the paint will be used on approximately one-fifth of the Pentagon's interior walls. . . .

"The bottom line is this technology uses castor oil, soybean oil or lesquerella oil to allow us to make latex polymers that have wide applications. Not just paints, but inks, adhesives, carpet backings and coatings for fibers and concrete steel," said Dr. Shelby Thames, leader of the research team. "According to specifications called for by the Green Seal Society, our [paint] far exceeded their expectations in terms of the amount of volatiles in it, the odor, the washability and the scrub-resistance values. So this has now become Green Seal-certified."[8]

Gensler and Associates Architects, one of the world's largest architectural and interior design firms, is taking a stand for environmentally sound design. One example is the design of the Los Angeles offices of HBO (Home Box Office). Gensler recycled all demolished materials, including wood, paper, glass, plastics, copper, and aluminum. Recycling bins were placed on each floor of the construction area. The carpeting was laid with low-toxicity carpet adhesive, and special solution-dyed, nontoxic carpeting was installed (carpet manufacturers accelerated the **off-gassing** process before installation). The carpeting was shipped off-site and was ventilated for 48 hours with massive amounts of fresh air. Linoleum, while more expensive, was used instead of vinyl composition flooring, and low-biocide, low-fungicide paints were also used. Where possible, existing furniture and ceiling tiles were reused and repainted with **nonbridging** paint.

ENERGY STAR PROGRAM

Energy Star is a dynamic governmental/industry partnership that offers businesses and consumers energy-efficient solutions, making it easy to save money while protecting the environment for future generations. . . . The Energy Star label is now on major appliances, office equipment, lighting, home electronics, and more. EPA has also extended the label to cover new homes and commercial and industrial buildings.[9] (See Figure 1.4).

Energy Star provides a benchmarking tool for buildings (found at www.epa.govnrgystar/about.html) that allows a comparison of energy expended with those of similar organizations. The website also helps companies to purchase products with the Energy Star label.

ENVIRONMENTALLY CONCERNED COMPANIES

The following companies, which manufacture products covered in this textbook, are all involved in recycling or preserving our planet in some way. Manufacturers of similar products may also be working on environmental concerns; those who are concerned about the environment should check with other manufacturers as well.

1. Aged Woods®, a trademark of Yesteryear Floorworks Company, has the following statement regarding its product:

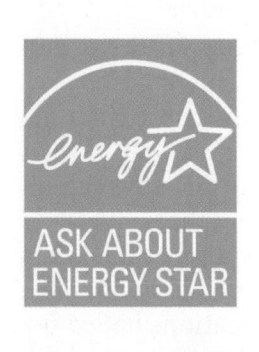

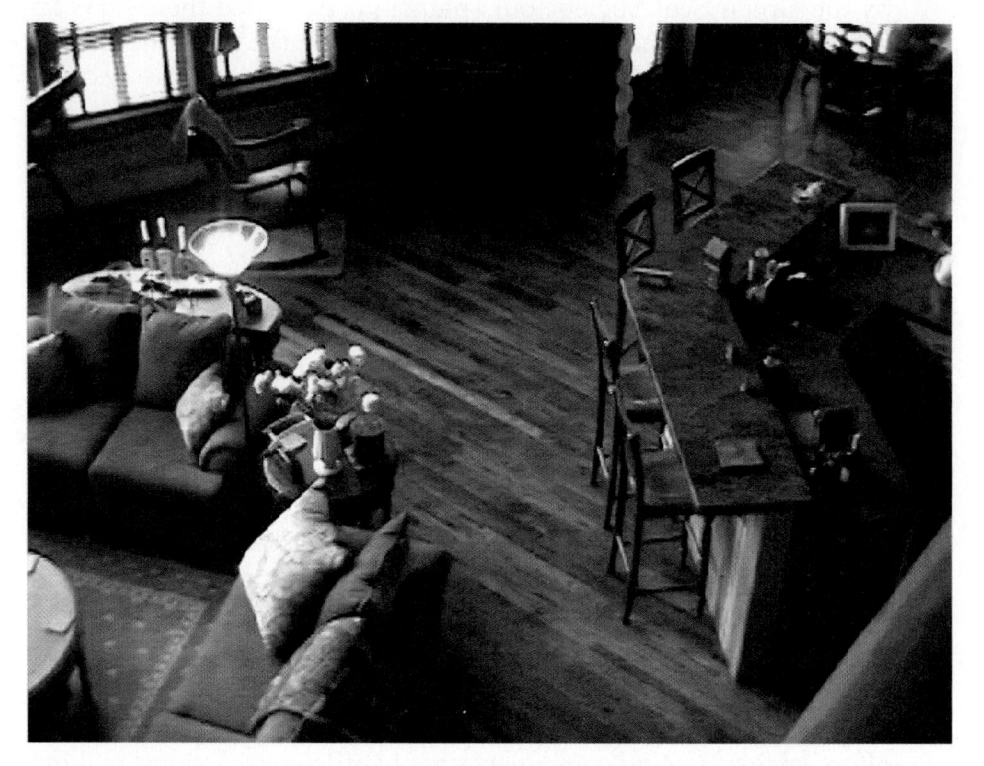

Aged Woods® brand flooring is precision-milled from old, destined-for-the-dump barn wood. Proper kiln-drying before milling assures a stable, bug-free floor. The look of these antique woods is natural resulting from a century or two of weathering and the signs of old-time craftsmen. Aged Woods® floors are warmly inviting adding the rugged feel of Early America to residences, retail stores, restaurants, casinos, country clubs, etc. The authentic rustic character is unobtainable with new wood.[10] (See Figure 1.5).

2. Avonite. Three patterns of Avonite's line are made from reclaimed solid surfaces, which contributes to the company's goal of zero waste from its manufacturing facility.

3. BASF, one of the companies supplying chemicals to make carpet, has a recycling program called 6ix Again, after the name for its nylon fiber, which is the basis of every Zeftron® nylon system. The 6ix Again program is based on the company's patented process for recycling old BASF Nylon 6ix carpet fiber into new carpet nylon. This is an innovation that for the first time allows the company to effectively reuse Nylon 6ix fiber recovered from used carpets that would have been landfilled or incinerated. Since the introduction

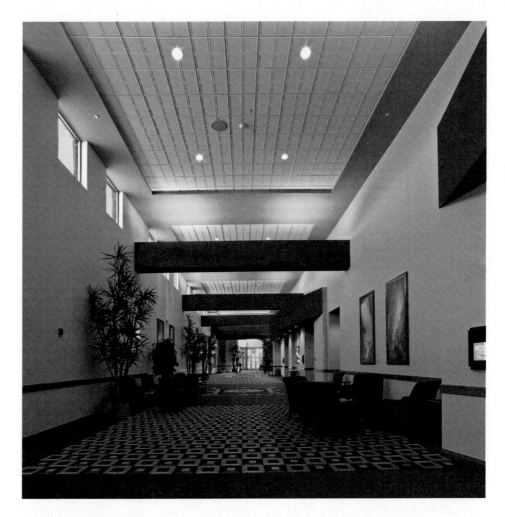

FIGURE 1.6
This EuroStone™ ceiling, in the Frisco Center Conference Center, Frisco, Texas, is a unique, nonfibrous, perlite blend, which offers the best defense against harmful mold and bacteria growth without coatings or biocides. (Photo courtesy of Chicago Metallic)

of the 6ix Again program, BASF has committed not to landfill or incinerate any BASF nylon 6ix fiber recovered from used carpets that qualities for the 6ix Again program.[11]

4. Chicago Metallic produces EuroStone™, a sustainable ceiling panel that is manufactured from expanded perlite, an inorganic material. EuroStone™ will not promote the growth of mold, **mildew,** and fungus, all of which threaten IAQ. It will not burn or contribute smoke in a fire situation. It will not warp or sag, and is dimensionally stable for the lifetime of the building.[12] (See Figure 1.6.)

5. Crossville tile has added two new colors to its Eco-Cycle series. Since reclaimed materials are used to manufacture Limestone and Pompeii Eco-Cycle tiles, the color and shade consistency may vary from production run to production run. In addition to being ecologically correct, Limestone and Pompei Eco-Cycle tiles are very affordable, yet offer all the plus features of high-fire porcelain tile: strength (it's stronger than natural stone; 30 percent harder than granite), durability (porcelain refuses to scratch, stain, or fade), and no special cleaners or sealers are required.[13]

6. ECOsurfaces™ from Dodge-Regupol is a commercial rubber flooring made from recycled tire rubber and postindustrial colored rubber.

This company converts 45 million pounds of old tires into a high-grade rubber flooring.

7. Lonseal has been awarded the GREENGUARD Environmental Institute (GEI) GREENGUARD Indoor Air Quality Certification for its GreenAir resilient flooring.

8. Syndecrete® is a restorative product consisting of reconstited of materials extracted from society's waste stream to create a new, highly valued product. The advanced cement-based composite contains natural minerals and recycled materials from industry and postconsumer goods that contain up to 41 percent recycled content. Such materials include metal shavings, plastic regrinds, recycled glass chips, and scrap wood chips, among others. These materials are used as decorative aggregates, creating a contemporary reinterpretation of the Italian tradition of terrazzo.

   Syndecrete's broad range of applications and its unique aesthetic qualities differentiate the product from other environmentally friendly building materials. The provision of custom Syndecrete products often introduces the use of recycled and environmentally friendly products to a high-end, design-oriented market segment that might not otherwise be predisposed to seek out recycled products. The company hopes that its own emphasis on the outstanding environmental qualities of Syndecrete will stimulate the growth of "environmental quality" as an important product selection criteria in the building and design industry.

   Syndecrete is an advanced cement-based composite using natural minerals and recycled materials as its primary ingredients. There are no resins or polymers. Syndecrete is a solid surfacing material that provides consistency of color, texture, and aggregate throughout. It is less than half the weight with twice the compressive strength of normal concrete and is available in a variety of densities ranging from 35 lbs to 100 lbs/c.f.

   Custom mix designs incorporating aggregates offer unlimited creative possibilities. Past uses include recycling of postconsumer and scrap materials from industry, such as plastic regrinds, wood chips, crushed glass, metal shavings, and stone fragments. Surfaces can be ground, polished, or textured to expose the natural porosity and aggregates. Form or mold surface finishes allow for exacting detail, from wood grain to glass.[14] (See Figure 1.7).

9. Tarkett has now become the first ever floor covering manufacturer to be awarded Building Research Establishment (BRE) Certification for vinyl floor covering, which recognizes the environmental credentials of its iQ homogeneous vinyls. This certification means that all the inputs and outputs from the manufacture of its products are independently verified and the effects over the whole life are measured for their environmental impact.[15]

10. Smith & Fong.

   Fast growing and long lived, our timber bamboo grows to a height of 40 feet with a diameter exceeding 6 inches and matures in 6 years. Bamboo is a grass and from an environmental standpoint, this is important. Unlike traditional hardwoods, bamboo when harvested does not require replanting. Mature bamboo has an

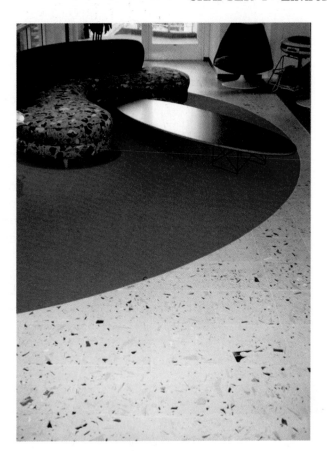

extensive root system that continues to send up new shoots for decades. Our bamboo is grown in managed forests in China. Harvesting is done by hand, minimizing the impact on the local environment. By working with bamboo and understanding its growth patterns, bamboo farmers are able to maximize timber production while maintaining healthy forests.[16]

11. Stark Carpet now has a bamboo rug. Bamboo seems to have come into its own in the last few years. It has always been used for furniture and window treatments, but is now finding applications in flooring.

12. tretford's secondary backing is made from 100 percent natural jute. "Indeed, the use of naturally renewable resources and environmentally friendly systems and processes has always been an important part of the Tretford ideal. Tretford improves the climate of your interior. Its natural fibers not only insulate to save energy, but also absorb and release moisture as the temperature and humidity change."[17]

13. UltraGlas®, Inc. All float glass in the production of UltraGlas® is composed of a minimum of 15 to 30 percent recycled glass (cullet). The company makes every effort to reuse scrap glass resulting from its manufacturing processes. UltraGlas® can detemper and reuse existing tempered glass to create new art glass, and the company is listed with local recycling agencies and local art schools to be notified when recyclable glass is available. Like most other manufacturers, all packing material used is re-

cyclable, and organic packing materials are used whenever possible.[18]

14. Wilsonart International's plant in Temple, Texas, has converted to Philips Lighting Co. brand ALTO low-mercury fluorescent lighting in its office areas. Other environmental choices made by the company include:

Recycle scrap cardboard, paper, and batteries.

Discharge no process waste to sanitary sewer.

Send flammable production waste to a fuel-to-energy process known as fuel-blending. This waste provides the energy needed to produce cement at cement kilns across the nation.

Recycle incoming steel raw material drums and complete the loop by purchasing only reconditioned steel drums for packaging of the company's own products.

Assist customers in complying with local, state, and federal regulations that apply to them by virtue of use of the company's adhesive products. This includes disposal of PVA adhesive washwater and outdated adhesives.[19]

GLOSSARY

EPA. Environmental Protection Agency.

HVAC. Heating, ventilating, and air conditioning; almost always written using the acronym.

IAQ. Indoor air quality. The result of measuring the air inside a building for toxic emissions.

mildew. Discoloration caused by fungi.

nonbridging. A paint that will not cover the small holes in acoustical tiled ceiling. See Chapter 6.

off-gassing. The process by which toxic fumes are emitted from carpet when it is newly laid.

OSHA. Occupational Safety and Health Administration.

SBS. Sick building syndrome. The symptoms of an illness caused by toxic emissions inside a building.

NOTES

[1]Joseph Milam, Principal at EDI Ltd. Consulting Engineers.

[2]Honeywell Inc. website, www.honeywell.com.

[3]Carpet and Rug Institute website, www.carpet-rug.com.

[4]Du Pont website, www.dupont.com.

[5]Carpet and Rug Institute website, www.carpet-rug.com.

[6]Green Seal website, www.greenseal.org.

[7]LEED website, www.leed.org.

[8]*Interior & Sources*, June 2001, p. 23.

[9]Energy Star website, www.energystar.gov.

[10]Aged Woods website, www.agedwoods.com.

[11]Zeftron website, www.infinitynylon.com.

[12]Chicago Metallic website, www.chicagometallic.com.

[13]Crossville website, www.crossvilleinc.com.

[14]Syndecrete website, www.syndesis.com.

[15]Tarkett website, www.tarkett-commercial.com.

[16]Smith & Fong website, www.plyboo.com.

[17]Tretford website, www.tretfordusa.com.

[18]UltraGlas website, www.ultraglas.com.

[19]Wilsonart International website, www.wilsonart.com.

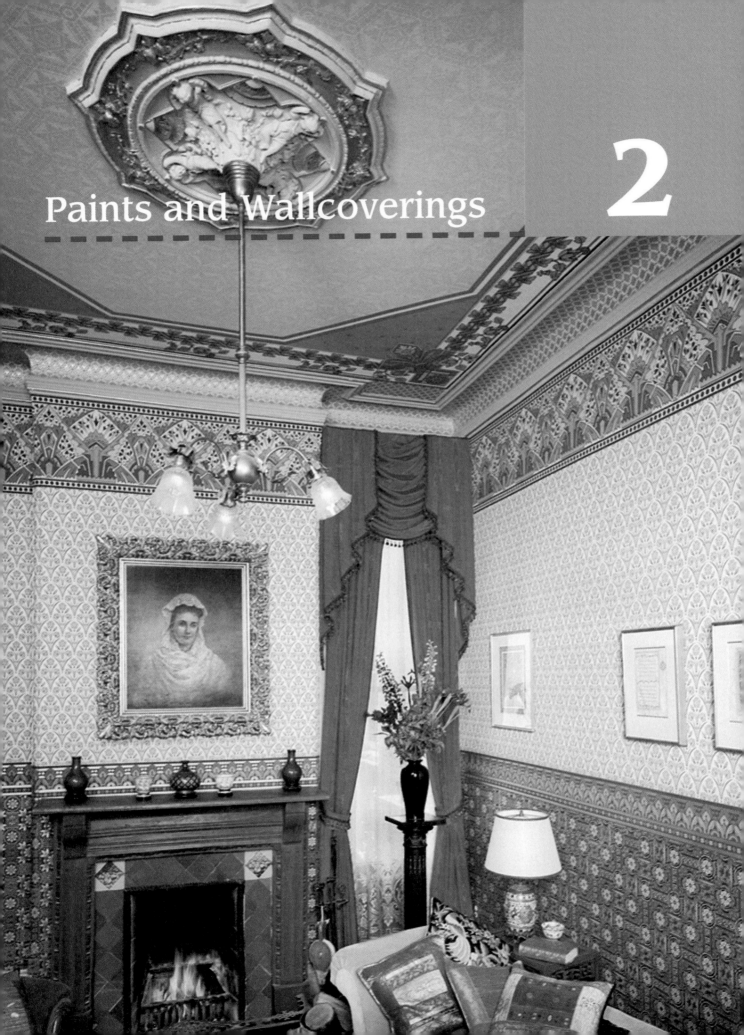

Paints and Wallcoverings

2

Paint—the group of emulsions generally consisting of pigments suspended in a liquid medium for use as decorative or protective coatings—made its earliest appearance about 30,000 years ago. Cave dwellers used crude paints to leave behind the graphic representations of their lives that even today decorate the walls of their ancient rock dwellings.[1]

The earliest known paintings were found in the Lascaux caves in France and in the Altamira cave in Spain and date from as early as 15,000 B.C. A thousand years later the Egyptians were making colors from soil and importing dyes such as indigo and madder. To this they added materials that are sometime found in paints used by artists: **gum** arabic, egg white, gelatin, and beeswax. The Egyptians also developed varnish from gum arabic around 1000 B.C.

It is only since 1867 that prepared paints have been available on the American market. Originally, paint was used merely to decorate a home, as in the frescoes at Pompeii, and it is still used for that purpose today. Modern technology, however, has now made paint both a decorative and a protective finish.

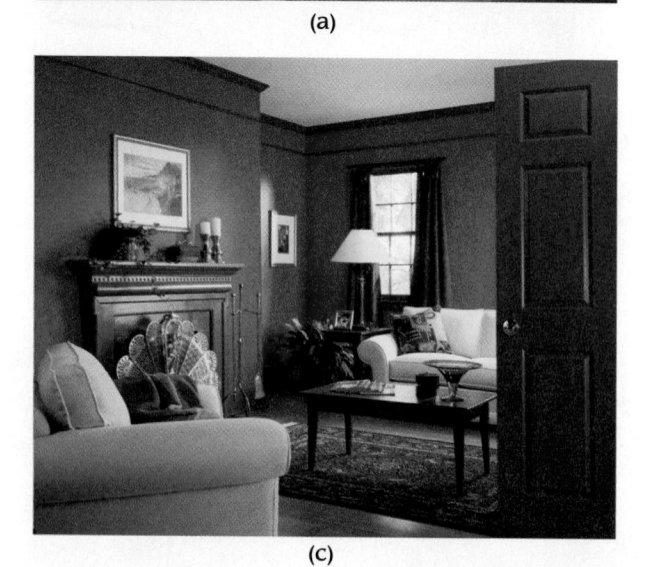

(a)

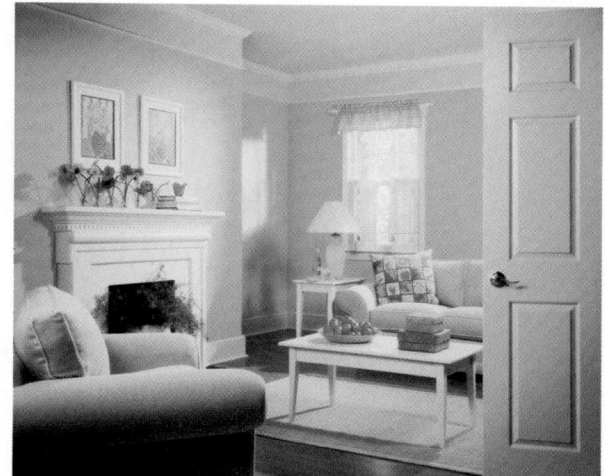

(b)

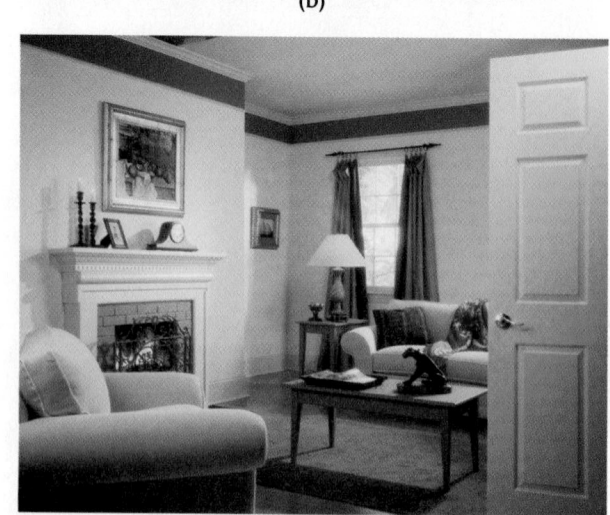

(c)

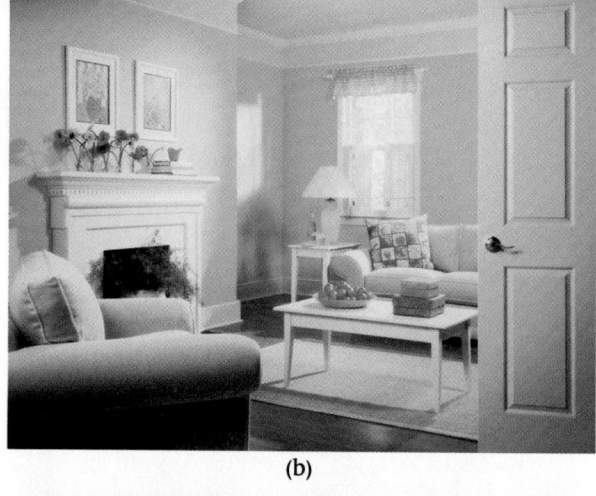

(d)

FIGURE 2.1

(a) The grey-blue gives a cool, neutral background. (b) The green room has a cool ambience. (c) These vibrant colors give an active feeling to the room. (d) Yellow prorides a warm, cheery atmosphere. (Photos courtesy of the Glidden Company)

The colors used are also of great psychological importance. A study by Johns Hopkins University showed that planned color environments greatly improved scholastic achievement. Most major paint companies now have color consultants who can work with designers on selection of colors for schools, hospitals, and other commercial and industrial buildings. Today, paint is the most inexpensive method of changing the environment. (See Figure 2.1).

Paint is commonly defined as a substance that can be put on a surface to make a film, whether white, black, or colored. This definition has now been expanded to include clear films.

COMPONENTS OF PAINTS

Household paints have not included any lead since its use was banned by the Consumer Product Safety Commission in 1978.[2] The four basic ingredients of coating ingredients are:

- **Pigments,** which give color to the coating.
- **Binders,** which act like glue to hold the pigment particles together and provide washability/scrubbability, chemical resistance, durability, and other properties.
- **Solvents,** which make the coating wet enough to spread on the surface.
- **Additives,** which perform special functions.

A typical coating product contains some or all of these ingredients.[3] (See Figure 2.2.)

Pigments

Pigments consist of powdered **solids** (such as *titanium oxides* and *silicates*) that give the coating its color and brightness qualities. These solids are important not only for their color, but also for their hiding ability. Generally speaking, the more pigment

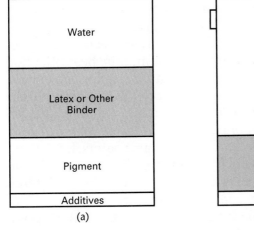
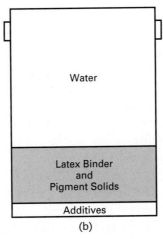
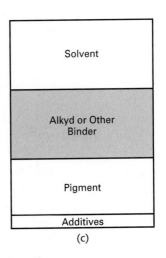

FIGURE 2.2

Components of paint. Ingredients in (a) quality latex paint, (b) low-cost latex paint, and (c) quality alkyd paint. (Drawings courtesy of *Builder's Guide to Paints and Coatings,* NAHB Research Center)

contained in a coating, the better it will hide, or obscure, the surface. [emphasis added][4]

Different pigments have different purposes. **Titanium dioxide** is the best white pigment **hiding power. Extender** pigments, such as **calcium carbonate,** are inert. Masonry paints have a larger percentage of calcium carbonate than other paints. In flat paints, extenders improve sheen, uniformity, and touch-up capability. In "eggshell" and semigloss paints they affect **gloss.**

Binders

Binders are liquid adhesives (such as **alkyd, resin,** latex, and **urethane**) that form a film of pigment particles on the surface. These sticky resins and other adhesives are the **vehicle** for binding the pigments to the surface, creating a strong and durable bond. Thus, the strength of the binder contributes to the useful life of the coating. [emphasis added][5]

Paints are generally classified as either solvent based or water based. Water-based coatings are usually called *latex*, and drying occurs when the water evaporates. Alkyds are coatings produced by reacting a drying oil with an alcohol. Drying of the surface occurs by the evaporation of the solvent; curing of the resin occurs by oxidation.

Solvents

Solvents are liquids (such as water and mineral spirits) that make the product easier to apply. Sometimes called thinners, solvents "carry" the other ingredients over the surface. Without solvents, the paint would be thick as molasses. The solvent helps the coating to penetrate the surface and then evaporates as the coating dries.[6]

Solvent-containing coatings can be used safely if overexposure is avoided and proper protective equipment is used. The disposal of all types of coating materials is controlled by government regulations. Benjamin Moore has some useful tips for dealing with and disposing of leftover paint. For example, do not order more paint than is needed. Use all the paint you buy—an extra coat will give more protection. Leftover paint can always be donated to a local charity, community beautification or service program, or neighborhood group that is assisting the elderly, disabled, or disadvantaged with the maintenance of their homes. Make sure the product you donate is in its original container with the label left intact. *Leftover paint should not be poured down the drain—neither household sinks, toilets, nor storm sewers.* To dispose of latex paints, leave them to dry completely by removing the lid and allowing the water portion to evaporate. This should be done in an area that is away from children and animals. In most states, the container can then be disposed of in your household trash. Leave the lid off the can so that the disposal hauler can see that the paint is hardened. For disposal of solvent-based paints (alkyds or oil-based paints), contact the local or state government environmental control agency for disposal guidance.

Additives

Additives are special purpose ingredients (such as thickeners and mildewcides) that give the product extra performance features. For example, mildewcides reduce mildew problems, and thickeners lengthen the drying time for application in hot weather.

The combination of these basic four ingredients is what creates a particular type and quality of coating.[7]

Mildew is a fungus that thrives in good growing conditions—an environment having food, moisture, and warmth. Mildew is a major cause of paint failure. Several mildew-cleaning solutions are available, the simplest of which is bleach and water.

Portersept® paints include chemicals called *mildewcides* that prohibit the growth of mildew on the paint film. Mildewcides slowly leach out of the paint to the surface and maintain their inhibition properties for many years. Portersept® is an EPA-registered antimicrobial and is guaranteed for a minimum of seven years.

To comply with the VOC emissions laws, more solids are being added, which makes the paint heavier bodied; and, therefore, it may take longer to dry. In many areas of the United States, the amount of VOC, expressed in pounds of VOC per gallon, is restricted. (See Figure 2.2.)

SOLVENT-BASED PAINT

Solvent-based paints use a petroleum derivative (e.g., mineral spirits) as the solvent. Alkyds and oils are often used as the binder in solvent-based paints. Some people refer to a paint by its binder, such as "oil" paint.

Solvent-based paints form a film through evaporation of the solvent and **oxidation** of the resins. Solvent-based paints take longer to dry, because the solvent takes between 24 and 48 hours to evaporate. [emphasis added][8]

Alkyds are coatings produced by reacting a drying oil acid with an alcohol. Drying of the surface occurs by the evaporation of a solvent; curing of the resin occurs by oxidation. The more oil the formula contains, the longer it takes to dry, the better the wetting properties, and the better the elasticity.

WATER-BASED PAINT

Water-based paints use water to make the paint easier to spread. Latex, **acrylic** latex, and vinyl acrylic are common binders found in water-based paints. When these paints are applied to a surface, the water evaporates and individual resin particles become closely packed together. These resins unite to bind the pigment particles into a continuous film. . . . Water-based paints dry when the water has evaporated, usually within four hours after application. [emphasis added][9]

Water-based latex paints adapt well to changing weather conditions. Microscopic pores allow water vapor to pass through the dried latex paint film. Because of this "breathing" ability, moisture is less likely to build up between the paint and the surface.

> Water-based paints are a good choice for someone who is having trouble with peeling paint. . . . Customers still need to eliminate the cause of the peeling, but they stand a much better chance of getting the long-lasting coating if they use a water-based paint such as latex.[10]

A note of interest about latex:

> Latex paint is not made with latex rubber; in fact the name "latex" is really just a decorative way to describe rubber-based paint. Latex paint is a carefully formulated polyvinyl material with acrylic resin and has never contained natural rubber. It is natural rubber that causes an allergic reaction. So people who have sensitivity to latex products are in no danger of having a reaction to latex paint.[11]

STAIN

Stains are coatings that also contain all four ingredients, but use a unique binder. The binder in stains causes the coating to penetrate deeply into the surface, leaving a thinner film on top. This extra-thin film allows the natural form of the surface to show through.

In addition to producing a thin film, stains have a low content of binder and pigment solids (in some cases as low as 14 percent) which results in a shorter life of the coating. Even so, stains are widely used on wood and other surfaces to show some of their natural beauty. Stains may be used for both interior and exterior applications. They are classified as either solid color or semitransparent.

- Solid color stain permits the texture of wood to remain visible while hiding the grains so that the surface appears uniform.
- Semitransparent stain allows both the texture and grain to remain visible.[12]

Non-grain-raising (**NGR**) stains are more of a surface type of stain than a penetrating one, but they do not require sanding before application of the final coat. Both alcohol stains and NGRs are used industrially because of ease of application and fast-drying qualities.

Stain waxes do the staining and waxing in one process, penetrating the pores of the wood and allowing the natural grain to show, while providing the protective finish of wax. Real wood paneling may be finished with a stain wax, provided that the surface of the wood will not be soiled.

CLEAR COATING

Clear coatings are a group of products that contain little or no pigments. Therefore, they do not hide the surface as does a paint or stain. However, clear coatings sometimes produce a wet or shiny appearance that makes the surface look slightly different than it did originally.

Clear coating products are important for a variety of applications that require an extra layer of protection. Varnish, for example can be used by itself on bare wood or as a protective finish coat over stained wood.

Urethane (polyurethane) coatings form tough, hard, flexible, chemically resistant films by of the following methods.

Moisture curing—moisture cured urethanes dry by solvent evaporation and cure by reacting with moisture/water vapor in the air. Generally, for this to occur, relative **humidity** levels must exceed 20 percent.

Urethanes are light stable, gloss retentive, and nonyellowing. [emphasis added][13]

Both the Occupational Safety and Health Administration (OSHA) and the Environmental Protection Agency (EPA) have strict rules governing not only the manufacture of paint, but also its application. Check the appropriate regulatory agency for the VOC limits in your area. Paint companies sell specially manufactured paints for sale in California, which has the strictest VOC regulations. Eight other states soon will be adopting the same regulations. Most paint companies have discontinued products that do not meet the new regulations, replacing them with VOC-compliant coatings.

Several paint companies have developed very durable acrylic latex paints. Scuffmaster™ Armor™, for example, is an extremely durable and cleanable multicolor or one-tone water-based paint system for walls. Scuffmaster™ Armor™ is the only wall finish product made with polyurethane plastic. The result is a paint finish that will withstand 25,000 ASTM (American Society of Testing Materials) scrub test cycles. This paint is very suitable for high-traffic commercial spaces such as corridors, lobbies, and restrooms.

Scuffmaster™ contains Microban® antimicrobial product protection. Whereas most very durable paints have an **enamel** high-gloss finish, ScrubTough™ from Scuffmaster™ is a solid-color eggshell paint that is up to 10 times more durable than residential-grade acrylic latex paint. ScrubTough™ is a longer-lasting finish that's easy to keep clean, making it the perfect paint for high-traffic areas where regular paint just isn't able to hold up.

Parma White® mildew-proof bathroom wall and ceiling paint from Zinsser, Inc., features a five-year mildew-proof guarantee. It is also scrubbable, and blister- and peel-proof. Figure 2.3 shows how the pigment volume concentration (**PVC**) affects light reflectance. The classification of paints according to gloss ratings depends on the ability of the surface to bounce back varying amounts of light beamed on it. These readings show the relative reflectance of the coated surface as compared with a smooth, flat mirror. The ratings in Table 2.1 measure the light reflectance of the surface only. Table 2.2 shows the percentage of light reflected by different hues and their different values.

Several finishes, or **lusters,** are available in both alkyds and latex:

Flat—These paints, with the highest PVC, provide a velvety appearance and a rich, soft-looking surface on walls where less glare is

FIGURE 2.3
An illustration of how pigment volume concentration affects light reflectance.
(Drawings courtesy of *Builder's Guide to Paints and Coatings,* NAHB Research Center)

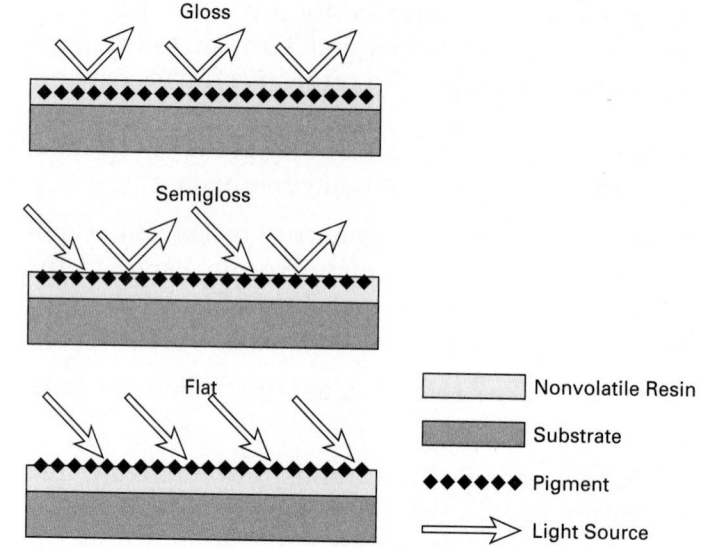

TABLE 2.1
Standard Gloss Range for Architectural and Special Coatings

Name	Gloss Range	Test Method (ASTM D-523)
Flat	Below 15	85° meter*
Eggshell	5–20	60° meter
Satin	15–35	60° meter
Semigloss	30–65	60° meter
Gloss	Over 65	60° meter

*Angle at which light is reflected.

Source: Consumerism Subcommittee of the NPCA Scientific Committee acting with the Subcommittee D01.13 of the American Society for Testing and Materials (ASTM).

TABLE 2.2
Percentage of Light Reflected by Colors

Color	Percentage of Light Reflected
White	89
Ivory	77
Canary yellow	77
Cream	77
Orchid	67
Cream gray	66
Sky blue	65
Buff	63
Pale green	59
Shell pink	55
Olive tan	43
Forest green	22
Coconut brown	16
Black	2

desired and little washing is required. Examples of rooms for which flat paint might be appropriate include the den, library, or adult or guests' bedrooms. *Eggshell, Pearl, or Satin,* are terms used by various manufacturers to denote a paint formulation of slightly lower PVC than flat paint, providing slightly higher light reflections. They combine this characteristic with moderate scrubability. Such paints can be used in areas of the home where

Interior		Exterior
Alkyd	*Latex*	*Alkyd*
Gloss	Gloss	Gloss
Semi-gloss	Semi-gloss	Flat
Eggshell	Eggshell	
Satin	Satin	
Flat	Flat	
Velvet		

FIGURE 2.4
Interior and exterior print.
(Chart courtesy of Sherwin
Williams, *Store Training and
Reference Text*)

    finger marks must from time to time be removed, but where frequent, heavy-duty scrubbing will not occur.

Semigloss—This is the next step down in PVC. Semiglosses provide a mid-range sheen, and have good scrubability. They can be used in kitchens, bathrooms, and children's rooms. Where a significant amount of scrubbing can be anticipated, it is important to choose a good-quality semigloss.

Gloss or High Gloss—These low-PVC paints provide a very shiny surface with easy washability. It should be noted that higher-gloss paints, with their low PVC count, are more likely to show surface imperfections. This is true with both walls and woodwork and explains the importance of proper surface preparation.[14] (See Figure 2.4.)

Enamel is a term whose meaning has become increasingly imprecise over time. It originally designated a hard, durable, high-gloss interior paint. However, some flat paints are now called "flat enamels." While enamel formulations run toward gloss or semigloss, a flat appearance can be produced through the use of appropriate additives. Enamels include both alkyd and latex paints. Today, manufacturers generally use the term *enamel* to indicate a higher quality paint with greater durability and smoother finish.[15]

Enamels and other paints should be applied to a properly prepared surface. A glossy surface will not have **tooth** and should be sanded with sandpaper or a liquid sanding material before application of another coat of paint.

    Because of the VOC laws, latex enamels have been greatly improved; one advantage is that latex enamels do not yellow.

PRIMERS

A primer is the first coat applied to the **substrate** to prepare for subsequent finishing coats, and it may have an alkyd or latex base. Some primers also serve as sealers and function on porous substrates, such as some woods, and particularly on the paper used on **gypsum board.** These nonpenetrating sealers prevent the waste of paint caused by absorption of the porous materials and provide a good base for the final coats. Other primers are specially formulated for use on wood surfaces on which the natural dyes in the wood might cause unsightly stains. Some finish coats are self-priming, whereas others require a separate primer. The manufacturers' specifications will provide this information.

> Benjamin Moore Fresh Start® QD-30® Stain Blocking Primer 202—A general purpose solvent-thinned primer, sealer and stain suppressor. Holds back water-soluble stains and most "bleeding" stains such as lipstick, crayon, and grease. Effectively primes and seals charred or smoke stained surfaces.

Manufacturers often formulate primers and finish coats that are intended to be used together as a system. Where such systems are offered, it is good practice to use them rather than choosing one manufacturer's primer and another manufacturer's topcoat.[16]

FLAME-RETARDANT PAINTS

Most conventional paint systems, when applied at normal film thicknesses, will develop a "Class A" (0-25) flame spread rating over a noncombustible, previously uncoated substrate. Substrates themselves can contribute significantly to the overall flame-spread rating of the substrate and the subsequent coatings. As a guide, the noncombustible substrates cement asbestos board, and plaster have a flame-spread rating of zero. Drywall will contribute to flame spread by a factor of approximately 10. On a substrate that burns readily, such as a wood surface that has not been treated to resist burning, standard coatings do nothing to prevent the substrate from burning. Wood will contribute significantly to the flame spread of the coating.[17]

Products from Flame Control® Coatings Inc. comply with federal, state, and local building and fire code requirements. They retard flame spread and penetration of heat through their intumescent-sublimative-ablative and synergistic flame-suppressing action. On contact with flame or excessive heat, Flame Control® Intumescent Fire Retardant Coatings decompose and puff up (intumesce), forming a thick, dense, spongy foam layer that checks flame spread and retards heat penetration. This company has a variety of **fire-retardant** paints, from clear varnishes to flat, low, and semi- and high-gloss sheens.

These paints are for use in schools, hospitals, offices, factories, warehouses, homes, farms, or wherever there is a need for greater fire protection and lasting beauty. Most major paint companies manufacture a flame-retardant paint.

Flame-retardant paints are specified for public buildings, especially offices and hotels. After the tragic hotel fires of the early 1980s, it became necessary to seriously consider the use of these paints. Although they are not fireproof, they do reduce the flammability of the substrate.

For many commercial painting contracts, a Class A fire rating, defined as a **0-25 flame spread,** is required by law. Included in some technical data are the amounts of smoke developed and fuel contributed. More people die in fires from smoke inhalation than from the flames, so perhaps the smoke-development figure is more important than the flame-spread figure.

VARNISH

Varnish is a transparent or pigmentless film applied to stained or unstained wood. Varnish dries and hardens by evaporation of the volatile solvents, oxidation of the oil, or both.

Where a hard, glossy finish that is impervious to moisture is needed, spar varnish is recommended for both outdoor and indoor use. In areas where moisture is not present, an alkyd varnish provides a slightly longer-lasting finish. Polyurethane is a synthetic resin used to make varnish resistant to both water and alcohol, thus making it usable as a finish on wood floors and tabletops. This type of varnish does not yellow or change color as much as conventional varnishes. The moisture-cured urethane varnishes are more durable but are also more expensive. Humidity must be rigidly controlled, because less than 30 percent humidity will result in too slow of a curing time, and too high humidity will result in too fast of a curing time, resulting in a bubbly surface.

Where a satin finish is needed, the gloss varnish surface may be rubbed down with steel wool, or a satin varnish may be used. Names of finishes do not seem to vary as much in opaque paints as they do in varnishes. One manufacturer will label varnish "dull" and another will call it "flat." Semigloss may also be called "satin" or "medium-rubbed-effect," and high gloss may be called "gloss." Remember that the paired names are synonymous.

Flame Control® Coatings Inc. has a Class "B" water-based fire-retardant varnish for new or previously coated wood surfaces (except floors). The varnish does not leach or turn white on aging or washing.

Varnish stains are pigmented and give a very superficial-colored protective surface to the wood. They are used when a cheap, fast finish is desired, but they never have the depth of color obtained with other stains. When the surface of a varnish stain is scratched, the natural wood color may show through.

SHELLAC

Shellac is a natural resin secreted by the lac bug. This secretion forms a protective cocoon for the developing lac bug larvae. The resin is harvested from tree branches, cleaned, and processed into dewaxed flakes that are then dissolved in denatured alcohol. It is available in clear, orange, and pigmented white. All varieties dry to clear transparent films—the clear dries to virtually colorless; the orange dries with an amber cast often preferred for antiques and for floors; and the pigmented white is sometimes used as an undercoat on wood that is to be painted. Shellac is often used as a sealer for knots and sappy streaks in new wood, porous surfaces before painting or papering, and priming hard-to-grip surfaces. To experienced finishers and restorers of fine furniture, shellac remains the finish of choice. One of the most elegant finishes for furniture, French Polish, is done with shellac. Conservators and restorers of antiques use shellac for refinishing antiques. And, most important, its low toxicity makes it a perfect choice for items that come into contact with food or children's toys. In addition, a pharmaceutical shellac is used to coat pills so that they will dissolve slowly. Another grade is used to coat apples.

Shellac was the original glossy, transparent surface finish for furniture and was the finish used on what are now considered antiques. On a piece of furniture, shellac will turn white when exposed to water and/or heat. The urethane and oil varnishes have replaced shellac because they are not as quickly affected by heat and water.

Old shellac should never be used because as it ages its water-resistance decreases and its drying time increases. When there is any doubt about the age of a particular shellac, it should be tested before it is used on a project. If the surface remains tacky, the shellac should be discarded in the proper manner because it may never harden.

LACQUER

Lacquer is a paint that dries by solvent evaporation only and is applied by a spray gun. Lacquer may or may not contain pigments and is used commercially in the finishing of wood furniture and cabinets. A fine built-up finish may be achieved by many coats of lacquer, each of which is finely sanded before the subsequent coats.

DANISH OIL

Danish oil hardens and reinforces the wood fibers beneath the surface. It forms a protective finish that will not peel, crack, or wrinkle. It resists alcohol, hot liquids, common stains, and chemicals. The clear oil gives a natural finish, whereas the stained oil contains a wood stain to achieve the colored effect. The main components of Danish oil finish are tung oil and boiled linseed oil, giving the wood a rich, penetrating oil surface while sealing the pores. Danish oil may have a protective clear coat applied over the wood finish after 72 hours. Danish oil is unique because its high linseed oil content and its colorant (gilsonite) allow it to penetrate and color, unlike pigmented stains.

NOVELTY AND FAUX FINISHES

Faux finishing is a painting technique used to create the illusion of texture on a wall. Faux finishes can be achieved by using sponges, special rollers, rags, and so on. The second color used is often of the same hue as the base but is darker or lighter than the base. Most paint stores sell kits with a basecoat and translucent color, opal or pearl **glaze,** or metallic such as gold, silver, or copper.

Several companies now manufacture commercial multicolored wall coatings. The finish consists of separate and distinct pigmented enamel particles suspended in an aqueous solution; the vehicle is a modified acrylate. These nonflammable coatings are sprayed over a special basecoat, with a two-step final coat.

FAULUX™ from Triarch is a seamless, interior acrylic finish that utilizes faux painting techniques made easy and high-performance materials. All finishes boast of over 2000 scrub cycles, making the finishes durable and abrasion resistant. All finishes are also washable. [These finishes have a] Class "A" Flame Spread and Smoke Contribution rating, and low VOCs.[18]

Plexture® is a low-profile, textured, seamless interior acrylic texture, and generally costs less than TYPE II vinyl wallcovering. Plexture® is many times more abuse resistant than conventional paint. Plexture® also contains Teflon® for increased cleanability. It is warrantied against mold and mildew growth and coating integrity for five years. A two-step spray process delivers a choice of four standard patterns. Eighty standard colors plus custom color and texture options provide a very wide range of design options.

Duroplex® coatings, from Triarch, are tough finishes applied exclusively by factory-trained installers who are in the painting trade. Use Duroplex interior textured acrylic wall finish for maximum longevity, abuse resistance, mold and mildew prevention, and lowest long-term maintenance. It has a 10-year performance warranty against mold and mildew, cracking, or delamination. Duroplex can be applied by spray or roller methods and cures to a surface hardness that is 80 percent as hard as mild steel and has a Class A flame-spread and smoke-contribution rating 19 times less toxic than vinyl wall covering. This product is suitable for hotel guestrooms. It is as tough as concrete and provides an improved performance dimension to drywall.

> Stenciling is a folk art form of wall painting that originated as an alternative to buying expensive wallpapers and rugs. Scenes of everyday life were cut into templates then stenciled on walls and wood floors to create decorative patterns that actually resembled upscale wallpaper and rugs.
>
> Now the technique has been revived along with other elements of country-style decorating and design. One advantage of stenciling today is that the modern plastic stencils don't tear, fray or fall apart like the paper versions did in the old days. Stencils may be used for wall and/or floor borders, highlight certain parts of a room, cover entire wall sections, or decorate furniture and fabrics.[19]

COLOR

Color is the least expensive way to dramatize, stylize, or personalize a home. Colors affect us psychologically, and they should be selected with this in mind. **Chroma** is the degree of saturation of a hue. A color at its full intensity has maximum chroma.

When studying paint chips, be sure to mask other colors on the same paint card. Otherwise, the eye will tend to blend all the colors rather than see them individually. Another point to remember is that when matching a color, select a hue several shades lighter and of less intensity.

The following information is from the Paint & Coatings Industry Information Center:

> If you want a room that generates energy or excitement, choose reds and oranges. If you want to warm up or brighten a shady or darker room, choose yellows, oranges and reds.

If you want to cool off a too-sunny southern exposure, choose greens, blues and purples.

If you want to open up a small, dark area and make it seem larger or brighter, choose white or yellow.

If you want to create a cozy, sophisticated feeling in a large room, choose dark blues, and dark brown.

If you want to create a calm, peaceful environment, choose blues and greens. [See Figure 2.1.][20]

The Sherwin-Williams website offers a very useful Color Visualizer. This can be used by homeowners and professionals alike. The visualizer allows the user to select from a broad palette of colors for different walls, trim, ceilings, accents, and upholstery selections. By just moving selected colors to these areas the color scheme for an entire room can be seen.

Glidden® Paint Visualizer works on the same principle with various styles of rooms. Accent colors have become popular over the last 10 years. Note that with these darker colors, additional coats may be required and tinted primers are recommended. Anytime a drastic color change is done, multiple-coat jobs should be expected. To calculate the amount of paint required for a job, Porter Paints and many other companies have handy paint calculators available on their websites.

APPLICATION METHODS

The four most common methods of applying paints are brush, roller, pad, and airless spray. Pads and rollers are do-it-yourself tools, although the roller may be used in remodeling if removal of furniture is impossible. The best available equipment should be used, since poor-quality tools will result in a poor-quality paint job.

Whatever the material used for the bristles (hog hair or synthetic), brushes should have **flagged bristles** that help load the brush with more paint while helping the paint flow more smoothly. Cheap brushes have almost no flagging, which causes the paint to flow unevenly. Brushes are used for woodwork and for uneven surfaces, whereas rollers are used for walls and flat areas.

Spraying is used to cover large areas such as walls and ceilings in new homes, but especially for commercial interiors, where large expanses of surfaces require paint. Airless spraying uses fluid pressure. Most airless spraying uses undiluted paint, which provides better coverage but also uses more paint. All surrounding areas must be covered or masked to avoid overspray, and this masking time is always included in the painting contractor's estimates.

Spraying is 8 to 10 times faster than other methods of application. These figures refer to flat walls, but spraying is an easier and more economical method of coating uneven or irregular surfaces than brushing, since it enables the paint to penetrate into the crevices. When spraying walls, the use of a roller immediately after spraying evens out the coat of paint.

Spraying is also the method used for finishing furniture and kitchen cabinets. For a clear finish on furniture and cabinets, heated lacquer is used, which dries quickly, cures to a hard film with heat, and produces fewer toxic emissions. Heated lacquer is formulated to be used without **reduction,** thus giving a better finished surface.

SURFACE PREPARATION

Surface preparation is the most important procedure to achieve a good paint finish. According to Sherwin-Williams "as high as 80% of all coatings failures can be directly attributed to inadequate surface preparation that affects coating adhesion. Selection and implementation of proper surface preparation ensure coating adhesion to the substrate and prolong the service life of the coating system."[21]

Until the late 1970s lead-based paints were used. Renovation of buildings painted before the late 1950s must be done by a professional contractor trained in proper handling of lead-based paints.

Wood

Moisture is the major problem when painting wood. Five to 10 percent moisture content is the proper range. Today most wood is **kiln-dried,** but exposure to high humidity may change that moisture content. Although knots in the wood are not technically a moisture problem, they do cause difficulties when the surface is painted, because the resin in the knots may **bleed** through the surface of the paint; therefore, a special knot sealer must be used. [See Table 2.3.]

All cracks and nail holes must be filled with a suitable wood putty or filler, which can be applied before or after priming, according to instructions on the can or in the paint guides. Some woods with open pores require the use of a paste wood filler. If a natural or painted finish is desired, the filler is diluted with a thinner; if the surface is to be stained, the filler is diluted with the stain.

If coarse sanding is required, it may be done at an angle to the grain; medium or fine sanding grits should always be used with the grain. Awkward places should never be sanded across the grain because the sanding marks will show up when the surface is stained.

Sherwin-Williams Chemical Coatings Division now offers an updated edition of its guide for selecting factory finishing systems

Softwood	Open Pores*	Color	Hardwood	Open Pores*	Color
Douglas-fir	No	Pale red	Chestnut	Yes	Light brown
Pine	No	Cream	Elm	No	Yes
Redwood	No	Dark brown	Hickory	Yes	Light brown
HARDWOOD	OPEN PORES*	COLOR	Maple	No	Light brown
Ash, white	Yes	Light brown	Oak	Yes	Brown
Birch, yellow	No	Light brown	Teak	Yes	Dark Brown
Cherry	No	Brown	Walnut	Yes	Dark brown

* All wood with yes requires a filler due to open pores.

Source: www.fpl.fs.Fed,us/documents/fplgtrl13ch15:pdf

TABLE 2.3
Wood Classification According to Openness of Pores

meeting Architectural Woodwork Industry (AWI) finishing standards. The guide was created to provide manufacturers and finishers of mouldings, panels, bookshelves, cabinets and furniture with information on the company's Sher-Wood Wood® Finishing systems.[22]

Plaster

When preparing a plaster wall for painting, it is necessary to ensure that the plaster is solid, has no cracks, and is smooth and level, since paint will only emphasize any problems. Badly cracked or loose plaster should be removed and repaired. *All* cracks, even if hairlines, must be repaired, since they will only enlarge with time. To achieve a smooth and level wall, the surface must be sanded with fine sandpaper, and before the paint is applied the fine dust must be brushed from the wall surface. Plaster is extremely porous, so a primer-sealer, which can be latex or alkyd, is required.

Gypsum Board or Drywall

On gypsum board, all seams must be taped, and nail or screw holes must be **set** and filled with spackling compound or joint cement; these filled areas should then be sanded. Care should be taken not to sand the paper areas too much because doing so causes the surface to be **abraded.** The abrasion may still be visible after the final coat has dried, particularly if the final coat has any gloss. Gypsum board may also have a texture applied, as described in Chapter 5, and the luster selected will be governed by the type of texture. Gypsum board must also be brushed clean of all fine dust particles before the primer is applied.

Metal

All loose rust, **mill scale,** and loose paint must be removed from metal before a primer is applied. There are many methods of accomplishing this removal. One of the most common and effective is sandblasting, in which fine silica particles are blown under pressure onto the surface of the metal. Small areas may be sanded by hand. For metals other than galvanized metal, the primer should be rust inhibitive and specially formulated for that specific metal.

Masonry

Masonry usually has a porous surface and will not give a smooth topcoat unless a block filler is used. Product analysis of a block filler shows a much larger percentage of calcium carbonate than titanium dioxide. A gallon of masonry paint does not cover as large an area as a gallon of other types of paint, because the heavier calcium carbonate content acts as a filler. One problem encountered with a masonry surface is **efflorescence,** which is a white powdery substance caused by an alkaline chemical reaction with water. An alkaline-resistant primer is necessary if this condition is present. However, the efflorescence must be removed before the primer is applied.

WRITING PAINTING SPECIFICATIONS

The specifier should learn how to read the technical part of the product guide, or find the same information on the label of the can. This is similar to the ingredients listed on food packaging. Some manufacturers state in the product description that it is a short-, medium-, or long-oil coating. A long-oil paint has a longer drying period and is usually more expensive. One property of a long-oil product is that it coats the surface better than a short-oil product because of its wetting ability.

The volume of solids is expressed as a percentage per gallon of paint. This percentage can vary from as much as 90 percent in some industrial coatings to the high teens and up to 40 percent in architectural paints. If, for the sake of comparison, a uniform thickness of $1\frac{1}{2}$ **mils** is used, the higher-percentage-volume paint would cover 453 square feet and the lower-percentage paint only 199 square feet. This, of course, means that more than twice as much paint of the lower volume would have to be purchased when compared with the higher volume. Thus, the paint that appears to be a bargain may turn out to cost more if the same result is to be achieved.

Painting specifications are a way of legally covering both parties in the contract between the client and the painting contractor. There will be no misunderstanding of responsibility if the scope of the paint job is clearly spelled out, and most major paint companies include in their catalogues sample painting specifications covering terms of the contract. Some of these are more detailed than others. Tables 2.4 and 2.5 will aid the designer in calculating the approximate time required to complete the painting contract.

A time limit and a penalty clause should be written into the contract. This time requirement is most important, because painting is the first finishing step in a project, and if it is delayed, the completion date is in jeopardy. The penalty clause provides for a deduction of a specific amount of money or a percentage for every day the contract is over the time limit. Information on surface preparation may be obtained from the individual paint companies. The problems created by incorrect surface treatment,

Method	Coverage per Hour
Brush	50–200 sq ft
Roller	100–300 sq ft
Spray	300–500 sq ft

TABLE 2.4
Coverage According to
Method of Application

Surface	Vehicle	Number of Coats
Woodwork	Oil gloss paint	2–3 coats
	Semigloss paint	2–3 coats
Plaster	Alkyd flat	2–3 coats
Drywall	Alkyd flat	2–3 coats
	Vinyl latex	3 coats
Masonry	Vinyl latex	3 coats
Wood floor	Enamel	3 coats

TABLE 2.5
Average Coat Requirements
for Interior Surfaces

priming, and finishing are *never* corrected by simply applying another coat of paint.

High-performance paints should be selected if budget restrictions permit, because high-performance paints last several times longer than regular paints. This longer durability means that business or commercial operations will not have to be shut down as frequently. Therefore, the increase in cost will more than offset the loss of business. The words *high performance* should be included in the product description.

The method of application should be specified: brush, roller, or spray. The method must suit the material covered and the type of paint used. Moreover, primers or base coats must be compatible with both the surface to be covered and the final topcoat. When writing painting specifications, excluded items are just as important as included items. If other contractors are present at the site, their work and materials must be protected from damage. One area should be designated as a storage for all paint and equipment, and this area should have a temperature at or near 77°F, the ideal temperature for application of paints. The painting subcontractor should remove daily all combustible material from the premises.

The specifier should make certain that inspections are made before the application of each coat, because these inspections will properly cover both client and contractor. If some revisions or corrections are made, they should also be *put in writing* and an inspection should be made before proceeding.

Cleanup is the responsibility of the painting contractor. All windows and glass areas must be free of paint streaks or spatters. The area should be left ready for the next contractor to begin work without any further cleaning.

Some states do not permit interior designers to sign a contract for clients, whereas other states do allow this. The designer should check state laws to see whether he or she or the client must be the contractual party.

USING THE MANUFACTURER'S PAINTING SPECIFICATION INFORMATION

All paint companies have different methods of presenting their descriptive literature, but a designer with the background material this chapter provides will soon be able to find the information needed. For example, first the material to be covered is listed, then the use of that material, and then the finish desired. Let us use wood as an example: The material is wood, but is it going to be used for exterior or interior work? Is it going to left natural, stained, or painted? If interior, will it be used on walls, ceilings, or floors? Each different use will require a product suitable for that purpose. Floors will obviously need a more durable finish than walls or ceilings.

Another category will be the final finish or luster—flat, semigloss, or gloss? Will you need an alkyd, a latex, or, for floor use, a urethane? This category is sometimes classified as the vehicle or generic type. The schedule then explains which primer or sealer will be used for compatibility with the final coat. After the primer, the first coat is applied. This coat can also be used for the final coat or another product may be suggested. Drying time for the different methods of application may also be found in the descriptive literature. Two different times may be mentioned, one being "dust free," "tack free," or "to touch," meaning the length of time it takes before dust will not adhere to the freshly painted surface. Sometimes a quick-drying paint will have to be specified because of possible contaminants in the air. The second drying time is recoat time; this is important so that the application of the following coat can be scheduled.

The spreading rate per gallon will enable a specifier to calculate approximately how many gallons are needed for the job, thereby estimating material costs. Sometimes, in the more technical specifications, an analysis of the contents of the paint is included both by weight and by volume. The most important percentage, however, is the volume amount, because weight of solids can be manipulated, whereas volume cannot. This is the only way to compare one paint with another. The type and percentage of these ingredients makes paints differ in durability, application, and coverage. Some paint companies now have these percentages printed on the label of paint cans, similar to the manner in which percentages of the daily requirements of vitamins and minerals are printed on food packages.

If paint will be sprayed, there is information on lowering the **viscosity** and, for other methods of application, the maximum reduction permitted without spoiling the paint job. Most catalogues also include a recommended thickness of film when dry, which is expressed as so many mils **DFT** (dry film thickness). This film can be checked with specially made gauges. The DFT cannot be specified by the number of coats. The film thickness of the total paint system is the important factor, not the film thickness per coat.

PROBLEMS WITH PAINT AND VARNISH AND HOW TO SOLVE THEM

The ideal temperature for application of paints and varnishes is 77°F, but effective application can be achieved at temperatures ranging from 50°F up. This includes air temperature, surface temperature, and paint temperature. Cold affects viscosity, causing slower evaporation of the solvents, which results in sags and runs. High temperature lowers viscosity, also causing runs and sags. High humidity may cause less evaporation of the solvent, giving lower gloss and allowing dirt and dust to settle and adhere to the film. Ventilation must be provided when paints are applied, but strong drafts will affect the uniformity of luster.

Today, most paints start with a base and the pigments are added according to charts provided to the store by the manufacturer. Sometimes it is necessary to change the hue of the mixed paint, and this can be done by judicious addition of certain pigments. It is vital that the designer be aware of the changes made by these additions. Any hue can now be matched by using a **spectrophotometer** connected to a computer, which can provide the necessary formula.

WALLPAPER AND WALLCOVERING

As wallpaper and wallcoverings are sold mainly in paint stores, this subject is now covered in this chapter.

The Chinese mounted painted rice paper on walls as early as 200 B.C. Although mention of painted papers has been historically documented as early as 1507 in France, the oldest fragment of European wallpaper, from the year 1509, was found in Christ's College, Cambridge, England. This paper has a rather large-scale pattern adapted from contemporary damask. Seventeenth-century paper, whether painted or block printed, did not have a continuous pattern repeat and was printed on sheets rather than on a roll, as is the modern practice. The repetitive matching of today's papers is credited to Jean Papillon of France in the late 17th century. In the 18th century, England and France produced hand-printed papers that were both expensive and heavily taxed.

Leather was one of the original materials used as a covering for walls. The earliest decorated and painted leathers were introduced to Europe in the 11th century by Arabs from Morocco and were popular in 17th-century Holland.

Flocked papers were used as early as 1620 in France. The design was printed with some kind of glue, which was then sprinkled heavily with finely chopped bits of silk and wool, creating a good imitation of damask or velvet. Flocked papers have been popular in recent decades, but are less popular now.

Scenic papers were used in the 18th century, many of them handpainted Chinese papers. Wallpapers were imported to the United States during the second quarter of the 18th century. Domestic manufacturing did not start until around 1800, and even then the quality was not equal to the fine imported papers.

After the Industrial Revolution, wallpaper became available to people of more moderate means and the use of wallpaper became more widespread. In the late 19th and early 20th centuries, William Morris stimulated interest in wallpapers and their designs. In the first half of the 20th century, papers imitating textures and having the appearance of wood, marble, tiles, relief plasterwork, paneling, and moiré silk were in demand.

In the late 1930s and 1940s, wallpaper was in style, but in the 1960s, 1970s, and 1990s, painted walls were in fashion.

Today, designers are more discriminating with the use of wallpapers or, as they will be referred to from now on, wallcoverings. This change of name results from the fact that although paper was the original material for wallcoverings, today these wallcoverings may be all paper, paper backed by cotton fabric, vinyl face with paper or cotton backing, or fabric with a paper backing. Foils or **mylars** have either paper or a nonwoven backing to ensure a smooth reflective surface. (See the section "Basic Wallcovering Backings" later in this chapter.)

The majority of wallcoverings have three layers, each of which performs an important function. Starting from the top surface and working to the back, the layers are:

The decorative layer—The thinnest layer in most cases, this is comprised of the inks applied to the top of the intermediate layer. This decorative layer is normally the major reason a wallcovering is chosen. The decorative layer may also have a protective polymer coating to provide added performance characteristics.

The intermediate layer—This layer, the ground, provides the surface upon which the decorative layer is printed. It also provides the background color that, though often an off-white, can be any color depending upon the design. This layer can range in thickness from less than 1 mil to as much as 10 mils as in heavier-weight, "solid-vinyl" products. Note that a mil is $\frac{1}{1000}$ of an inch.

The third layer—The substrate or backing is the portion of the wallcovering that goes against the wall. This backing can be of a wide variety of materials ranging from woven and nonwoven fabrics to lightweight paper products.

Characteristics of Wallcoverings

Many different grounds and substrates can be used to make wallcoverings. These various materials provide the characteristics typical in wallcoverings. These features include degrees of strength or durability, scrubbability, washability, stain resistance, abrasion resistance, and colorfastness. A listing of the most important or common characteristics and definitions is as follows:

Washable means that a wallcovering can withstand occasional sponging with a prescribed detergent solution.

Scrubbable means that a wallcovering can withstand scrubbing with a brush and a prescribed solution.

Stain resistance is the ability to show no appreciable change after removal of different types of stains such as grease, butter, coffee, and so on.

Abrasion resistance is the ability to withstand mechanical actions such as rubbing, scraping, or scrubbing.

Colorfastness is the ability to resist change or loss of color caused by exposure to light over a measured period of time.

Peelable means that the decorative surface and ground may be drypeeled, leaving a continuous layer of the substrate on the wall that can be used as a liner for hanging new wallcovering. It must, however, be scraped off to prepare the wall for paint. Peelable wallcoverings today are usually paper-backed vinyl products in which a layer of solid vinyl is adhered to a substrate.

Strippable means that the wallcovering can be drystripped from the wall, leaving a minimum of paste or adhesive residue and without damage to the wall's surface. Be sure to note the difference between strippable and peelable.

Prepasted means that the substrate of the wallcovering has been treated with an adhesive that is activated by water.

Whether a particular wallcovering is strippable or peelable will be marked in the sample book or on the label of the wallcovering bolt.[23]

Patterns

Today's wallcovering manufacturers produce pattern collections based on market research concerning consumer response to specific patterns and demand for certain styles. Thus, designers can use these collections to create the desired atmosphere in a client's installation.

Many of the early American designs were inspired by valuable brocades and tapestries that adorned the homes of wealthy individuals. Several contemporary companies have made arrangements with museums to produce historical designs. For example, Bradbury & Bradbury Art Wallpapers have meticulously researched historical collections from the last quarter of the 19th century through the art deco period. Brunschwig & Fils has arrangements with the Historic New England collection of SPNEA (Society for the Preservation of New England Antiquities), the Musé des Arts Décoratifs in Paris, the Antiquarian and Landmarks Society of Connecticut, the Benaki Museum in Athens, the Winterthur Museum, and a number of other American museums and historic houses. Scalamandre produces wallpaper for the Preservation Society of Newport County and Prestwould Plantation. F. Schumacher & Company's licensors include Colonial Williamsburg, Historic Natchez, the National Trust for Historic Preservation, the Library of Congress, the Edith Wharton Restoration, and the Victorian Society. Thibaut Wallcoverings issues the Historic Homes of America collections based on samples from actual homes. Because Thibaut's papers are produced in large quantities, they are less expensive than the **hand-screened** prints mentioned previously, which are printed in smaller quantities. (See Figure 2.5.)

Murals are large-scale, nonrepeat, hand-screened papers done on a series of panels, usually installed above a chair rail. They may be scenic, floral, architectural, or graphic in nature. **Chinoiserie** murals are the perfect background for English-style furniture. Murals are sold in sets, varying from two to six or more panels per set. Each panel is normally 28 inches in width and is printed on strips 10 to 12 feet in length. The height of the designs varies greatly, but most fall somewhere between 4 and 8 feet. Some graphics go from ceiling to floor. Murals for recreation rooms are also available.

For a French ambience, wallcoverings with delicate scrolls or lacy patterns are suitable for a formal background, whereas **toile-de-Jouy** and checks are appropriate for the French Country look. Wallcoverings for a formal English feeling range from symmetrical damasks to copies of English chintzes and embroideries.

Geometrics include both subtle and bold stripes and checks, as well as polka dots and circles. The colors used will dictate where these geometrics can be used.

Trompe l'oeil patterns are three-dimensional designs on paper. Examples of realistic designs are a cupboard with an open door displaying some books, a view from a window, or a niche with a shell top containing a piece of sculpture. These trompe l'oeil patterns are sold in a set.

Dye Lots

A pattern number and dye-lot or "run number" is printed on each roll. A pattern number identifies a particular design and color way of a pattern. The dye-lot number represents a particular

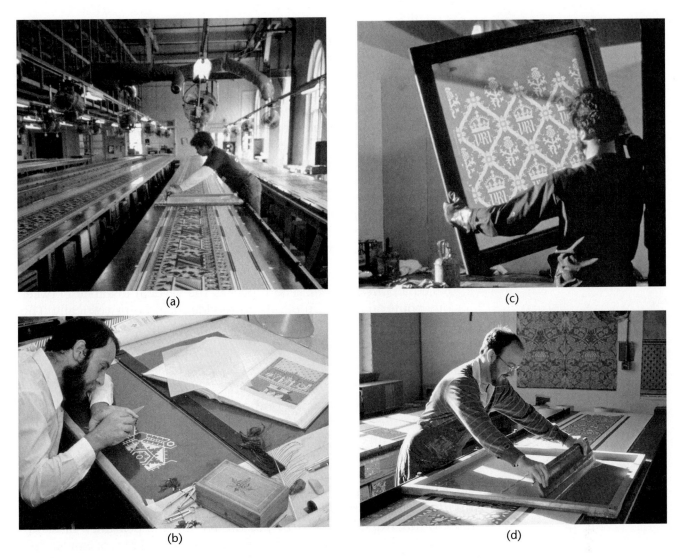

FIGURE 2.5
The process of silk screening. (a) Printing table. (b) Artwork done by hand. (c) An actual silk screen. (d) Paint being forced through the screen. (Photos courtesy of Bradbury & Bradbury Art Wallpapers)

group of rolls that are printed on the same print run. Different dye-lot numbers could signal variables such as a possible tonal change of color, a change in the vinyl coating or a change in the embossing process.

Because of this, it is very important to check each individual roll in your wallpaper job to ensure uniformity in color and pattern. It is also important to record pattern numbers and dye-lot or run numbers in case additional rolls are needed to complete a project.[24]

It is important to find out if the wallcovering to be hung has a pattern match. There are three major types of pattern matches:

Random match—the pattern matches no matter how adjoining strips are positioned. Stripes are the best example of this type of match. It is recommended to reverse every other strip to minimize visual effects such as shading or color variations from edge-to-edge. Note also that stripes, or random match, will produce much less waste since there is no repeat distance to take into account.

Straight-across match—in which the design elements match on adjoining strips. Every strip will be the same at the ceiling line.

Drop match—which has several different types:

Half-drop match—every other strip is the same at the ceiling line and the design elements run diagonally. It takes three strips to repeat the vertical design. If you numbered the strips consecutively, the odd-numbered strips (1, 3, 5, and so on) would be identical and the even-numbered strips (2, 4, 6, and so on) would match one another.

Multiple-drop match—a match that takes four or more strips before the vertical design is repeated. These are similar to half-drop match except it takes more strips to repeat the first strip.

Note that all wallcoverings, except textures and murals, have what is called a *pattern repeat.* The repeat is the vertical distance between one point on a pattern design to the identical point vertically. This pattern repeat is an integral part of the design.[25]

Types

Wallcovering textures include **embossed** papers, which hide any substrate unevenness; solid-color fabrics; and grasscloths. Embossed papers have a texture rolled into them during the manufacturing process. Care should be taken not to flatten the texture of embossed papers when hanging them.

Anaglypta® is an embossed product made from paper that has been imported from England since the turn of the century. Designed to be painted, this wallcovering provides the textured appearance of sculptured plaster, hammered copper, or even hand-tooled Moroccan leather. Anaglypta® is a highly textured wallcovering that is applied to the wall like any other product. Once painted, the surface becomes hard and durable. The advantage of Anaglypta® is that not only is it used on newly constructed walls in residential and commercial interiors, but it may also be applied after minimal surface preparation. In older dwellings and Victorian restoration projects, Anaglypta® provides the added advantage of stabilizing walls while covering moderate cracks and blemishes. **Friezes,** with ornate embossed designs, are part of the heavier Lincrusta® line, the original extra-deep product. Low-relief and vinyl versions are also available.

Fabrics should be tightly woven, although burlap is frequently used as a texture. Walls are pasted with a nonstaining paste and the fabric, with the selvage removed, is brushed onto the paste. Custom Laminations, Inc. can apply a backing of paper to fabrics for wallcoverings. Its VKC™ Vinylizing is a clear film that is factory applied to the surface of your wallpaper. The colors, tone and surface of your wallpaper are permanently locked in and protected forever. This means you can use the most beautiful wallpapers in the harshest of environments. Delicate, expensive papers can be used in bathrooms, kitchens, hallways, restaurants, or anywhere. This patented process comes with a three-year limited warranty. For all the benefits of VKC™ Vinylizing for Wallpaper with a built

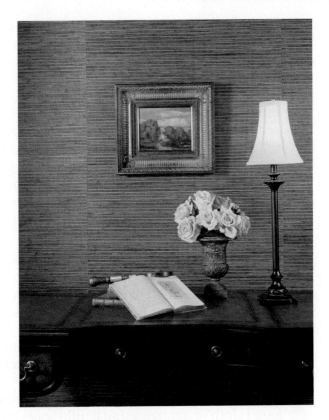

FIGURE 2.6
Grasscloth wallcovering
adds interest and texture to
the wall. (Courtesy of MDC
Wallcoverings)

in flame retardant, use VKC-FP™ Vinylizing for Wallpaper. Wallcoverings processed with VKC-FP™ Vinylizing for Wallpaper will pass most flammability requirements.

Grasscloth is made of loosely woven vegetable fibers backed with paper. (See Figure 2.6.) These fibers may be knotted at the ends and are a decorative feature of the texture. Because the fibers are of vegetable origin, width and color will vary, thus providing a highly textured surface. In addition, because of the natural materials from which grasscloth is made, it is impossible to obtain a straight-across match, so seams will be obvious. Woven silk is frequently included in grasscloth collections; its finer texture gives a more refined atmosphere to a room.

Grasscloth, bamboo, and paper weaves are the natural choices for today's environmentally sensitive designers. With a wide array of textures, patterns, and color shadings, this sophisticated and elegant selection offers a style to complement any décor. The designs truly harmonize pattern and texture with a quality that stimulates multiple sensory perceptions at once. These unique, very high-end wall treatments are ideal for specialty commercial projects such as boutiques, hotels and resorts, hotel ballrooms, restaurants, casinos, spas, cruise ships, conference or meeting rooms, executive offices, reception rooms or atriums, and high-end retail environments. All patterns are crafted on 36 inches paper backing and meet Class A fire rating.[26]

Flocked papers, as mentioned previously, are one of the oldest papers on record. They are currently manufactured by modern methods but still resemble pile fabrics. One problem with flocked papers is that through abrasion or constant contact with the face of the paper, the flocking may be removed and a worn area will appear. A seam roller should never be used to press down seams because this also flattens the flocking.

Foils and mylars provide a mirrored effect with a pattern printed on the reflective surface; because of this high shine, the use of a lining paper is suggested to provide a smoother substrate. Foils conduct electricity if allowed to come in contact with exposed wires. Some older foils had a tendency to show rust spots in moist environments. This is why most "metallic" wallcoverings are presently made of mylar. Foils are used to best effect in well-lit rooms because the light reflects off the foil surface and enhances the effect of the wallcovering.

Kraft papers are usually hand-printed patterns on good-quality kraft paper similar to the type used for wrapping packages. Unless specially treated, these kraft papers absorb grease and oil stains, so care should be taken in placement (e.g., it might not be a good idea to use them in kitchens).

A new dry erasable wallcovering from OMNOVA Solutions Inc. is MemErase™. This product is made with PolyFox® material. This proprietary patented technology has proved ideal in developing an innovative dry erasable material that resists stains, scratches and abrasion. It is available in nine different colors, 62" wide. MemErase is suitable for presentations and idea generation, for schedules and time lines. This type II wallcovering has a full 2-year warranty. The suggested installation is railroading to avoid any seams. Ordinary dirt and stains may be removed by rubbing lightly with a moistened cloth or sponge using a mild soap, detergent or non-abrasive cleaner. All dry erase marks should be removed and the MemErase wallcovering cleaned monthly.[27]

Leather is cut into designs or blocks (much like blocks of Spanish tiles) because the limited size of the hide prohibits the use of large pieces. The color of the surface varies within one hide and from one hide to another; therefore, a shaded effect is expected.

Coordinated or companion fabrics are used to create an unbroken appearance where wallcovering and draperies adjoin. When using coordinated paper and fabric, the wallcovering should be hung first; then the draperies can be adjusted to line up with the pattern repeat of the wallcovering. (See Figure 2.7.) The tendency is to call these companion fabrics "matching fabrics," but this is incorrect. Paper or vinyl will absorb dyes in a different manner than will a fabric, and many problems will be resolved by strict avoidance of the word *matching*. One way of avoiding color differences is to use the actual fabric and have it paper backed for the wallcovering.

Lining paper is an inexpensive blank paper recommended for use under foils and other fine-quality papers. It absorbs excess moisture and makes a smoother-finished wall surface. A heavier canvas liner is available for "bad walls."

Printing of Wallcoverings

The most widely used print processes are surface, flexographic or flexo, gravure and screen. It is important to recognize that each process is capable of yielding attractive, stylized and salable products. Each process enables the manufacturer to produce a specific characteristic look.

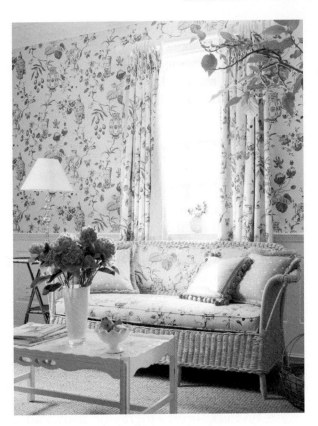

FIGURE 2.7
This is a good example of coordinating wallcovering and fabric. This is the Sweet Life Collection from Thibaut. (Photograph courtesy of Thibaut® Wallcoverings)

Surface printing is a mechanized form of block printing. Instead of using flat blocks, the design is engraved on rollers or cylinders. The raised area of the cylinder prints the ink, much like a rubber stamp. Most surface printing machines can print 12 colors, with each cylinder printing a different color. Surface printing is beautiful and very recognizable—the inks are thicker than most printing processes and often appear to be hand painted. This process adds an historical quality because it simulates the look of block printing—the oldest form of printing for wallcovering.

Flexographic printing is a machine printing process that utilizes rollers or cylinders with a flexible rubberlike surface that prints with the raised area, much like surface printing, but with much less ink. This means the ink dries quickly and allows the machine to run at high speed. The finished product has a very smooth finish with crisp detail and often resembles rotary screen printing.

Gravure printing is a machine printing process used for wallcovering. The copper printing rollers are engraved with a design and then plated with chrome for hardness. The engraved or recessed areas of the rollers pick up the ink and deposit it on the wallcovering surface. There is a separate roller for each color, and the depth of the engraving determines the strength of the color. This means that each roller or cylinder is capable of printing tones of that color. Gravure machinery usually allows up to eight printing rollers/cylinders which print the wallcovering as it passes through the machine. The machinery runs at high speed and the ink is applied and then runs through a dryer before the next color is printed. This process allows for very fine detail and reproduction of images of photo quality.

Rotary screen is a mechanized version of hand screen printing. This process uses hollow screen mesh and squeegee blades located inside the cylinders that force the ink onto the wallcovering as it travels through a press. There is a separate screen for each color. Rotary screen printing allows for a heavy application of ink and a rich look—very similar to hand screen prints but at a lower cost.[28]

There are several means by which a wallcovering can be hand printed. First, it may be silk screened. A brief history of silk screening is supplied by Bradbury & Bradbury:

> Silk screening originated in Japan, evolving from the traditional art of stencil printing on fabric. Cutting intricate patterns was a highly prized skill in Japan, but it was hindered by the inherent fragility of paper stencils, and their tendency to tear during handling and printing.
>
> The problem was solved by glueing strands of silk (or human hair) to the stencil to increase its strength and durability.
>
> New levels of intricacy were achieved using this technique, and stencils became covered with an ever-expanding mesh of supporting threads.
>
> The next logical step was to stretch a piece of woven silk on a wooden frame and then glue the stencil directly onto the silk mesh: the first "silk screen."
>
> The art of silk screen printing moved to the West in the early 20th century, first as a commercial printing method, and then as a fine art form: *serigraphy*. It was adapted by the wallpaper industry as a method for making the highest quality handprints. [See Figure 2.5.][29]

The following information is adapted from Bradbury & Bradbury and explains the process of custom silk screening. Printing tables are 90 feet long and each holds six rolls of wallpaper. Metal rails along the side of the table have adjustable knobs that are set to the particular repeat of the pattern to be printed. A complex pattern for an average-size Victorian room can require over 1,000 individual impressions. (See Figure 2.5a., 2.8)

Artwork is done by hand in the traditional manner by painting on acetate or cutting a stencil using a graphic arts film, as shown in Figure 2.5b. A separate stencil must be prepared for each different color in the pattern, and all must align perfectly. Once a full repeat has been cut or painted by hand, computers aid in replicating the artwork.

Screen making is done by coating a silk screen with a photosensitive emulsion, essentially creating a large piece of film. The screen and artwork are sandwiched in a large vacuum frame and exposed to light. Areas exposed to the light become impervious; the other areas can be washed out. In the early days, silk on a wooden frame was used; today monofilament polyester is used on a titanium frame. (See Figure 2.5c.)

Paint is forced through the stencil using a plastic-bladed squeegee. The printer must skip every other repeat to prevent the silk screen frame from falling in wet ink. Each screen lays down one color—if a pattern has eight colors it must be printed eight times with eight different colors.[30] (See Figure 2.5d.)

Block printing is the process of producing a pattern on a wallcovering by means of wood blocks into which the design is cut.[31] (The block printing method is similar to the process used to make potato blocks in

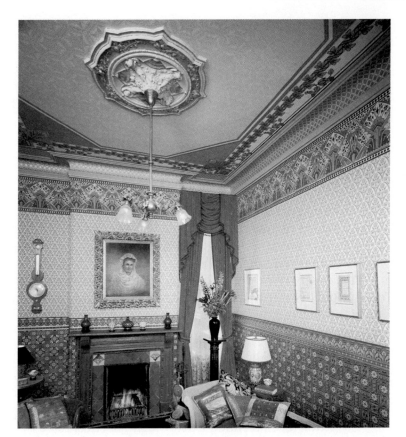

FIGURE 2.8
This photo is part of the Dresser collection (1834–1904). Dresser was one of the most startlingly original designers of the Victorian era. (Photo courtesy of Bradbury & Bradbury Art Wallpapers)

grade schools.) Because silk screening and block printing are hand processes, a machinelike quality is not possible or perhaps even desirable. The pattern does not always meet at the seams as positively as does the roller-printed pattern. Matching should be exact in the 3- to 5-foot area above the floor, where it is most noticeable.

One of the best characteristics of the Duraprene-based line from Blumenthal is its great absorption of inks and surface dyes in patterning. The coverage and saturation is much deeper and better than standard vinyl printing, and printing is much more stable. The feel of the product is also an added bonus. It is sumptuous and soft to the touch, like brushed leather.

Basic Wallcovering Backings

The surface of wallcovering products usually commands the majority of attention paid to wallcoverings, but the backing of these products is just as important from a functional value. The various types of backing are:

Paper backings—used on paper-backed vinyls, vinyl-coated papers, and specialty products.

Woven fabric backings—commonly referred to as scrim or **osnaburg.** Scrim is used mostly in light construction areas whereas osnaburg is installed in medium- to heavy-usage areas such as commercial corridors.

Nonwoven fabric backings—in different grades offer improved wallcovering printing techniques while maintaining the tear-strength qualities necessary for commercial installations.

Latex acrylic backings—used on fabric wallcoverings to allow for stability and improved handing qualities.[32]

Most machine-printed wallcoverings are **pretrimmed** at the factory, but the majority of handprints and hand-made textures are untrimmed. "This selvage (excess trimmed edge) should be removed from the wall and seams closed within one hour."[33]

Packaging

Wallcovering comes in many different lengths and widths and, although usually priced by the yard or single roll, it is packaged in either double- or triple-roll bolts. Double- and triple-roll bolts provide more usable wallcovering than single rolls.

Although most designers and contractors use commercial (contract) wallcoverings, many designers are using residential products, especially in extended care and corporate environments. Following are some facts about residential wallpaper:

Residential wallcoverings vary in width from $20\frac{1}{2}$ to 28 inches and range from $13\frac{1}{2}$ to $16\frac{1}{2}$ feet in length, which yields a metric size single roll between 27 and 30 square feet. The primary reason is due to different equipment.

Metric, also called Euroroll single rolls, have between $27\frac{1}{2}$ and 29 square feet. It is generally sold in double rolls.

Residential wallcoverings may be priced by the single roll, but are generally packaged in double or triple rolls. American single rolls, which are being phased out, are packaged with almost 25 percent more wallcovering than a metric roll. American single rolls, regardless of their lengths and widths, usually have about 36 square feet of surface.[34]

When ordering handprints from a retail store, there are a few things one must know: There is a cutting charge if the wallcovering order requires a cut bolt. Because the shading and even the positioning of the pattern on the roll may vary between dye lots or runs, SUFFICIENT BOLTS SHOULD ALWAYS BE ORDERED when the order is placed. The particular dye lot, which is stamped on the back of the roll, may not be available if it is necessary to order more in the future. Opened or partially used bolts are not returnable, and unopened bolts may be subject to a restocking charge.

Commercial Wallcoverings

Commercial, or contract, wallcoverings are manufactured specifically for commercial use and are 52 or 54 inches wide and are sold by the lineal yard. A lineal yard is any width by the length of 36 inches.[35]

These wider coverings require a highly skilled professional paperhanger and a helper. The final appearance of the walls depends on the ability of the paperhanger.

Commercial wallcoverings are produced specifically for use in hotels, apartments buildings, office buildings, schools, and hospitals. They are manufactured to meet or surpass minimum physical and performance characteristics set forth in federal guidelines (Federal Specifications CCC-W408). The guidelines focus on requirements for flammability, tear strength, abrasion resistance, washability, scrubbability, and stain resistance. Examples of various types of commercial wallcoverings are:

> **Vinyl coated paper**: This wallpaper has a paper substrate on which the decorative surface has been sprayed or coated with an acrylic coating. The proper name for this type of paper should be acrylic coated paper, but the inaccurate name has caught on and is used in its stead. These wallpapers are classified as scrubbable and strippable, and are suitable in most any area. These papers are better resistant to grease and moisture than plain paper, and are good for bathrooms and kitchens....
>
> **Cork and cork veneer**: They have a variegated texture with no definite pattern or design. Cork veneer is shaved from cork planks or blocks and laminated to a substrate that may be colored or plain. Cork naturally absorbs sound, insulates, provides visual contrast and can be used as a bulletin board.[36]

Tensile strength is the single most important performance feature in commercial wallcovering. Abrasion resistance is important but mainly in key areas such as outside corners. As mentioned previously, mildew is a problem with walls and whether using paint or wallcovering, the walls should be washed with a mixture of equal parts of household bleach and water. The correct paste or adhesive will help prevent mildew from forming under newly hung wallcovering. If proper precautions are not taken, any mildew that forms will permanently discolor the wallcovering. As noted, most adhesives contain an antifungal protection.

> ESSEX 54" wallcoverings last three times longer than paint and may be specified in both Type I and Type II. Perfect for protection of healthcare environments, all ESSEX vinyl wallcoverings incorporate germicidal additives, inhibiting the growth of bacteria on the product. Our easy-to-clean PreFixx® coating, a valuable option, provides invisible, hygienic protection against stains while preserving textural and design detail.[37]

With plain textures, grasscloths, and suedes, it is advisable to reverse the direction of every other strip of wallcovering. This will provide a better finished appearance, particularly if one side of the wallcovering happens to be shaded a little more than the other.

Commercial wallcoverings are no longer limited to using only textures for style diversity. JM Lynne manufactures a decorative overprint on its plain Renaissance texture. The print and the texture may be used in the same area for a touch of elegance.

As mentioned, commercial wallcovering usually comes in 52- to 54-inch wide bolts. Milliken & Company has introduced 180 Walls™, a revolutionary self-adhesive textile wall covering that hangs without paste; experiences no wet movement, shrinkage or corner peel; and can be removed years later without damage to walls.

The proprietary pressure-sensitive adhesive component of 180 Walls™ is carefully engineered to adhere to a prepared surface and then remove cleanly even after years of service. Since 180 Walls™ will remove without damaging the walls, the surface will be ready for the next product without additional preparation. The adhesive-textile construction has passed performance hang tests beyond seven years.[38]

Quantex™ from MDC Wallcoverings is a one-of-a-kind textile wallcovering which creates totally seamless rooms and corridors. The roll is 108 inches tall and endless in length in that the total width of all the walls is the length ordered. The only seam is at the chosen point of origin. This woven textile has the best characteristics of olefins, such as durability and cleanability, but because of its extreme width provides seamless installations and avoids panel shading. The current Quantex collection is Teflon coated.

RJF International was first to begin work on perfecting the use of water-based inks in our processes and discontinued the use of cadmium-based inks.[39]

Koroseal®, a division of RJF International, pioneered the Early Warning Effect®, a process by which a colorless, odorless, harmless vapor is released, setting off an ionization smoke alarm when the wallcovering is heated to a temperature of 300°F. This temperature can occur as early as 45 minutes before actual combustion takes place. Koroseal® is also top-coated with KoroKlear®, a water-based acrylic coating that enhances wallcovering cleanability. These vinyls are also UL approved to Class A federal standards and contain antimicrobial and mildew-resistant elements. The UL label is recognized on products as a measure of safety and assurance for the customer.

Texturglas® from Roos International Ltd. is a wallcovering system that combines the versatility of paint, from latex to **epoxy,** with the strength and benefits of woven glass textile yarns to meet the most demanding wall finish requirements. The glass textile yarns are made from all natural materials—sand, lime and clay. The yarns are woven into various textures and patterns and treated with a natural starch binder for dimensional stability during the hanging process. All glass textile wallcovering textures come unfinished from the factory.

It is available in many textures of timeless designs that are designed to be finished with a paint coating or decorative finish after installation. With its inherent characteristics, glass textile wallcovering is a natural choice where durability, safety and health are a concern. It will not shrink or stretch; exceeds Class A fire ratings and toxicity requirements; is highly breathable to reduce the risk of mold and mildew; environmentally friendly; highly durable and long lasting; can be renewed/repainted on the wall many times thereby reducing landfill waste; and paintability means color and finish options are virtually unlimited. [emphasis added][40]

All textile wallcoverings have good acoustic qualities and good energy-saving insulation qualities. Textiles may be backed by paper, and the fiber content may be 100 percent jute or a combination of synthetics and wool and jute and/or linen and cotton. These textiles usually have a flame-spread rating of 25 or less.

Tretford Broadloom, a concentric ribbing in 38 colors from Eurotex, is mainly used in Europe for floors, but in the United States it is also used on walls. Face yarns are 80 percent wool/mohair and 20 percent nylon, with a primary backing of PVC and a secondary backing of jute. With a flame spread of 5, Tretford Broadloom is very suitable for contract work, absorbs sound, cushions impact, insulates to save energy, and is an excellent display surface that accepts Velcro® and push pins. Tretford can be installed on any dry, smooth surface, such as concrete, drywall, plaster, wood paneling, or particleboard. Installation on cinder or cement blocks or on surfaces covered with wallpaper or vinyl wallcovering is *not* recommended. Tretford is installed with an adhesive applied with a notched trowel, and maintenance involves brushing lightly in the direction of ribs and periodically vacuuming the surface.[41]

Sisal is another wallcovering that has high sound absorption and is static free. Rolls are either 4 or 8 feet wide and 100 feet long. Sisal has an extremely prickly texture, as opposed to the other textiles, but this roughness can be an asset, as in the following case: A school found that when students lined up outside the cafeteria, the wall against which they were standing became dirty and defaced by graffiti. Installation of sisal prevented both problems and reduced the noise level.

One of the special surface treatments for wallcoverings is DuPont Tedlar®, which is a tough, transparent fluoride plastic sheet that is very flexible, chemically inert, and extremely resistant to stains, yellowing, corrosive chemicals, solvents, light, and oxygen. Most commercial wallcovering manufacturers produce wallcovering products that are, or may be, surfaced with Tedlar. Another stain-resistant product is PreFixx®, which protects invisibly with no loss of texture.

Some companies offer special-order printing of wallcoverings for minimum orders of 50 rolls or more. These prints may be designs already in a company's line or custom designs. Because such special orders involve hand printing, they are expensive; but they may solve a particular design problem.

In large public buildings, different colors of vinyl wallcovering are often used as a path-finding aid for patrons. The different colors can indicate certain floors, or areas or departments within that floor.

Installation

Before hanging any wallcovering, the walls must be sized. Sizing is a liquid applied to the wall surface that serves several purposes: It seals the surface against alkali, also known as hot spots, reduces absorption of the paste or adhesive to be used, and provides tooth for the wallcovering. The sizing must be compatible with the paste or adhesive used. There are many types of wallcovering adhesives, each formulated for various performance characteristics. Some adhesives are formulated for lightweight and delicate fabrics whereas others are designed to adhere heavyweight vinyl and acoustical coverings.

Adhesives vary in level of wet-tack, solids, open-time, strippability and ease of application. All wallcovering adhesives contain a biocide system. These systems are designed to prevent bacteria contamination and mildew/fungal infestation both "in-the-can" and in the dried adhesive. Wallcovering adhesives are generally applied on the back of the wallcovering either by roller or pasting machine.[42]

The manufacturer will always specify which type of adhesive is to be used. If fabric or grasscloth is hung, a nonstaining cellulose paste should be used. Adhesives on the surface of textile wallcoverings is difficult or impossible to remove.

There are four main categories of adhesives: prepasted activators, mainly used for do-it-yourself use; clear adhesives for both retail and commercial installers; clay adhesives, which increase the wet-tack and level of solids, for use by professional installers; and vinyl-over-vinyl, for use when pasting vinyl or vinyl borders to other vinyl-faced materials.

Paste or adhesive is applied by means of a wide brush to the back of the wallcovering. Particular attention should be paid to the edges because this is where any curling will occur. The wallcovering is folded or **booked,** without creasing. This allows the moisture in the adhesive to be absorbed by the fabric substrate or backing, thus allowing for any shrinkage before the wallcovering is applied to the wall surface. Booking also makes an 8- or 9-foot strip easier to handle and transport from the pasting table.

Maintenance

All stains or damage should be corrected immediately. Paper-faced wallcoverings should be tested to ascertain if the inks are permanent before cleaning fluids are applied. Vinyls may be scrubbed with a soft brush and water if they have been designated scrubbable. Foils are washed with warm water and wiped with a soft cloth to avoid any scratching. Hard water tends to leave a film on the reflective surfaces of foil.

Grasscloths, suedes, fabrics, sisal, and carpeting may be vacuumed to remove dust. Again, always follow the manufacturer's instructions for maintenance. Vinyl-covered walls should be washed at least once or twice a year. Grease and oils, in particular, should not be allowed to accumulate.

Koroseal recommends the following maintenance procedures:

1. For routine dirt and grime, use a mild detergent dissolved in warm water.
2. For severe dirt conditions, use a concentrated solution of a mild detergent applied with a stiff brush. Remove the grimy suds by padding with a damp sponge. The wall should be rinsed with clean water to remove detergent residue.
3. For surface stains such as lipstick, ball-point ink, heel marks, shoe polish, carbon smudges, and the like: use anhydrous isopropyl alcohol as an efficient cleaner for removal of such stains from vinyl wallcoverings. Ethyl alcohol or denatured alcohols are also efficient. Do not use strong alkaline or abrasive cleaners.[43]

BIBLIOGRAPHY

Builders Guide to Paints and Coatings. Upper Marlboro, MD: NAHB Research Center in co-operation with Sherwin-Williams, 1993.

Entwisle, E. A. *The Book of Wallpaper, A History and an Appreciation.* Trowbridge, England: Redwood Press Ltd., 1970.

50,000 Years of Protection and Decoration, History of Paint and Color. Pittsburgh, PA: Pittsburgh Plate Glass Company, 1995.

Morgans, W. M. *Outlines of Paint Technology. Painting and Coating Systems Guide.* Cleveland, OH: Sherwin-Williams, 2004–2005.

Schumacher Co. *A Guide to Wallcoverings.* New York: Schumacher.

S.T.A.R.T. *Paint, Stains and Clear Coatings.* Sherwin Williams.

GLOSSARY

abrade. To scrape or rub off a surface layer.

acrylic. A synthetic resin used in high-performance water-based coatings.

alkyd. Synthetic resin modified with oil.

binder. Solid ingredients in a coating that hold the pigment particles in suspension and attach them to the substrate. Consists of resins (e.g., oils, alkyd, latex). The nature and amount of binder determines many of the paint's performance properties—washability, toughness, adhesion, color retention, etc.

bleed. When color penetrates through another coat of paint.

booked. Wallpaper that has been folded with the pasted sides together in order to carry it from the cutting table to the wall.

calcium carbonate. An extender pigment.

chinoiserie. (French) Refers to Chinese or Oriental designs or themes.

chroma. A measurement of color; the degree of saturation of a hue.

DFT. Dry film thickness. The mil thickness when coating has dried.

efflorescence. A white alkaline powder deposited on the surface of stone, brick, plaster, or mortar, caused by leaching.

embossed. Paper covered with raised designs.

enamel. Broad classification of paints that dry to a hard, usually glossy finish.

epoxy. Extremely tough and durable synthetic resin used in some coatings.

extenders. Ingredients added to paint to increase coverage, reduce cost, achieve durability, and alter appearance. Less expensive than prime hiding pigments such as titanium dioxide.

faux. French for "false" or "artificial"; pronounced *fo*. Includes marbling or other imitation finishes.

fire retardant. A coating that (1) reduces flame spread, (2) resists ignition when exposed to high temperature, or (3) insulates the substrate and delays damage to the substrate.

flagged bristles. Split ends.

frieze. A type of wallcovering popular in the early 1900s. Generally a pictorial border that ran above the door height or, in dining rooms, above the plate rail.

glazes. Clear mediums that, when added to paint, make the paint more transparent, giving depth to the desired faux finish.

gloss. Luster. The ability of a surface to reflect light. Measured by determining the percentage of light reflected from a surface at certain angles.

gum. A solid resinous material that can be dissolved and that will form a film when the solution is spread on a surface and the solvent is allowed to evaporate. Usually a yellow, orange, or clear solid.

gypsum board. Thin slabs of plaster covered with heavy-weight, 100 percent recycled paper covering.

hand screened. Hand-printed wallcovering, especially silk screen designs.

hiding power. The ability of paint film to obscure the substrate to which it is applied. Measured by determining the minimum thickness at which film will completely obscure a black-and-white pattern.

humidity. The amount of water vapor in the atmosphere.

intumescent. A mechanism whereby fire-retardant paints protect the substrates to which they are applied. An intumescent paint puffs up when exposed to high temperatures, forming an insulating, protective layer over the substrate.

kiln-dried. Lumber dried in an oven to a specific moisture content.

luster. Same as *gloss*.

mill scale. An almost invisible surface scale of oxide formed when iron is heated.

mils. Measurement of thickness of film. One one-thousandth of an inch. One mil equals 25.4 microns (micrometers).

mural. A scene made up of several panels in sequence.

mylar. A hard plastic film that offers an impressive appearance along with durability.

NGR. Non-grain-raising; a type of stain.

osnaburg. Coarse linen or cotton woven fabric.

oxidation. Chemical reaction upon exposure to oxygen.

pigments. Insoluble, finely ground materials that give paint its properties of color. Hiding capabilities.

pretrimmed. Selvages or edges have been removed.

PVC. When used in connection with paint, pigment volume concentration; in wallcoverings, indicates polyvinyl chloride.

reduction. Lowering the viscosity of a paint by the addition of solvent or thinner.

resin. A solid or semisolid material that deposits a film and is the actual film-forming ingredient in paint. Can be natural or synthetic. See *gum*.

set. Countersunk below the surface of the gypsum board.

solids. The part of the coating that remains on a surface after the vehicle has evaporated. The dried paint film.

solvent. Any liquid that can dissolve a resin. Generally refers to the liquid portion of paints and coatings that evaporates as the coating dries.

spectrophotometer. An instrument used for comparing the color intensities of different spectra.

substrate. Any surface to which a coating is applied.

tensile strength. Resistance of a material to tearing apart when under tension.

titanium dioxide. A white pigment providing the greatest hiding power of all white pigments. Nontoxic and nonreactive.

trompe l'oeil. French for "fooling the eye." A design that creates a three-dimensional illusion.

tooth. The slight texture of a surface that provides good adhesion for subsequent coats of paint.

urethane. An important resin in the coatings industry.

vehicle. Portion of a coating that includes all liquids and the binder.

viscosity. The resistance to flow in a liquid. The fluidity of a liquid such as water has a low viscosity and molasses a very high viscosity.

0-25 flame spread. Lowest acceptable rating for commercial and public buildings.

VOC. Volatile organic compound. Topic emissions from solvents in paints and other ingredients used in manufacturing.

NOTES

[1]History of Paints and Coatings, National Paint and Coatings Association, www.paint.org/ind_info/ history.htm.

[2]Website, www.paint.org.

[3]S.T.A.R.T. *Paints, Stains and Clear Coatings,* Sherwin Williams, p. 2.

[4]Ibid, p. 3.

[5]Ibid, p. 3.

[6]Ibid, p. 3.

[7]Ibid, p. 3.

[8]Ibid, p. 5.

[9]Ibid, p. 6.

[10]*Builders Guide to Paints and Coatings.* Upper Marlboro, MD: NAHB Research Center, 1993, pp. 10, 12.

[11]Website, www.paint.org.

[12]*Paints, Stains and Clear Coatings,* p. 6.

[13]Ibid, p. 6.

[14]*Builders Guide to Paints and Coatings,* pp. 12, 13.

[15]Ibid, p. 12.

[16]Ibid, p. 13.

[17]Ibid, p. 13.

[18]Website, www.triarcinc.com.

[19]Hometime Video Publishing Inc., "Stenciling."

[20]Paint & Coatings Industry Information Center, www.paintinfo.org/articles/newpaint.htm.

[21]Morgans, W. M., *Cultures of Paint Technology*. *Painting and Coatings Systems* Guide. Cleveland, OH: Sherwin-Williams, 2004–2005, p. 5.

[22]Sherwin-Williams website, www.sherwin-williams.com.

[23]Wallcovering Association website, www.wallcovering.org, "Contract Wallcovering Guide: Grounds & Substrates."

[24]Ibid.

[25]Ibid, "Types of Pattern Matches."

[26]MDCoverings website, www.mdcwallcovering.com.

[27]OMNOVAR Solutions Inc. website, www.omnova/com.

[28]Website of Seabrook Wallpaper, www.srabrookwallpaper.com.

[29]Website, Bradbury.

[30]Wallcovering Association website, www.wallcoverings.org, "Contract Wallcovering Guide.

[31]Website, www.doityourself.com.

[32]Ibid, "Basic Wallcovering Backings."

[33]Ibid.

[34]Ibid.

[35]Ibid.

[36]Ibid.

[37]Website, www.omnova.com.

[38]Milliken Co. website, www.milliken.com.

[39]Website, www.koroseal.com.

[40]Website, www.roosintl.com.

[41]Website, www.tretfordusa.com.

[42]Website, www.dlcouch.com.

[43]Koroseal, "Suggested Specifications, Installation Instructions, Care and Maintenance." New Jersey, n.d.

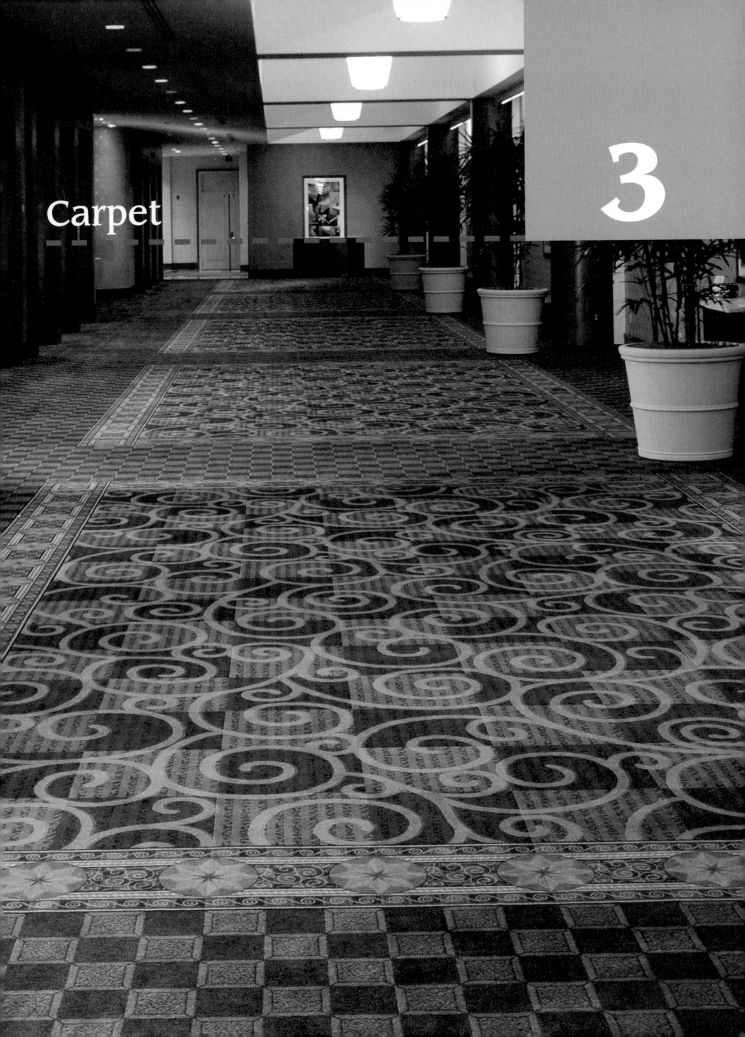

Carpet

3

HISTORY OF CARPET

When and where carpets were first knotted is unknown, but it is generally believed that nomadic tribes in central Asia were some of the first rug weavers in areas known today as Turkey and Iran (Persia). The climate was very cold and the mountain ranges in these areas are perfect for raising sheep, the source of carpet wool. We know very little of early weavings as the materials used were all perishable, and only a few rug fragments woven before the 15th century have survived.

Fortunately, while archeological excavations were ongoing in a valley of the Altai mountain range in lower Siberia during 1947–49, a Russian archeologist, S. J. Rudenko, made an exciting discovery. He found an extremely well-preserved rug in a burial tomb that belonged to the prince of Altai who lived in the 5th century B.C.

This rug, today called the Paxryk carpet, survived in good condition due to a lucky combination of circumstances. It appears that shortly after the prince's grave-mound was completed, it was plundered by robbers who tunneled into the mound and removed all the precious objects. They had no interest in the Paxryk carpet and left it behind. Later, a torrent of water rushed into the opening the robbers made into the grave-mound and filled the chamber. The huge volume of water turned into ice, freezing the Pazryk carpet until it was discovered 2,500 years later. Incredibly, the rug was well preserved. The design, dyes and construction were all of the highest quality, indicating that the weaver was knowledgeable and experienced, and that rug weaving was at quite an accomplished level in the 5th century B.C.

The Pazyrk carpet measures 6' × 6'6" and is exhibited in the Hermitage Museum in St. Petersburg. The design has a large geometric center field area composed of squares and is framed by two main borders. In one border are deer, in the other warriors are featured on horseback.

There are several other famous carpets woven between the 16th and 18th centuries that have survived. Most of these are now in museums throughout Europe. Many of the over-sized pieces were commissioned for the palaces of royalty. These carpets are truly breathtaking when one considers their exquisite detail and the thousands of hours devoted to their weaving.[1]

No royal support for carpet weaving was given until Henry IV set up a workroom for weaving in the Louvre in 1604. Royal support not only meant the development of carpets that reflected courtly taste, but also ensured the protection and growth of the industry. The Spanish were the first Europeans to make hand-tied **pile** rugs. Often credited with the "invention" of the weaving industry is Englishman Thomas Whitty of Axminster, who in the 1700s developed the first machine loom that could weave carpets, which resulted in **Axminster** carpets. Frenchman Joseph-Marie Jacquard devised a mechanism for figured or patterned weaving in 1800, and it was first used in Wilton, England.

In colonial America, the first floor coverings were herbs, rushes, or sand spread on the floor. Later, rag rugs made from clothing scraps and hooked or braided mats were used. Affluent settlers, however, introduced America to prized oriental rugs, which they brought with them to the New World. Oriental rugs may have as many as 500 to 600 knots per square inch and are named for the pattern and district where they are woven.

The first U.S. carpet mill was started in Philadelphia in 1791. America's most important historic contribution to the industry was the invention of the power loom by Erastus Bigelow in 1841. Years later, the first Brussels (looped-pile carpet) was made here, utilizing the **Jacquard** method of color pattern control, and with further modification the first **Wilton** carpets were also woven in the United States. By the later 19th century, a great deal of machinery and skilled labor found its way to the United States, and the roots of many of today's major carpet manufacturing firms were established.

For centuries, a hand-made wool rug has been a status symbol. In the past the high price of a wool rug or carpet was probably due to the tremendous labor involved; an ancient weaver needed 900 days to complete an oriental carpet.[2] It is interesting to note that whereas Europeans buy old oriental rugs, Americans prefer to buy new ones.

Thus, carpets were originally for the wealthy. Today, because of modern technology, carpet is one product that gives more value for the money than in the past.

This chapter deals with carpet, defined as fabric used as a floor covering, rather than rugs (carpet cut into room or area dimensions and loose laid). Area rugs also include oriental rugs, **kilims, rya** rugs, **dhurries,** and American Indian rugs. (Note: According to historians, American Indians developed weaving traditions independently from other civilizations.) Much of the information on weaves, pile, etc. may also apply to area rugs.

Area rugs are gaining in popularity because of the mobility of our population. Rugs can be used in many ways: as accents over existing carpet, to highlight a wood floor, or to spotlight area groupings.

Much of the information presented in this chapter is taken, with permission, from the Carpet and Rug Institute's *Specifier's Handbook*, a detailed and informative book available from the CRI. All interior designers should have a copy of this handbook in their design library.

FUNCTIONS OF CARPET

According to the CRI, the following are the primary features of carpet:

Acoustical—Carpet absorbs 10 times more airborne noise that any other flooring material and as much as most other types of standard acoustical materials. It virtually eliminates floor impact noises at the source. . .

Beauty—Carpet provides a tremendous choice of colors, textures, and designs to suit every taste. Custom-designed carpet for commercial installation is also available at reasonable prices. Carpet has a way of framing the furnishings in a room or office that makes them look more important and distinctive.

Atmosphere—Carpet dramatically enhances the feeling of quality in interior design—a major consideration in hotels and motels.

Carpet also has the ability to "de-institutionalize" a building—a significant factor in improved patient morale in hospitals, and in student attitudes in school.

Thermal Insulation—Physically, the pile construction of carpet is a highly efficient thermal insulator. Mechanical demonstrations have shown that over a cold cement slab, carpet's surface temperature is substantially higher than that of hard surface tile. Thus, carpet relieves coldness at foot and ankle levels and lends a psychological warmth as well. . .

Safety—The National Safety Council reports that falls cause most indoor injuries. . . . Carpet's ability to cushion falls and prevent serious injuries means savings in medical costs, and man-hours to businessmen.

Comfort—Carpet reduces "floor fatigue". . . . This characteristic is important to salespeople, teachers, nurses, waiters—all those who spend many hours on their feet during the course of their work.[3]

CONSTRUCTION METHODS

It is important to understand carpet construction in order to apply the variables that affect performance of a specific installation. Tufted carpet consists of the following components: the face yarn, which can be cut pile, loop pile, or a combination of cut and loop pile; primary backing fabric; a binding compound, usually **SB** latex, but may be polyurethane, PVC, or fabric; and (often) a secondary fabric.

The development of the broadloom tufting machine and the introduction of synthetic carpet yarns in the early 1950s transformed American carpet industry from low-volume production of woven luxury products to mass production of high-quality and comfortable, yet popularly priced, goods. The explosive growth of carpet sales in the United States in the ensuing years paralleled the development of tufting technology, the proliferation of high-speed tufting machines, and the development of synthetic carpet fibers and alternative backing systems. As a result, today's carpet is both better and less expensive.[4] (See Figure 3.1.)

In the beginning, carpet looms were only 27 inches wide. Most carpet is usually 12 feet wide, although some carpets come in 15-foot widths and carpet may be custom sized for large installations. However, according to the CRI:

6-foot width carpet is increasing in use and is available in many designs with a variety of backing systems to accommodate performance

FIGURE 3.1
Annual fiber consumption. (Courtesy of the Carpet and Rug Institute, Carpet Primer)

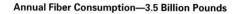
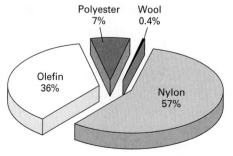

Annual Fiber Consumption—3.5 Billion Pounds

Polyester 7%
Wool 0.4%
Olefin 36%
Nylon 57%

The largest manufacturer alone uses over 2 million pounds of fiber per day.

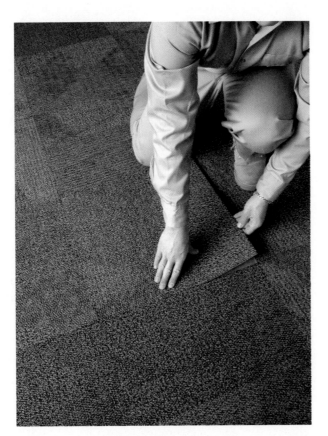

FIGURE 3.2
Installation and removal
of carpet modules is
easy, as shown in this
photo. (Courtesy of
Interface FLOR, LLC.)

needs. This narrow carpet roll is often a benefit in high-rise buildings where transporting a 12-foot roll is difficult or expensive. The narrow width may also provide a cost savings where many hallways or other narrow spaces exist. However, careful planning is needed to avoid more seams.[5]

Another production output is *modular carpet tiles*, available in 12-inch × 12-inch and 18-inch × 18-inch sizes, although 24-inch × 24-inch is occasionally used. Tiles 36-inch × 36-inch are rarely used. (See Figure 3.2.)

Lees' Self Lock® is a patented, factory-applied, releasable adhesive system, available exclusively on Lees Squared® modular carpets. . . . The adhesive is manufactured directly to the back of each module, so carpet tiles go down quickly, cleanly and economically.

The Self Lock system prevents shifting even at pivot pints, on ramps and under rolling chairs. Chair pads are not required.

FirstStep® from Lees Carpet is an 18-inch × 18-inch modular carpet tiles designed specifically for entryways. FirstStep is engineered with heavy "scraper" yarn that provides for ideal soil removal and collection. FirstStep can reduce the amount of soil and moisture entering a facility by up to 91 percent, resulting in lowered maintenance costs and extended life for all floor coverings beyond the entry to the building.

Carpet tile construction is also advancing because of performance. Continually changing configuration of open plan systems office furnishings have demanded advanced technologies in carpet

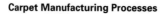

Carpet Manufacturing Processes

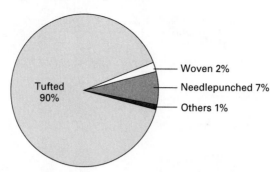

Tufted 90%

Woven 2%

Needlepunched 7%

Others 1%

Most carpet today—90%—is tufted, the process that
grew out of the chenille bedspread industry.

tile, or modules, for increased functional benefits. . . . The possibility of rotation of tiles where paths or soiling occur is sometimes a better alternative than a complete replacement.[6]

The main manufacturing processes in order of quantity of carpet produced are tufting, woven, needle-punch, and others, some of which are shown in Figure 3.3.

Tufting

It is interesting to note that the art of tufting started in Dalton, Georgia, with hand-tufted bedspreads. This process gradually became mechanized and looms were widened to make tufted carpet. In a tufted piece of carpet, the back is woven first and then the face is tufted into it and backed with additional material. Tufting is a much faster process than the traditional weaving method and has greatly reduced the cost of carpet, thereby making it available to more buyers. The technique is fast, efficient, and simple. More than 90 percent of all carpet sold in the United States is tufted and 70 percent is made in Dalton, the "Carpet Capital of the World."

Weaving

Weaving is a fabric formation process used for manufacturing carpet in which **yarns** are interlaced to form cloth. The weaving loom interlaces lengthwise (warp) and widthwise (filling) yarns. **Pitch** is measured by the number of lengthwise warp yarns; in a 27-inch width, the higher the number, the finer the weave. Carpet weaves are complex, often involving several sets of warps and filling yarns. The back and the face are produced simultaneously and as one unit. When describing an area rug, the term *tapestry weave* is sometimes used, but sisal is always woven. According to the DuPont Company, "When a woven carpet backing is used, specify 100% moisture-resistant warp, filling and stuffer yarns for this construction to eliminate shrinkage during wet cleaning or where installation is on or below grade."[7]

Velvet carpets are the simplest carpets to weave. They are made on a velvet loom that is similar to the Wilton loom but without the Jacquard unit. The rich appearance of velvets is due to their high pile density. Velvets can be cut or looped pile.

Knitted

Knitted carpets were not made by machine until 1940. Their quality is generally high, depending on the yarns used and their density. Knitting a carpet involves at least three different facing yarns and perhaps a fourth for backing. Face yarns are knitted in with warp chains and weft-forming yarns in a simple knitting process. Variations of colors, yarns, and pile treatment (cut or looped, high or low) create design choices for knitted carpets. Knitting today is a speedy process that produces fine-quality carpet. Most knitted carpet is solid colored or tweed, although some machines have pattern devices. Both loop and cut-pile surfaces are available.

Needle Punching

Needle-punched carpet is a durable, felt-like product manufactured by entangling a fiber fleece with barbed needles. . . . A latex coating or attached padding is applied to the back. . . . Technological advances in machinery now allow a diverse range of designs, including ribs, sculptured designs, and patterns. Needle-punched carpet is almost always glued down when installed.[8]

Aubusson

Aubussons are flatly woven tapestries and carpets in silk or wool, named for the French town where they originated (circa 1500). Tapestries bear narratives or portraits, whereas carpets feature architectural designs in rich colors or flowers in muted pastels.

Axminster and Wilton

Axminster and Wilton carpets both are woven, and although their appearance may be similar, their construction is very different. In an Axminster, pile tufts are inserted from colored yarns arranged on spools, making possible an enormous variety of colors and geometric or floral patterns. The Wilton looms have Jacquard pattern mechanisms that use punched cards to select pile height and yarn color. In a Wilton, unwanted yarn colors are buried under the surface of the carpet, limiting the color selection to five or six colors. The carpets are often patterned or have multilevel surfaces. The traditional fiber in Axminster and Wilton construction is wool, but a blend of 80 percent wool and 20 percent nylon is sometimes used. One way to distinguish between the two types is to roll them across the warp and weft. A Wilton will fold in both directions, an Axminster only in one.

It is critical when cleaning Axminster cut-pile carpet not to use spin bonnets, rotary brushes, or rotary extractors. The rotary action of this equipment can severely distort the pile yarn. In addition, the

FIGURE 3.4
Construction methods.

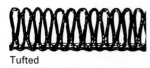
Tufted

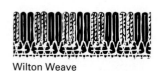
Wilton Weave

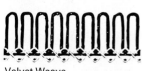
Velvet Weave

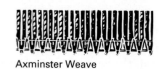
Axminster Weave

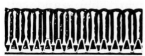
Knitted

spin bonnet method can leave chemical residue which builds up in the carpet.[9]

See Figure 3.4 for examples for carpet construction methods.

The three Cs—**c**olor, **c**omfort, and **c**ost—are probably the major factors in residential carpet choice, whereas in commercial and institutional projects durability, traffic, cost, and ease of maintenance are more important features. The properties considered in carpet selection also include type of fiber, density of pile, depth of pile, method of construction, pattern, and cleanability.

FIBERS

Fiber type is the major decision in selecting a carpet. Each fiber has its own characteristics, and modern technology has greatly improved the features of synthetic fibers. The cost and characteristics of the fiber need to be considered together so the final selection will fulfill the client's need.

The most prevalent natural fiber used in carpet is wool, but in some rare instances silk, linen, and cotton may be used. Other natural fibers gaining in popularity are sisal and coir. Synthetic fibers are always more colorfast than natural fibers because to produce colored fibers, the dye can be introduced while the fiber is in its liquid state. Wool, in its natural state, is limited to off-white, black/gray, and various shades in between.

Carpet manufacturers do not produce the actual fibers described in this section, but rather buy the fibers from various chemical companies. Honeywell Nylon Inc. has been sold to Shaw Industries Group, Inc., a subsidiary of Berkshire Hathaway, Inc. Honeywell will supply Shaw with caprolactum and nylon resin, the chemicals used in the production of nylon fibers for carpeting. Zeftron is their name brand for commercial carpet. Du Pont sells the fibers. Solutia only makes 6,6 nylon, in brands such as Wear-Dated and Ultron; the other companies produce both type 6 and type 6,6.

Nylon

Nylon was introduced by DuPont in 1938 and accounts for nearly 90 percent of all carpet sold today. In the past, nylon was designated by the generations, which basically went from 1 to 5. Each generation had some type of improvement in the manufacturing process. However, nylon producers no longer use the generation label. Type 6 and type 6,6 do not have the same chemical composition. Type 6,6 has a tighter molecular structure with more hydrogen bonding, better resistance to stains, enhanced resilience, and better resistance to crushing and matting.

Antron® Legacy nylon from DuPont has a square, four-hole hollow **filament** shape, which diffuses light to hide soil. Ideal for heavy traffic/soiling areas, it has DuPont's patented fluorochemical treatment, DuraTech®, which is applied only to Antron nylon fibers during the carpet manufacturing process. According to DuPont, DuraTech can lower maintenance costs. Testing at a busy New York school has shown that the cost of hot water extraction cleaning can be reduced by 30 to 50 percent as compared to carpet not treated with DuraTech®. It is an integral part of the Antron® system and does not need to be specified. Antron® products are **antistatic** and suitable for office environments with electronic information systems.

Duracolor® is Lees' patented stain-resistant dye technology that is integrated into the fiber—rather than applied topically—to provide permanent stain resistance. In addition, Milliken has created Carpet for Extreme Conditions, or cXc™. This 6-foot, high-performance carpet, with proprietary finish technologies, was specifically engineered to succeed in 24/7 facilities where durability, maintainability, and infection control are major operational concerns.

> Solutia makes Ultron® VIP nylon, which the various companies use to manufacture their own carpet under that brand name. Solutia offers the ChroMatix™ color system for Ultron® VIP solution nylon, with 116 colors. Using a patented process, which modifies the surface properties of nylon fiber, DyeNamix™ triggers an innovative chemical reaction when color is applied in printing or space-dyeing processes.
>
> A gel-like concentrate of color is formed on the fiber surface that allows controlled, uniform absorption of dye by literally holding the rich color right where it's needed until it's set with steam.
>
> Once inside the steamer, the gel rapidly dissolves and bonds the dye to the fiber. So you get noticeably brighter, deeper shades and much sharper pattern definition. Plus, DyeNamix™ is environmentally friendly requiring significantly less dye and natural resources.[10]

Solutia's fibers are sold under the WEAR-DATED® brand for residential carpet and the ULTRON® brand for commercial carpet.

Solutia's fibers are engineered to match the wool-like luster that specifiers desire. It uses 3M™ Carpet Protector, which keeps dirt as well as water- and oil-based soils from adhering to the fiber and makes the carpet easier to clean.

> When it comes to durability, there is little difference between bulked continuous fiber **(BCF)** or staple (spun) fibers. The difference lies in the length of the fibers in the yarn, with staple having

shorter lengths, giving the yarn more bulk (sometimes described as being more like wool). [emphasis added][11]

As a synthetic fiber, nylon absorbs little water. Therefore, stains remain on the surface rather than penetrate the fiber itself. Dirt and soil are trapped between the filaments and are removed by proper cleaning methods. In addition, nylon has excellent abrasion resistance. The reason for worn or thin spots is that the yarn has been damaged physically by grit and soil ground into the carpet. This problem can be taken care of with proper maintenance. (See Table 3.1).

Wool

For many years, wool has represented the standard of quality against which all other carpet fibers are measured; this is still the case today to some degree. Most important are the aesthetics and inherent resilience of wool. The best wool for carpet comes from sheep that are raised in colder climates, such as New Zealand (domestic wools are too soft and fine for carpets). Although wool has a propensity for high static generation, treatments are available to impart static-protection properties. Wool retains color for the life of the carpet, despite wear and cleaning. It has good soil resistance because of its naturally high moisture content and has excellent pile resilience.

Wool gives good service. When price is no object, the best carpet fiber is wool. Wool blends, usually 80 percent wool and 20 percent nylon, currently have a larger market segment than they did a decade ago. Wool will stain or bleach in reaction to some spills, however, and is not as easy to clean as nylon. "Wool is naturally flame resistant, forming a char that will neither melt nor drip."[12]

A combination of 80 percent goat hair and wool is used in Tretford USA cord carpet. (See Chapter 1.) This product uses fusion-bonded construction, which can be cut in any direction without fraying or raveling, making it suitable for great floor graphics. (See Table 3.1).

TABLE 3.1
Fiber Performance
in Carpet

	Nylon (filament)	Nylon (staple)	Olefin (filament)	Polyester (staple)	Wool (staple)
Fiber Strength	Excellent	Excellent	Excellent	Excellent	Good
Appearance Retention	Excellent	Excellent	Fair	Fair	Excellent
Stain Resistant*	Very Good	Very Good	Excellent	Very Good	Very Good
Soil Resistant**	Very Good	Very Good	Fair	Good	Very Good
Cleaning	Very Good	Very Good	Very Good	Good	Very Good
Available Colors	Excellent	Excellent	Fair	Very Good	Fair
Pilling & Fuzzing	Excellent	Fair	Very Good	Fair	Fair
Resistance to Household Cleaners	Very Good	Very Good	Excellent	Very Good	Good

*Assuming nylon is treated with a stain-resistant chemical.

**Assuming treatment with a soil-resistant chemical.

Source: Fiber Performance chart courtesy of Mowhawk Industries.

Acrylic

Acrylic is the synthetic fiber that most feels like wool. Acrylic carpets have a low soiling rate, clean well, are highly static resistant, and have very good to excellent abrasion resistance and excellent colorfastness. In properly constructed carpets, pile resilience is good. "Acrylics are always used in **staple** form, and sometimes can be found in blends with other fibers." [emphasis added][13]

In the 1960s and early 1970s, acrylic was a popular fiber for commercial and residential carpet because of its good performance. New dyeing processes introduced in the 1970s, however, favored nylon due to its high dyeing rate and resistance to deformation under hot and wet conditions. In 1990, acrylic fibers were used in Berber styling to take advantage of their wool-like appearance. Now, producer-dyed acrylic is being offered, which should again make acrylic a viable fiber for commercial and residential installations. One disadvantage of acrylic is that it is less abrasion resistant and not as resilient as nylon.

Polyester

> Polyester has excellent color clarity and retains its color and luster. It is resistant to water soluble stains, and is noted for a luxurious "hand" when used in thick **cut pile** textures. Polyester is offered for carpet in staple form only. Polyester is an important carpet fiber, but more in residential styles than for commercial carpet applications. [emphasis added][14]

Polyester is a soft fiber with good soil and wear resistance, but it has a tendency to crush with wear; therefore, it should not be used in heavy-traffic areas. Polyester is often blended with polyamide in needled carpets. The CRI notes that:

> *Polypropylene* is classified as an olefin . . . and is the lightest commercial carpet fiber, with a density of 0.905. It has excellent strength, toughness, and chemical resistance. The fiber is offered as both **continuous filament** and a staple. It is sold as a **solution dyed** fiber or yarn. Because of its very low moisture absorbency and the fact that the color is sealed into the fiber, olefin has excellent resistance to stains. It has resistance to sunlight fading, and generates low levels of static electricity. [emphasis added][15]

Olefin is used for indoor and outdoor carpets, carpet backing, and wall coverings. However, olefins have fair to poor resilience of pile. (See Table 3.1).

Cotton

Cotton is an expensive natural fiber most often used for flat woven rugs such as Indian dhurries.

Sisal and Coir

Sisal, the world's strongest natural fiber, has its origins in Mexico, where the fiber is harvested from the leaves of the Henequin plant. Coir is also a natural fiber taken from the tough fibrous husk that surrounds the coconut. Because sisal and coir are natural fibers, there will be color variations when left undyed; however, several companies are dyeing, painting, or stenciling these fibers. Regardless of whether the color is natural or dyed, it may change with direct sunlight. Both of these materials have bound edges.

Seagrass

Seagrass, the perennial grass of saltwater marshes, is cut from the plant. The plants are native to the monsoon climate of the Pacific basin. Reeds are thick and rigid. The nonporous skin is smooth to the touch and gives a slight natural sheen. Seagrass, as a natural fiber, characteristically absorbs atmospheric humidity or releases it, depending on climate conditions. This will cause the material to expand slightly in damp air and contract slightly in dry conditions. Waves and curling occur when the carpet is loosely laid. To eliminate curling of the carpet, roll the corners backward, allow the carpet to lay flat, and place a few heavy books on the corners overnight. Little or no matting occurs due to the flat weave construction. The hard skin will not allow footmarks to develop. All seagrass carpets are backed with a natural rubber mat.

Paper

Merida Meridian's twisted paper cord uses pulp from conifers grown in cold, northern climates. Coniferous softwoods produce stronger paper than hardwoods because their fibers are longer. The flat woven designs combine color, weave, and texture to create textiles with visual depth and distinction. Merida uses only virgin paper because the use of recycled fibers can yield weak paper. (Of course, paper carpeting can be completely recycled after use.) When the pulp is blended, resins are added to coat the fibers, producing a high-wet strength paper, which is extremely durable. Like other carpet, this product comes 12 foot wide with a natural latex backing, and is suitable for home and light contract. This material may also be used for wall and window treatments.

Jute

Jute is the softest among the plant fibers. It comes in natural colors ranging from creamy whites to browns. It can be dyed or bleached to get other colors. Jute carpets are very economical. Although jute makes an excellent base for inexpensive, handwoven Persian kilim (rugs), it is not durable. Jute is prone to staining. It is advisable to use jute for low- and medium-traffic rooms such as bedrooms and guest rooms. Jute should not be used on stairs because the surface becomes slippery with wear.

Jute is particularly sensitive to direct sunlight; though exposure to sunlight speeds up deterioration of any plant fiber, in jute this process is hastened. West Bengal in India and Bangladesh are pioneers in jute carpets.[16]

DYEING

Color is the most important aesthetic property of carpet. Designers should be familiar with the major methods of color application to carpet. This increases their ability to specify the most appropriate carpet for a given application.

Solution Dyed—The fiber is dyed in its liquid state before it is spun into yarn. The color becomes a permanent part of the fiber and will not fade or bleach out. The precolored fibers are supplied to the carpet mills by the fiber manufacturers. This method is common for olefins (polypropylenes), nylons, and polyesters.

Stock Dyeing—After the fibers are made, they are dipped into a bath of dye where heat and pressure force color into the fiber before it is spun into yarn. There is a wide range of color choices, but fibers dyed with this process are more susceptible to fading, bleaching out, and staining. This method is used in dyeing wool, acrylics, polyesters, and some nylons.

Skein Dyeing—Yarns are spun into skeins, which are stored and dyed as orders are obtained. This method can be used for spun yarns, bulked continuous filament yarns, **heat set** yarns, and non-heat-set yarns of almost any fiber type.[17]

Piece Dyeing—is the application of color from an aqueous dyebath onto unfinished carpet (called **greige goods**) consisting only of primary backing and undyed yarns. . . . Piece dyeing is generally for solid colors. However, two or more colors can be produced in tweed, Moresque, or stripe patterns in the same carpet from a single dyebath. This is achieved by using fibers of modified and/or altered dye affinity. [emphasis added][18]

Most residential carpet today is dyed using the piece-dyeing method, since manufacturers can store the plain or undyed carpet until a particular color is needed.

Beck Dyeing The beck dye process is a method of batch dyeing carpet. This process is used for solid color carpets and carpets that use yarns of different dyeabilities. Beck deing achieves excellent color uniformity throughout the carpet.[19]

Carpet Printing is accomplished with machinery that is essentially enlarged, modified textile printing equipment. . . . Printed carpet is available in a wide variety of patterns or textures ranging from low-**level loop** carpet to **Saxony,** cut-loop, and shag. Printed carpets can simulate woven patterns at much lower cost.

Jet printing machinery consists of rows of color jets arranged across the width of the carpet. The jets are closely spaced, about an eighth to a tenth of an inch apart. Each jet may be opened or closed by computer-controlled valves as the carpet moves under the row of jets. Controlled patterns are produced without screens or physical contact of machinery against carpet. Each row of jets applies a different color. Pattern changes are rapid, requiring only computer program modifications. The jets squirt color onto the carpet surface, but unlike screens, do not crush the pile, resulting in superior texture. . . . The machinery is costly, but the obvious advantages suggest that various types of the jet printing technology may gain importance in the carpet industry.[20]

Space Dyeing (Random Printing) is the technique used to place color continuously in varied combinations of colors and spacing to avoid formulation of a discernible design repeat. How the color is imparted varies with the technique used. Space dyeing is primarily used on BCF nylon and produces different color segments along the length of the yarn. Currently there are several major space dyeing techniques: knit-de-knit, multicolor skein, warp sheet printing, and the newer continuous processes.

The knit-de-knit process or "knits" forms the yarn into a tube shape and then horizontal or diagonal color stripes are printed on both sides. The tube is steamed and dried, then unraveled (deknitted), and wound onto cones.

This process is modified from the skein dyeing technique. Various portions of the skein are dyed different colors. The colors are less random than other space dyeing techniques but can be used on multicolored cut and loop products.

A tufting type creel supplies a sheet of yarn for warp-sheet printing. A computerized printer applies colors in various lengths along the yarn axis, which is then steamed, rinsed, dried and wound onto cones. [emphasis added][21]

The Easy Change™ program from Milliken allows the designer to: (1) Select a pattern; (2) decide on the changes, such as base, background, and accent colors; (3) request a computer image; and (4) request a carpet sample and then place the order.

Although floorcloths are mentioned in the section on wood floors in Chapter 4, the manner in which they are designed and constructed is appropriate for discussion here. In the past, heavy canvas was stretched and cut to size, then primed and stenciled or hand painted in a variety of patterns, and then sealed with oil. Today, extra-heavy canvas up to 12 feet wide is used and treated with a custom-developed flexible, nonyellowing protective coating to ensure longevity and prevent cracking. Several contemporary companies and designers have stock patterns and also make floorcloths on commission.

FABRIC PROTECTORS

When discussing the different types of fabric protectors, it is important to keep in mind that some manufacturers are not anxious to divulge the contents of their protector. You may find some catchphrases that can be confusing when trying to decide what type of protector is used. Words such as *polymer, copolymer, hydrocarbon, alaphatic, chlorinated*, and even *metal cross-linked* have been used in describing fabric protectors. Although these words may have some relationship to protectors, you really only need to understand the three basic types of fabric protectors:

1. *Colloidal silica*, which fill pores, thus preventing soil from becoming embedded.
2. *Silicones*, which provide a water-repellent coating.

3. *Fluorochemicals*, which form an invisible shield on the fibers that helps prevent soil and stains from sticking. Fluorine is a very reactive, but when it once reacts or combines with something, it becomes very stable or nonreactive to the point of being repellent to just about everything.[22]

The chemistry used in Scotchgard® from the 3M Company was changed in May of 2000. The new Scotchgard treatment for carpet has been provided to carpet manufacturers to replace previous formulations. DuPont allows for the private labeling of its products. Therefore, many products containing DuPont Teflon® have appeared in the marketplace. Make sure the recommended concentration of Teflon® is being used.

Another factor to consider for computer rooms and electronic offices is a backing engineered for control of electrostatic discharge, or **ESD.**

Fire-retardant products are also used, especially in commercial installations where fire codes require such products. Wool self-extinguishes when the source of ignition is removed and merely chars, leaving only a cold ash that can be easily brushed away with no permanent scars; in contrast, synthetic fibers melt.

ANTIMICROBIAL ISSUES

For a carpet manufacturer to claim a carpet is antimicrobial, the carpet must be registered with the EPA. Registration, however, is a lengthy and expensive process. EPA registration currently has no established test methods to support antimicrobial claims on carpet. However, in order to help identify which carpet will exhibit antimicrobial efficacy, the GSA (not the EPA) uses the procedures outlined in AATCC 174 and AATCC 138 as a guideline for testing carpets. Currently, the GSA accepts any carpet that shows greater than 90% reduction in bacterial growth after 24 hours and no visible fungal activity after three days. If there is a need for antimicrobial protection in the carpet, specifiers may use the AATCC test methods when writing a specification to determine if the carpet meets their criteria.

Since the test for antimicrobial efficacy is performed on finished carpet, the carpet manufacturer must determine how to engineer their product to meet antimicrobial specifications.[23]

Intersept®, mentioned in Chapter 1, is a patented antimicrobial preservative against molds, mildews, bacteria, and odor-causing microorganisms, as shown in Figure 3.5.

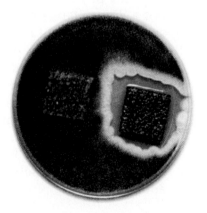

FIGURE 3.5
Intersept antimicrobial preservative. (Photo courtesy of Interface FLOR, LLC.)

FLAMMABILITY TESTING

It is extremely important for designers to realize the legal ramifications of flammability specifications because of possible damage and liability lawsuits. Designers should require carpet suppliers to submit written documentation of fire code compliance.

All carpet sold in the United States must meet the federal flammability standards, but local and regional standards also exist. The local fire marshal has the authority to establish additional specific criteria, and should be consulted prior to writing specifications or purchasing carpet for a particular installation.

Monsanto Contract Fibers has prepared a special report on flammability resistance, part of which follows:

> With the Federal regulations which govern the manufacturing of all carpet, it is now against the law to make or sell any carpet which does not pass the Methenamine Tablet Test (DOC FF 1-70). (There are additional tests required if for a commercial installation.)
>
> All fires have three distinct stages: ignition, flashover, and expansion. In the ignition stage, the fire has started but is contained in a small area of one room. Flashover occurs when the fire spreads beyond its point of origin and everything in the room is burning. In the expansion stage, the fire leaves the room and spreads over into other rooms or down a corridor. If the fire can be contained during the ignition stage, minimal damage will occur.
>
> This is the rationale behind the Methenamine Tablet Test, or pill test, as it is more commonly known. In this text eight identical carpet specimens are placed in a draft-free environment. A methanamine tablet is positioned in the center of each specimen and ignited. If two or more of the specimens burn for three inches in any direction, the carpet fails the test and cannot be sold in the United States.
>
> Another method for testing the flame resistance of carpet is the Steiner Tunnel Test (ASTM E-84). . . .
>
> This test is being replaced by the Radiant Panel Flooring Test in most states because of greater accuracy.
>
> A more accurate test is the Radiant Panel Flooring Test (ASTM E-648), which simulates conditions that could cause flame-spread in a carpet system, but applies only to carpet installed in corridors. In this test, the carpet sample and underlayment are positioned inside a test chamber. A radiating heat panel, not a direct flame, is placed at a 30° angle above one end of the sample. This panel generates heat at the carpet surface ranging from 1.1 watts/cm^2 directly beneath the panel to about 0.1 watts/cm^2 at the far end of the sample. The total distance the sample burns is measured and then converted to watts/cm^2. This number is called the critical radiant flux **(CRF).** Each sample is tested three times and an average CRF is derived. The higher the CRF, the more resistant a carpet system is to flame-spread. For example, oak flooring has a CRF of about 0.35 to 0.40 in comparison to carpet, which may have a CRF above 1.1. [emphasis added][24]

TYPES OF PILE

The CRI notes the following information pertaining to the Americans with Disabilities Act (ADA) requirements:

> The requirements by the ADA allow carpet having a pile height of $\frac{1}{2}$" or less (measured from the bottom of the tuft). Exposed edges should be fastened to floor surfaces with trim along that edge. Carpet with a pile height over $\frac{1}{2}$" must have a transition ramp between surfaces.

Today's carpets feature any of several types of pile:

Loop pile has an even surface consisting of uncut loops. Variations include high and low loops, **multilevel loops,** colors, and highly twisted yarns.

Cut pile (plush) may be made from unset yarns (frizzy ends) for an even, velvety texture or from **set yarns** (firm ended) to give a velour texture with tuft definition. These carpets look more luxurious than loop, but they also tend to show footsteps or flaws more readily. Patterned wovens or printed tufteds will offset such characteristics. Area rugs, particularly those with borders or a colored pattern, often use a **sculptured** cut pile. Where two colors meet, the pile is cut in a V shape to delineate the pattern and produce a three-dimensional effect. Plain carpet may also be carved in any design.

Frieze (hard twist) is cut pile from a highly twisted yarn set in a snarled configuration. It will hide footsteps, **shedding** and the **shading** which occurs when pile lays in opposite directions.

Semishag (splush) is soft, cut pile with shorter piles than shags. Ends of yarn stand up so that the carpet has a pebbled look.

Shag is soft carpet with long pile. An example is the Scandinavian rya rug in which different yarns may be used, but always with the side of the yarn exposed to give a shaggy look.

Tip-sheared is loop-pile carpet with some loops sheared on the surface to create areas of cut pile and a luxurious, sculpted look.

Berber was named after the original hand-woven wool squares made by the North African tribes. It is now made by machine but features a country, homespun effect and natural colors. Usually coarse loop pile, but also made in cut pile, shags, and a variety of designs, Berber is most often used in contemporary rooms. The Berber weaving system is the oldest in the history of rug making; it may be as old as the second millennium B.C. Flat, hand-loomed woven rugs are still being produced by the American Indians, as well as in India, China, Iran, and elsewhere.

Along with the quality of the fiber, the amount of fiber is crucial to a carpet's durability. The depth of pile is not as important as its **face weight** (i.e., the density of fiber in the pile). If asked, sales staff will disclose (if sometimes reluctantly) the face weight of a carpet. In terms of durability, carpets are often divided into four grades:

1. Grade One is intended for residential or domestic use;
2. Grade Two is for normal contract (commercial) use;

3. Grade Three is for public areas such as lobbies where face weight is especially important;
4. Grade Four is for stairs, offices containing chairs with casters, and institutions. Many Grade Four carpets have uncut loop pile for greater resilience.[25]

CARPET CUSHIONING

A firm and resilient carpet cushion is necessary to form a good foundation for your carpet, increasing its comfort and extending its life by absorbing the impact of foot traffic. Cushion also adds insulation and reduces noise. For most residential carpet applications, choose cushion not more than $7/16$" thick. If the carpet is a Berber or a low-profile carpet, choose a cushion no more than $3/8$" thick.

Selecting Cushion/Pad

The appropriate carpet cushion, or "pad," provides additional resilience, acoustical and thermal qualities, comfort underfoot, and can extend the life of the carpet. Cushion should be selected according to the carpet manufacturer's requirements for thickness and density. Improper selection of carpet cushion can accelerate loss of carpet surface appearance, cause wrinkling and buckling, cause separation of the carpet seams, and cause a breakdown of the carpet structure itself. Improper cushion selection also may void applicable carpet manufacturer's warranties.

Carpet cushions are now available that will block spills from penetrating the cushion and soaking into the subfloor, as well as eliminate odors in your carpet.[26]

Carpet cushion is made primarily from polyurethane foam, fiber, or rubber and is available in a variety of styles and constructions to fit your needs. The type and thickness of cushion you need varies according to traffic levels and patterns. For example, bedrooms, dens, lounge areas, and other rooms with light or moderate traffic can use thicker and softer cushion, whereas living rooms, family rooms, hallways, stairs, and other heavy-traffic areas require thinner, firmer cushion.

- Residential cut pile, cut and loop, or high-level loop carpet requires a resilient, firm cushion with a thickness of $7/16$ inch or less. Types of cushion may be various polyurethane foams, including the very common bonded foam product often referred to as "re-bond," fiber, or rubber.
- Berber carpet, or thinner loop or cut-pile carpet. Berber carpet is made with large, wide loops and it has been found that a stable, low-flexing cushion foundation is necessary. A thicker, softer cushion is not acceptable. Cushion thickness should not exceed $3/8$" for these types of products. Again, check with the carpet manufacturer to see if a specific cushion is required.[27]

The following information is adapted from the Carpet Cushion Council website:

There are three basic types of cushion:

- *foam* (short for "polyurethane foam")
- *rubber* (short for "sponge rubber")
- *fiber* (short for "felted fiber")

Each type is further subdivided into two or three varieties. Each variety has characteristics that make it useful in particular types of carpet installation. Each variety also has *grades*, which vary by weight (also called *density*), thickness, and the amount of force it takes to compress the cushion.

Density is one of the most important parameters of any type of cushion. Density equals weight divided by thickness, and it is measured in pounds per cubic foot. All types of cushion can be made dense (more material), or light (more air), or any grade in between, so they can be soft or firm, resilient or supportive, according to the type of room and expected traffic on the carpet they support.

Foam

Generally speaking, foam cushion comes in three recognized, clearly different varieties:

Prime polyurethane foam is a firmer version of the same cushioning used in upholstered furniture, mattresses, and automobile seats. Two liquid ingredients are combined to form a large mass of foam, which is then sliced into sheets for use as carpet cushion.

Bonded polyurethane foam (sometimes called *rebond*) is quite unique. You cannot mistake it when you see it, because it is formed by combining chopped and shredded pieces of foam, in different sizes and usually different colors, into one solid piece. It frequently has a surface net for ease of installation and improved performance.

Bonded foam is one of the most amazing recycling products of all time. Nearly all the scrap foam in the United States, and some from other countries as well, is utilized to make bonded cushion. This recycles waste and it eases the strain on our landfills. Moreover, bonded foam is itself recyclable.

Froth polyurethane foam is made with carpets-backing machinery. Liquid ingredients are applied, either directly to the backs of some carpet styles or to a nonwoven material (for making separate cushions). They react and form a thin, dense foam that is particularly useful in commercial applications with wide expanses of carpet.

Sponge Rubber

There are two basic types of sponge rubber carpet cushion:

Waffled rubber cushion is made by molding natural or synthetic rubber. Heat cures the rubber and forms a waffle pattern. This variety produces a soft, resilient cushion whose luxurious feel is particularly useful for residences.

Flat sponge rubber is a firm, dense cushion that has a flat surface and is normally used in large-scale commercial applications and with loop-type (or Berber) carpet.

Rubber cushion manufacturing processes can be varied to produce different levels of density and firmness. The usual measurement is the weight in ounces per square yard.

Fiber

Foam and rubber cushions are produced from new and recycled materials. Fiber cushion, on the other hand, uses existing fibers (both virgin and recycled, and either natural or man-made fibers) that are interlocked into a useful sheet of felt. There are two distinct varieties of fiber cushion:

Natural fibers include felt, animal hair, and jute (the material used to make some kinds of rope and heavy burlap bags). This is one of the oldest types of carpet cushion, dating back to the earliest days of machine-made carpet.

Synthetic fibers include nylon, polyester, polypropylene, and acrylics, that are needle punched into relatively dense cushions that have a firm feel and, as with other types of cushion, can be made in virtually any weight, to stand up under *light*, *medium*, or *heavy* traffic, which is how they are usually classified.[28]

SPECIAL NOTES

Berber carpet is becoming increasingly popular, and needs a thin, firm cushion. When using this type of carpet, be sure that the accompanying cushion has been specified by the manufacturer as suitable for Berber carpet.

Radiant heating is becoming more widely used in certain sections of the country. In the case of radiant heating, you do not want a cushion that is an exceptionally effective insulator, but one that allows the heat from the subflooring to penetrate the carpet system and heat the room. A relatively thin, flat cellular sponge rubber or synthetic fiber cushion works well under these circumstances. Be sure to ask your customers if their room(s) have radiant heating.[29]

The heavier the traffic, the thinner the cushion. In heavy-traffic areas such as hallways, stairs, rooms with lots of activity, and rooms with heavy furniture, such as dining rooms, choose thinner ($^3/_8$ inch and less) and heavier cushion to better protect the carpet.

For bedrooms, dens, and areas where a more luxurious feel is desired, thicker and more resilient cushion can be used. But again, it's best to go with higher ounce weight or higher-density products to help make the carpet last longer. Visual appearances of cushion are nice, but remember, once it's installed, it will never be seen again. Pay more attention to ounce weights, densities, and thickness when buying.

Don't scrimp—Remember, the new floor covering is a system of both carpet and cushion. If you cut corners on cushion, you could be cutting the usable life of your carpet.

Ask about the installers—Most stores use their own professional installers or a reputable installation firm to make sure your new floor covering is properly installed. It doesn't hurt to make sure that your new carpet will be put down right by people who know how.[30]

As can be seen from Table 3.2, the Carpet Cushion Council (CCC) has established recommended minimum contract cushion criteria for three levels of traffic. Any cushion type and grade certified as meeting the CCC's guidelines can be expected to perform satisfactorily at that level under normal conditions, when used with a carpet made for the same specified traffic. To make proper selection easier, the various categories of cushioning have color-coded labels: red label—commercial to moderate traffic; green label—heavy traffic; blue label—commercial to extra-heavy traffic.

CARPET SPECIFICATIONS

Certain issues must be addressed to specify carpet, regardless of the installation site. Most of the critical decisions made during specification, including those for installation and maintenance, will determine the life cycle of the carpet. The specifier should determine the expectation for the carpet and what the most important selection criteria are. A proper specification covers the key technical aspects—from subfloor preparation, to choosing the proper cushion and method of installation, to postinstallation cleanup—none of these can be overlooked in a successful installation. Consider the following basic issues to create a carpet specification:

Aesthetics—texture, design/pattern, luster, appearance or the "look"

- Business type: hospitality, retail, office, etc.
- Desired ambience
- Color selection parameters
- Flexibility and functionality
- Restricted: must match or blend with other furnishings
- Dark or bright ambient lighting
- Nature of lighting: fluorescent, incandescent, etc.
- Psychological/motivational factors

Functional considerations—value, acoustics, ergonomics, safety, thermal insulation, low maintenance costs, flammability, static propensity, indoor air quality, life-cycle value

Appearance—durability, wearability, cleanability, installability, color retention and colorfastness, texture retention, appearance retention

Primary end-use considerations:
- Traffic levels and patterns
- Wheeled traffic and ADA requirements
- Nature of regional soil
- Projected life span
- Projected quality of maintenance
- Government or building code requirements

Types of Cushion	Class I Moderate Traffic
Commercial Application	**Office Buildings:** Executive or private offices; conference rooms **Health Care:** Executive, administrative **Schools:** Administration **Airports:** Administration **Retail:** Windows and display areas **Banks:** Executive areas **Hotels/Motels:** Sleeping rooms **Libraries/Museums:** Administration

Minimum recommended criteria for satisfactory carpet cushion performance in contract installations

Fiber

Rubberized Hair	Wt. 40 oz.	Th: .27"	D = 12.3
Rubberized Jute	Wt. 32 oz.	Th: .25"	D = 12.3
Synthetic Fibers	Wt. 22 oz.	Th: .25"	D = 7.3
Resinated Recycled Textile Fiber	Wt. 24 oz.	Th: .25"	D = 7.3

Rubber

Flat Rubber	Wt. 62 oz.	Th: .150"	CR @ 25% = 3.0 psi min.	D = 21
Rippled Waffle	Wt. 56 oz.	Th: .270"	CR @ 25% = 0.7 psi min.	D = 15
Textured Flat Rubber	Wt. 56 oz.	Th: .220"	CR @ 25% = 1.0 psi min.	D = 18
Reinforced Rubber	Wt. 64 oz.	Th: .235"	CR @ 25% = 2.0 psi min.	D = 22
			CR @ 65% = 50.0 psi min.	

Polyurethane Foam

Grafted Prime Polyurethane*	D = 2.7	Th: .25"	CFD @ 65% = 2.5 psi min.
Densified Polyurethane*	D = 2.7	Th: .25"	CFD @ 65% = 2.4 psi min.
Bonded Polyurethane**	D = 5.0	Th: .375"	CFD @ 65% = 5.0 psi min.
Mechanically Frothed Polyurethane***	D = 13.0	Th: .30"	CFD @ 65% = 9.7 psi min.

Footnotes: Maximum thickness for any product is 3/8"

D - Denotes Density in lbs./cu.ft.

Oz. - Denotes weight in ounces/sq. yd.

CR - Denotes Compression Resistance in lbs./sq. in as measured by ASTM D-3676

CFD - Denotes Compression Force Deflection as measured by ASTM D-3574

All thicknesses, weights and densities allow a .5% manufacturing tolerance

* = Polymer densities

** = Particle size not to exceed 1/2"

*** = Ash content = 50% max.

TABLE 3.2
Minimum Recommended Criteria for Satisfactory Carpet Cushion Performance in Contract Installations

Class II Heavy Traffic	**Class III Extra Heavy Traffic**
Office Buildings: Clerical areas, corridors (moderate traffic)	**Office Buildings:** Corridors (heavy traffic), cafeterias
Health Care: Patients' rooms, lounges	**Health Care:** Lobbies, corridors, nurses' stations
Schools: Dormitories and classrooms	**Schools:** Corridors, cafeterias
Retail: Minor aisles, boutiques, specialty	**Airports:** Corridors, public areas, ticketing areas
Banks: Lobbies, corridors (moderate traffic)	**Retail:** Major aisles, checkouts, supermarkets
Hotels/Motels: Corridors	**Banks:** Corridors (heavy traffic), teller windows
Libraries/Museums: Public Areas (moderate traffic)	**Hotels/Motels:** Lobbies and public areas
Convention Centers: Auditoriums	**Libraries/Museums:** Public Areas
	Country Clubs: Locker rooms, pro shops, dining areas
	Convention Centers: Corridors and lobbies
	Restaurants: Dining areas and lobbies

Wt. 40 oz.	Th: .3125"	D = 12.3	Wt. 50 oz.	Th: .375"	D = 11.1
Wt. 40 oz.	Th: .25"	D = 12.3	Wt. 40 oz.	Th: .34"	D = 10.1
Wt. 28 oz.	Th: .3125"	D = 7.3	Wt. 36 oz.	Th: .35"	D = 8.0
Wt. 30 oz.	Th: .30"	D = 7.3	Wt. 38 oz.	Th: .375"	D = 8.0

Wt. 62 oz.   Th: .150"   CR @ 25% = 3.0 psi min. D = 21   Wt. 62 oz.   Th: .150"   CR @ 25% = 4.0 psi min. D = 26
       Not Recommended for Use in This Class   Not Recommended for Use in This Class
Wt. 64 oz.   Th: .235"   CR @ 25% = 1.5 psi min. D = 22   Wt. 80 oz.   Th: .250"   CR @ 25% = 1.75 psi min.D = 26
Wt. 64 oz.   Th: .235"   CR @ 25% = 2.0 psi min. D = 22   Wt. 54 oz.   Th: .200"   CR @ 25% = 2.0 psi min. D = 22
                    CR @ 65% = 50.0 psi min.   CR @ 65% = 50.0 psi min.

D = 3.2	Th: .25"	CFD @ 65% = 3.5 psi min.	D = 4.0	Th: .25"	CFD @ 65% = 5.0 psi min.
D = 3.5	Th: .25"	CFD @ 65% = 3.3 psi min.	D = 4.5	Th: .25"	CFD @ 65% = 4.8 psi min.
D = 6.5	Th: .25"	CFD @ 65% = 10.0 psi min.	D = 8.0	Th: .25"	CFD @ 65% = 8.0 psi min.
D = 15.0	Th: .223"	CFD @ 65% = 49.9 psi min.	D = 19.0	Th: .183"	CFD @ 65% = 30.5 psi min.

To help you compare various types of cushion, the Carpet Cushion Council has established recommended minimum contract cushion criteria for three levels of traffic. Any cushion type and grade certified as meeting CCC's guidelines for cushion being installed at a particular traffic level can be expected to perform satisfactorlly at that level under norm conditions, when used with a carpet made for the same specified traffic. Red Label; Commercial - Moderate Traffic • Green Label; Commercial - Heavy Traffic • Blue Label; Commercial - Extra Heavy Traffic.

Source: Table reprinted by permission of the Carpet Cushion Council.

AESTHETIC CONSIDERATIONS

Carpet is widely recognized for its excellent "first impression" of beauty, prestige, and dignity in any business or facility. Well-chosen carpet dramatically enhances the feeling of quality buildings. Carpet also has the ability to "de-institutionalize" a building, creating a "homelike" factor and improving patient and staff morale in healthcare facilities, and improving student and teacher attitudes in schools. Carpet gives inhabitants a psychological "uplift."[31] For example, see Figure 3.6.

A realization in healthcare facilities that Alzheimer's patients can remember color differentiation better than numbers (according to the Alzheimer's Association) may be a consideration in any public facility. Color can provide an easily remembered visual link to a specific hall or wing. Brighter colors also aid in depth perception and differentiation of areas such as registration desks or main offices. Color is also a good way to differentiate a group or team area, or to differentiate between departments.[32]

Complete specifications for installations can be found on the CRI website in PDF format. They are contained in CRI 104—Standard for Installation Specification of Commercial Carpet and CRI 105—Standard for Installation of Residential Carpet.

Performance

To clarify the difference between performance and construction specifications, performance specifications define what characteristics the carpet must deliver in use. . . . In other words, performance specifications tell the manufacturer what the carpet must do

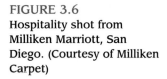

FIGURE 3.6
Hospitality shot from Milliken Marriott, San Diego. (Courtesy of Milliken Carpet)

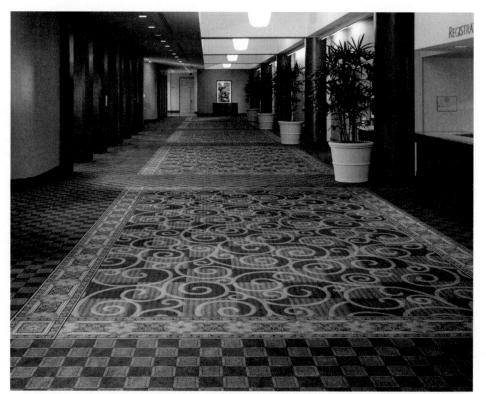

without detailing how it must be made. By contrast, a construction specification tells the manufacturer, in very precise terms, how the carpet is to be manufactured without stipulating performance needs. Specifying performance rather than construction can also take other important pressures off the specifier. For example, if the specifier does not regularly deal with carpet products, the latest technology and materials may be overlooked. The best, most economical product to ensure the desired performance may not be chosen . . .

Special requirements for different types of installation sites can be very complex and technical. For example, in window-wall architecture, fade resistance could be a matter of primary concern. In a hospital medical dispensary, stain resistance might be placed high on the list of performance priorities. Special static protection properties may be necessary for computer and data-processing areas . . .[33]

MEASURING

Before estimating the amount of carpet needed for a particular job, the designer needs to remember several points. First, if carpet is available in widths other than the usual 12 feet, then all the carpet must be of that width. **Do not combine different widths** because of differences in dye lots. Second, the **nap** or pile of the carpet must be considered, and all pieces must have the nap running in the same direction (toward the entrance unless otherwise specified) or the seams will be obvious. Third, seaming and nap direction must be shown on all carpet seaming plans. Placement of furniture will often decide where seams should be placed. Seams should never be in the middle of high-traffic areas, such as at right angles to a doorway, across a hallway, or in front of often-used office features such as copiers and drinking fountains. In residential seaming layouts, seams must not be placed directly in front of seating areas. Carpets that have to be seamed at right angles will also have an obvious seam; however, seams placed under a door are often necessary. The nap on stairs should run downward. The warp (nap) should always run in the longer direction.

The precise measuring of the carpet should be done by the installer on-site, and a carpet seaming diagram should be submitted to the designer for approval. Nevertheless, the designer should understand how carpet measuring is done.

Carpet usually comes in 12-foot widths, but 6-foot, 9-foot, and 15-foot widths are sometimes available. Whatever width is selected, it will be necessary to piece or seam the carpet. This may entail purchasing slightly more yardage, because the fewer the seams, the better the appearance will be.

Although carpet comes in widths measured in feet, the amount ordered is always in square yards, so a square-foot figure must be divided by 9 to arrive at the square yardage needed. (From experience, the author finds that when taking exams design students commonly make this error and as a result specify too much carpet.) However, the CRI has proposed a change to square feet because if carpet were sold by the square foot, it would be easier to make comparisons among other types of flooring materials that are priced by the square foot.

All measurers seem to have their own method of calculation. Some suggest using templates; others have complicated formulas. Some answers are very close with little waste, and others have few seams and much waste. The number of seams depends on each job. A master bedroom may have a seam 1 foot in from a wall where a dresser, bed, or other piece of furniture is to be placed, because there the seam will not be visible, but in an art gallery the same seam placement would be unacceptable. Whichever method is used, the installer is responsible for the accuracy of the measurements.

In today's computerized design offices, programs are available to assist the designer in producing an economical yet viable plan. Some programs actually produce a floor plan with measurements, nap directions, and seam placements. The program can provide an estimate needed with the 12-foot width going across the room or at right angles. A pattern repeat can be programmed so that the repeat is considered.

PROBLEMS

The following problems are associated with carpet:

Corn rowing—The tufting machine is set to insert the prescribed number of face yarns in the back. As the carpet or rug is made, the face yarns will stand erect. After the carpet or rug is placed on the floor and is subjected to use, there will be considerable pressure placed on the individual face yarns. If the density is high enough, the surrounding tufts help to hold each other erect; however, if the density is too low, there is less support from the adjacent tufts and some of the tufts may be pushed over. With some tufts standing, and others crushed, the cornrow appearance is created. This is not considered a manufacturing defect.

Depressions or indentations—The weight of heavy pieces of furniture can cause indentations in carpet. Some depressions may be permanent. Use furniture glides or cups under the legs of heavy pieces, or move your furniture a few inches backward or sideways so that the weight is not concentrated in one place. To remedy depressions, work the carpet pile back into place with your fingertips or the edge of a spoon, and then dampen the area and heat with a hair dryer, working the fibers with the fingers or a spoon.

Fluffing and shedding—The balls of fluff, or loose fibers, found on carpet or in the vacuum cleaner bag are the normal result of fiber left in the carpet during the manufacturing process. Removing these loose fibers does not affect the carpet life or appearance. Because of their size, these fibers are too large to become airborne or respirable. With proper vacuuming, using a quality vacuum cleaner, most shedding disappears within the first year after installation.[34]

Mildew—Mildew can be a problem on carpet and rugs, but it does not have to be. If a carpet is going to be used where mildew or other bacteria-growing conditions are present some or all of the time, then a carpet with all synthetic fibers (both front and back) should be used.[35]

Moth and beetle control—Most wool and wool-blend carpet made in the United States is permanently treated to prevent moth damage. Carpet and rugs made of man-made (synthetic) fibers are naturally resistant to insects. Synthetic carpet fiber is not a food source, and is resistant to beetles, commonly called carpet beetles. However, beetles already in the home may lay eggs in the carpet pile and hatch in 8 to 15 days. For assistance in removing beetles or other insects, contact a professional pest control specialist.

Ripples and buckles—Ripples and buckles in carpet are most often caused by the failure to adequately stretch the carpet using a power stretcher, the use of an inappropriate or failed cushion, or excessive temperature and/or humidity. Ripples can be caused by a combination of any of these deficiencies. If ripples or buckles develop, consult your carpet retailer. Generally, the problem can be corrected by a qualified carpet installer restretching the carpet with a power stretcher.

Shading or pile reversal. Shading is not a change in color, but a change in pile direction (pile reversal) that sometimes appears randomly in a carpet or rug. If you look at the shaded area in one direction, it will appear darker, but from another direction, it will appear lighter in color. Solid color, cut-pile carpet may show shading more than patterned styles and textured surfaces. Shading is not considered a manufacturing defect.

Pile reversal can also be classified as shading and is sometimes called "watermarking" or "pooling." This condition is usually permanent and has no known cause and no known remedy.[36] Some changes can be expected after the carpet is used. The traffic areas will appear a little different from the adjacent, unwalked-on areas. This difference is because the carpet pile has been compressed by the pressure from footsteps. Vacuuming and brushing will help to raise the crushed pile. An occasional vacuuming, however, cannot equalize the continual compressing of the carpet. The end user will have to work to keep the pile erect. Sometimes these shaded spots will occur even in areas with little or no traffic and may be called shading, watermarking, pooling, highlighting, or pile reversal. Vacuuming and brushing the pile all in one direction, or professional cleaning, may temporarily improve the condition. This changes only the top portion of the pile, however, and shading will soon redevelop. With some plush carpet, vacuum cleaner marks and footsteps may show after the carpet has been freshly cleaned.

Sprouting—Occasionally, a tuft will rise above the pile surface of a carpet. Just snip off these tufts level with other tufts. **Do not pull them out!**

Stain-resist carpet—Almost all of the carpet manufactured today finishes. This is a more stain- and soil-resistant. Although stain-resist carpet is easier to maintain, it still requires care. Remove spots as soon as something is spilled or tracked on the carpet. If spills or soil are allowed to remain, they may become permanent.[37]

Static electricity—Static electricity is caused by the rubbing together of two different types of materials, which results in a transfer and a buildup of electrical charges. Most carpets have some type of treatments built into them that will eliminate the static electricity problem. Moisture in the air will help the problem but may produce condensation on window glass in colder climates.

Yellowing—Yellowing in light-colored carpet can be caused by a variety of outside influences, such as pollutants from heating fuels, changes in alkalinity, cleaning solutions, and atmospheric or environmental contaminants. All carpet yellowing may not be removable; however, the use of acetic acid (white vinegar), citric acid, or tartaric acid is often successful in reversing yellowing. In some cases, the use of an alkaline detergent solution prior to the use of these acid rinses may cause permanent yellowing. A solution of one part white vinegar mixed with one part water is recommended for consumer use. If yellowing persists or is widespread, contact a carpet cleaning professional.

It is difficult to determine the exact causes of yellowing. With so many factors contributing to the problem, the potential for yellowing always exists. The problem can occur on all types of fibers and may not be limited to specific areas. It does seem to be more prevalent in coastal areas with high humidity and in colder climates, when homes are sealed up for the winter and air flow is restricted.[38]

INSTALLATION

The International Certified Floorcovering Installers Association is an organization that certifies carpet installers and provides training for installers in all flooring surfaces.

In 2002, Associates Armstrong, Pergo, Tarkett and the Ceramic Tile Education Foundation developed programs that engage the hard surface Installers as members of CFI. The [carpet] certification and training covers five different categories.

Residential I (R-1)—Minimum two years experience. Possesses the ability to install residential entry-level carpets.

Residential II (R-2)—Minimum four years experience. Possesses the ability to install residential carpets and patterns of a more difficult level.

Commercial I (C-1)—Minimum of two years experience. Possesses the ability to install commercial entry-level carpets.

Commercial II (C-2)—Minimum of four years experience. Possesses the ability and knowledge to install commercial carpets and patterns of a more difficult level.

Master-II Installer—Minimum of 10 years experience. Excels in all levels of certification; Possesses the ability to install woven carpets, handsew, and work with the most difficult products.

The Association's certification test also covers written OSHA, EPA, and CRI-104 and CRI-105 knowledge.[39]

The best carpet installer available should always be used.

Installations

Stretch-in Installation

In some situations the specifier will wish to utilize the stretch-in method. Its selection may be for one of the following reasons:

Provides enhanced underfoot comfort, acoustical properties (i.e., higher noise reduction coefficients and higher impact noise ratings) when installed with separate cushion
Increases thermal insulation (R-value)
Can be used over floors that are unsuitable for glue-down
Patterned carpet may be more easily matched
Corrective measures, such as seam repair, may be easier to perform
Removal costs usually are less than removal of an adhered installation

However, stretch-in installations should be avoided:

On ramps and inclines
Where office systems furniture and demountable partitions are utilized
Where heavy rolling traffic is likely
Where there is excessive humidity
When carpet has a unitary backing or other backing systems designed only for glue-down installation

Direct Glue-Down Installation

- Suitable for rolling traffic and ramp areas
- Seams are more durable since there is no vertical flexing
- Minimized buckling in buildings that have HVAC systems turned off for extended periods of time
- No restretch situations
- Facilitates access to electrical and telephone lines under floor
- Practically eliminates incidences of seam peaking
- No restrictions to area size
- Intricate border and inlay possibilities
- Usually less expensive

Double Glue-Down Installation

- Combines the stability of direct glue-down carpet with the cushioning benefits of a separate cushion, stretch-in installation
- Improves carpet appearance retention, foot comfort, and overall performance
- Simplifies carpet bordering and inlaying
- Suitable for wheeled traffic areas
- No restrictions to size of area[40]

The TacFast® Carpet System was the first product introduced by TacFast® Systems International to the carpet industry and is widely used in North America and Europe. The system is based on a hook-and-loop fastening system using wide-width carpet that has a loop material covering its entire underside. Hook tapes are fastened to the subfloor by means of a pressure-sensitive adhesive. The hook and loops "engage" and form a mechanical bond, which holds the carpet in place. The TacFast®

Carpet System provides to both carpet manufacturers and their customers a solution to address the many end-use and installation-related problems faced by both commercial and residential users. It is available through licenses from TacFast® Systems International to the carpet industry.[41] (See Figure 3.7.)

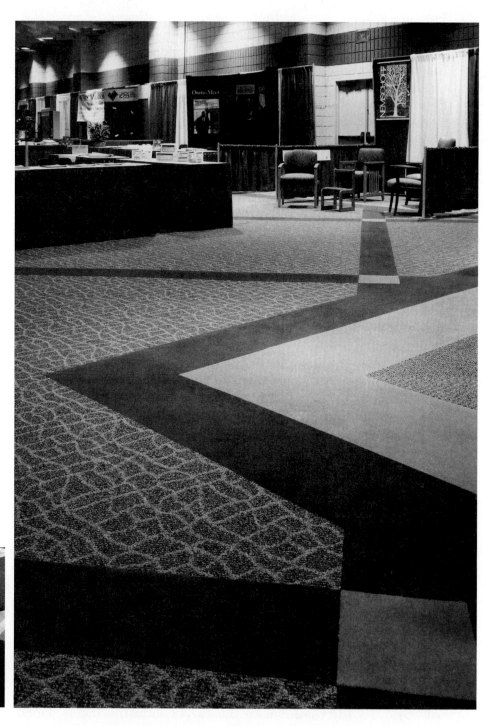

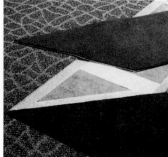

FIGURE 3.7
The Hyatt Regency, Dearborn, used the TacFast® Carpet System in its Great Lake Convention Center. Over 2400 square yards featuring a custom design pattern were used because of TacFast®'s design capabilities and ability to stay in place during the constant set-ups and tear-down of convention displays. The small photo shows a design section of the TacFast® carpet that has been lifted off the hook tape positioned on the floor. The large photo shows the finished installation. (Photo courtesy of TacFast® Systems International)

Lees' Self Lock® is a patented, factory-applied, releasable adhesive system, available exclusively on Lees Squared® modular carpets. . . . The adhesive is manufactured directly to the back of each module, so carpet tiles go down quickly, cleanly and economically. The Self Lock® system prevents shifting even at pivot pints, on ramps and under rolling chairs. Chair pads are not required.[42]

The Carpet and Rug Institute finds that most complaints about wrinkling or buckling in **tackless** installations result from inadequate stretch during initial installation or from cushion that does not provide adequate support for the carpet. . . . Adequate stretch can only be obtained by the use of power stretchers.

Another problem is the separation from the floor in a glue-down installation caused by an insufficient amount of carpet floor adhesive.

Because of their heavy backing, carpet tiles may also be loose laid. Carpet modules can be freely rotated and/or replaced without detracting from overall like-new appearance of the installation, particularly in the health care, institutional, retail, and hospitality areas, with their heavy use and traffic. This type of installation also eliminates restretching problems, with no movement of pattern-type carpet or bordering. It is also useful in furnishing the upper floors of tall buildings, where delivering heavy, cumbersome rolls of broadloom may present a problem. (This is particularly true in the case of refurbishing when construction cranes and elevators used to lift the original carpets are no longer available.)

Coir and sisal are highly absorbent, and therefore for at least 24 hours prior to installing they should be allowed to acclimate to the humidity and temperature of the room in which they will be placed. The direct glue-down procedure is the best method of wall-to-wall installation for coir and sisal if there are no great fluctuations in humidity or temperature. If these conditions exist, then loose laying is suggested.[43]

Intercell is an underfloor wire and cable management system that utilizes only 3 inches of your floor-to-ceiling height. Intercell uses a steel understructure and removable steel plates to provide a stable yet highly flexible below-floor grid for routing data, power, and telephony cable. Intercell is the ideal choice for a technology retrofit of an existing space. Intercell is available carpeted with your choice of Interface Flooring Systems carpet tile.[44] (See Figure 3.8.)

MAINTENANCE

Carpet is the only textile product on which people walk. This is why carpet construction, or performance, and installation specifications are so critical. The third critical specification is maintenance.

Specification of any one of these three elements without knowledge or consideration of the other two increases the risk that the carpet will not perform up to potential or expectation. Even properly specified carpet can wear out or appear to be worn out if it is not maintained adequately. Dirt is unsightly but it can also be abrasive. As foot traffic deposits soil and causes the pile yarns to flex, embedded grit cuts the face fibers. The carpet begins to lose density and resilience. Threadbare spots appear and the carpet wears out. Moreover,

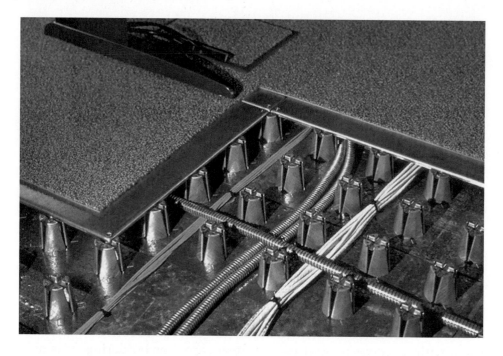

allowing soil to build up and to spread may give the carpet a worn out appearance even if the face fibers are essentially intact.

If carpet is not vacuumed regularly, the dirt builds up and begins to spread. To guard against buildup, a well-planned program is essential in commercial installations with their high-traffic loads. Planned maintenance is the key to extending the life expectancy of carpet. The maintenance plan is no less important than the initial carpet specification and installation.

Planning the Maintenance Program

The maintenance plan should be developed as the carpet specifications are being considered. (In fact, a plan should be prepared in case the carpet is installed prior to completion of construction.) One point that is often overlooked in carpet maintenance is minimizing the immediate sources of soil around the perimeter of the building by keeping sidewalks, parking lots, and garages adjacent to the building as clean as possible.

When preparing the maintenance plan, keep in mind that one of the advantages of carpet compared to hard floors is that carpet localizes soil. Carpet tends to catch and hold soil and spills where they occur instead of allowing them to spread quickly.

This feature of carpet suggests that the best maintenance plan will identify in advance the most likely areas for soiling and spilling. The plan will specify maintenance schedules and procedures for these areas, as well as the remainder of the carpet.

Specifically, heavy-traffic areas, entrances and lobbies, will not only require the most substantial carpet, they will probably have to be vacuumed once a day. In some instances, greasy motor oil from parking lots should be anticipated.

Kitchen smoke in restaurants and cafeterias will contribute heavily to overall soiling. Stains and spills in restaurants and hospitals will be very common. Routine procedures for attending to these as quickly as possible are necessary.

Whatever the nature of the installation, it is wise to anticipate dealing with soil from the very first day the carpet is installed. Otherwise, abrasive dirt may build up faster than it can be handled.[45]

For seagrass, periodic cleaning of the surface with a high-suction vacuum is recommended. The nonstatic, no-pile surface does not trap dirt and dust. Remove liquid spills immediately to avoid spots. Fiber seal is recommended in high-spill areas. For spot and overall cleaning use dry cleaning powder such as the Host Carpet Cleaning System, which is readily available.

Daily and Periodic Procedures

Two elements essential to an efficient maintenance program include daily procedures encompassing both regular vacuuming and spot cleaning, and scheduled overall cleaning to remove discoloring grime and to refresh the pile.

Overall grime not only causes discoloration, it presents another undesirable quality. Carpet that is not cleaned and reconditioned regularly, no matter how faithfully it is vacuumed, will tend to permanently crush and mat down. As greases present in smoke or pollutants in the air settle on the carpet, pile yarns may become gummy enough to stick to each other and flatten in use. Matted carpet appears to be worn out, even if there is no real pile loss. Obviously, carpet that must be replaced because it *looks* worn out is no less costly than carpet that must be replaced because it *is* worn out!

Color as a Maintenance Factor

The color of the carpet can contribute significantly to minimizing the appearance of dirt, particularly for entrances and lobbies, which get the bulk of tracked-in soil. If possible, colors should be chosen that blend with the color of the dirt brought in from outside.

Since the most common dirt colors are greys, beiges, browns, and reds, carpet colors for entrances should be chosen from these tones. The best choice would be a tweed coloration combining two or more of the colors. Another choice might be a multicolored, patterned carpet that would add visual interest while helping camouflage dirt and spills until they can be removed. Such highly patterned carpet is a popular choice for hotel lobbies and restaurants.

Lighter, more delicate colors are best reserved for inside spaces—offices, guest rooms, lounges—where soiling rates are obviously lower and the danger of accidental spills is more remote.

Walk-Off Mats

As a matter of preventative maintenance, **walk-off** mats should be installed in all entrances to collect dirt before it reaches the carpet inside. Walk-off mats can be constructed of stiff bristles, pieces of the carpet used

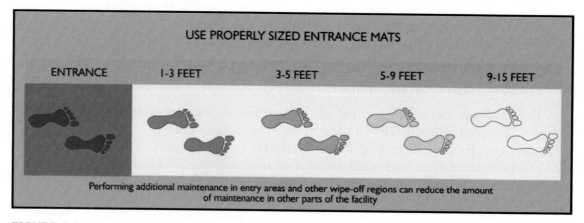

FIGURE 3.9
Properly sized entrance mats. (Courtesy of Carpet and Rug Institute)

inside, or they can be one of a variety of types specially made for commercial use. Some have aluminum strips between the carpet. (Sometimes pieces of carpet used as walk-off mats can, if the backing is rough enough, cause as much wear as walking on the carpet itself.) (See Figure 3.9.)

Mannington Commercial has an entryway system called Ruffian and Ruffian Ridgework as a two-step system. Upon entering, entrants first encounter the rugged grooves of Ruffian Ridge. Ruffian Ridge is a molded bi-level scraper tile designed with a network of deep channels that act as reservoirs to catch and hold water, dry soil and larger debris. Next, Ruffian's smooth, brush-like surface finishes the cleaning and drying process by trapping oil and finer dirt particles and storing them until cleaning.[46]

Elevators should also be carpeted, even if the entrance lobby is not. "Elevators take the brunt of foot traffic and soiling. Adding removable elevator carpets, fastened with Velcro® or double-sided tape for easy cleaning, helps capture accumulated dirt before it reaches the carpeted floors."[47] It is wiser to have soil wiped off on the elevator carpet rather than having it tracked over the carpet elsewhere.

It is common to have two sets of walk-off mats and removable carpets available. Because they take such heavy abuse, one set is kept in place while the other is being cleaned.[48]

Another method of dirt control in commercial buildings is to use a recessed mat or grating inside exterior doors. These gratings feature a system of self-cleaning recessed treads that are closely spaced to prevent the smallest heel from catching, yet allow dirt and sand to collect below the surface. The grate removes easily for cleaning.

In the residential carpet industry, soiling problems may occur related to products used by family members. For example, in a teenager's room acne medicine may spill on the carpet; in another room plant food, aerosols, or furniture polish may be the culprit. In bathrooms a toilet bowl cleaner or a dandruff shampoo can cause a dark brown stain, often with a blue fringe. Urine is also a culprit in small-area discoloration. These spots begin at the backing and progress upward over a period of time. They may be dull yellow or even red. The characteristic ammonia-like odor will be present for only a few hours, and it is replaced by a musty odor. Bleach can be a problem in the laundry area, or it may be tracked in from the swimming pool. Dimethysulfoxide, otherwise known as DMSO, is widely used for relief of pain from arthritis, back problems, athletic injuries, and other muscular aches. It is a clear liquid with an odor similar to garlic and causes rapid loss of color on carpet due to its solvent action.

Vacuuming Schedules and Equipment

For years, the CRI heard complaints about carpet being hard to maintain. So naturally, it did what any professional association would do; it began asking, "Why?"

Upon testing a few vacuum cleaners in a closed, stainless-steel chamber with carpet on the floor and a measured amount of soiling, they found that most vacuum cleaners didn't harm the carpet, but neither did they trap and retain soil very efficiently. Many of those vacuums were removing soil from the carpet, where it was doing no harm in terms of human health, and were flinging it into the air, where it became part of the airborne soil burden.

The CRI contacted the equipment manufacturers and told them what was found. The vacuum manufacturers—most of them—reengineered their equipment to make it more efficient. Today, the CRI has a listing of Green Label Seal of Approval vacuums on its website.

Further, closed-chamber tests conducted by Lees Commercial Carpets demonstrate that using a CRI Green Label vacuum on carpet for only four minutes results in a 10-fold reduction in airborne dust burdens compared to a non-Green Label vacuum. Think about the implications of that statement—less dust to breathe and less dust spread over furnishings and fixtures that has to be removed. That's a win-win situation for professionals.[49]

According to the Carpet and Rug Institute,

Of all the carpet maintenance procedures, vacuuming takes the most time and attention, yet is the most cost effective. The carpet should be inspected for spots during vacuuming. Spots should be removed as soon as possible. The longer they are allowed to set, the more permanent they may become.

The following is a normal vacuuming schedule:

High Traffic—Vacuum daily
Medium Traffic—Vacuum twice weekly
Light Traffic—Vacuum weekly

This broad guide recommends minimum schedules only. To reduce this general rule to specifics, some definitions will be useful. Track-off areas are where a carpet collects foot soil tracked in from the outdoors or from hard surfaced floors indoors. . . . Funnel areas are where foot traffic is squeezed into or through a concentrated area, such as a doorway, stairwell, in front of drinking fountain, vending machine, etc. . . . These areas can be identified in advance of soiling. Planned vacuuming in these areas, **even when soil is not visible,** will help prevent soil buildup. Also it will help focus maintenance attention on the places where it is known that soil will be tracked.

In the final analysis, an adequate schedule must be based on the individual installation and its own traffic load and soiling rate. For example, soil may accumulate so rapidly at entrances (track-off areas) that carpet at those locations will have to be vacuumed several times a day. In another instance, rooms may be entered directly from an uncarpeted corridor. Under those circumstances, even light traffic may cause heavy soiling, and the carpet may have to be vacuumed several times a week. Only experience will tell whether more frequent vacuuming is indicated.

Spot Removal

Identification and immediate action are the keys to effective spot-removal procedures. To minimize time and effort, it is helpful to know what causes a spot so that treatment can begin without guesswork. In most installations, spot identification may not be difficult because the possibilities are limited. In others, it could be a real problem.

A drug-dispensing area in hospitals, for example, is susceptible to hundreds of spotting and staining agents. Employees must be instructed to report spills as they occur and to identify the spilled material.

It is also important to clean up spills as quickly as possible. The longer a spot sets, the more difficult it may be to remove. If it sets too long, it might react with the carpet dyes and cause permanent discoloration. Hence, an alert staff and a well-stocked spot-removal kit are important to a good carpet maintenance program. Always test a cleaning agent to determine its effect upon the carpet dye, fibers, and the spot before applying larger amounts.

Importance of the Maintenance Plan

There are many factors that will influence the frequency of cleaning, but a maintenance plan should be in effect before the traffic areas start to show discoloration. If the traffic areas are allowed to become excessively soiled, on-location cleaning may not remove sufficient soil to restore them to an acceptable level. The high-use areas must be cleaned more frequently in order to maintain a satisfactory overall appearance.

Deep Cleaning

Periodic deep cleaning is required to remove oily materials that have become bonded to the carpet fibers, and to collect dirt particles that have been pushed into the space between fibers and onto the fibers by the pressure of foot traffic. Five main methods are used to clean carpet. There are many variations on the basic methods, multiple names for the same processes, and various combinations of methods. Operator training and experience are needed to use any of the methods successfully.

Absorbent Compound—This method uses the least moisture. A preconditioner may be applied before the main treatment in heavily soiled areas. Powder is poured over the surface of the carpet, then worked in with a stiff brush or mechanical agitator. The dirt particles are knocked off the carpet fibers. The chemicals in the powder break the oil bonds and adhere to the dirt particles. The absorbent compound is then removed by vacuuming. The carpet will normally take between one to three hours to dry completely.

Absorbent Pad or Bonnet (Dry)—This is another minimum moisture system. A solution of detergent and water is sprayed onto the carpet, a rotating pad agitates the carpet tufts, and the dirt is collected in the pad, which is washed out and reused as needed. The pad or bonnet must be replaced as it becomes saturated with soil in order to prevent resoiling. The cleaning agents should dry to a powder so that they do not leave a sticky residue that acts as a soil collector. Drying time is normally one to three hours, after which the carpet needs to be thoroughly vacuumed. This method is not recommended for cut-pile carpet.

Dry Foam Cleaning—A dry foam detergent solution is produced by means of an air compressor or mechanical agitation device. This foam is then forced down through or around a revolving cylindrical brush, which combs the foam through the carpet pile so each fiber is individually cleaned. The cleaning compounds dissolve oil bonds and encapsulate the dirt particles. Dirt is removed in the foam that is vacuumed from the carpet. Follow-up vacuuming when the carpet is dry gets loosened dirt particles out of the pile. The cleaning agents dry to a powder so that they do not leave sticky residue.

Shampoo Cleaning—A shampoo solution is fed through a brush into the carpet. A rotating brush agitates the solution into the carpet pile, knocking dirt particles off the fibers and opening up matted carpet pile. The cleaning compounds dissolve the oil bonds and help prevent dirt particles from reattaching to the fibers. Drying time may run from 1 to 12 hours and up to 24 hours in extreme cases. The cleaning agents should dry to a powder so they do not leave a sticky residue. Follow-up vacuuming is required to remove loosened dirt particles from the pile.

Hot Water Extraction (Steam Cleaning)—Hot water and detergent are driven down into the carpet under pressure. The cleaning chemicals dissolve oil bonds and prevent dirt particles from reattaching to the fibers. The flushing action of the water gets the loosened dirt particles out of the carpet pile. Maximum drying time is 24 hours.[50]

Beware of the bargain carpet cleaning companies that will clean a whole house for a ridiculously low price. They often hire untrained people and, in the case of water extraction, may soak the carpet so that it takes a long time to dry completely, especially in high-humidity areas. The time invested in developing a plan for carpet maintenance will pay off in longer use from the carpet. *Cleaning should be done before the carpet shows signs of soil.* It is essential that the manufacturer's recommendations be followed, especially if guarantees and liabilities are involved.

BIBLIOGRAPHY

Bridgepoint Corporation. *Protector Course*. Salt Lake City, UT: Bridgepoint Corporation, 1990.

Burlington Industries, Inc. *Carpet Maintenance Guide for Hospitals and Health Care Facilities*. King of Prussia, PA: Burlington Industries Inc., Carpet Division, 1987.

Carpet and Rug Institute. *Carpet Specifier's Handbook*. Dalton, GA: The Carpet and Rug Institute, 1987.

Monsanto Contract Fibers. *Concepts, Ideas for Specifiers*. Atlanta, GA: Monsanto Fiber and Intermediates Co.

Revere, Glen. *All About Carpets*. Blue Ridge Summit, PA: TAB Books Inc.,1988.

Reznikoff, C. S. *Specifications for Commercial Interiors*. Whitney, New York: Library of Design, an imprint of Watson-Guptil Publications, a division of Billboard Publications, 1989.

GLOSSARY

antistatic. Some nylon fibers introduce a conductive yarn bundle to conduct or dissipate static charges from the human body.

Axminster. Pile tufts are inserted from spools of colored yarns, making possible an almost endless variety of geometric or floral patterns.

BCF. Bulked continous filament. The name given to continuous strands of synthetic fiber that are first spun into yarn and then texturized to increase bulk and cover.

Berber. A looped-pile rug from North Africa. May be patterned or natural colored. Today, Berbers are mostly textured natural earth tones.

Carpet modules. Carpet precut into 18- or 24-inch squares or other suitable dimensions.

continuous filaments. Continuous strand of synthetic fiber extruded in yarn form without the need for spinning that all natural fibers require.

corn rowing. A characteristic that should be expected in carpet with higher tufts and lower density pile, resulting in the pile laying flat.

CRF. Critical radiant flux.

cut pile. A pile surface created by cutting the loops of yarn in a tufted, woven, or fusion-bonded carpet.

dhurrie. A reversible, tapestry-woven flat rug with no pile. Originally from India; today it comes mostly in pastel colors.

ESD. Electrostatic discharge; to be considered around computers.

face weight. Density of fiber in the pile.

filaments. A single continuous strand of natural or synthetic fiber.

Frieze. A yarn that has been very tightly twisted to give a rough, nubby appearance to the finish.

greige goods. Pronounced "gray" goods. Term designating carpet in an undyed or unfinished form.

heat set. After the fiber is twisted, it is treated with heat to lock in the twist. The result: carpet fibers that won't easily unravel or crush under heavy foot traffic.

indentations. Marks left in the carpet from heavy pieces of furniture remaining in one place.

Jacquard. An apparatus on a carpet weaving loom that produces patterns from colored yarns. The pattern information is contained on perforated cards. The holes in the cards activate the mechanism that selects the color to be raised to the pile surface.

kilim. A flat-woven, or pileless rug.

level loop. A carpet style having all tufts in a loop form and of substantially the same level.

mildew. A discoloration caused by fungi.

multilevel loops. A carpet with some tufts that are substantially longer than others. Gives a sculptured appearance or pattern.

nap. Carpet or rug pile surface.

noise reduction coefficient (NRC). The average percentage of sound reduction at various Hertz levels.

pile. The soft, velvety, raised surface of carpet.

pitch. Number of lengthwise warp yarns in a 27-inch width.

plenum. An air compartment maintained under pressure and connected to one or more distributing ducts.

ripples. Waves caused by either improper stretching or humidity.

rya. A Scandinavian hand-woven rug with a deep, resilient, comparatively flat pile. Usually of abstract design.

Saxony. A cut-pile carpet texture consisting of heat-set plied yarns in a relatively dense, erect configuration, with well-defined individual tuft tips. The tip definition of a Saxony is more pronounced than in single plush carpets.

SB. Styrene butadiene.

sculpturing. A patterned carpet made by using high and low areas.

set yarns. Straight yarns.

shading. Apparent color difference between areas of the same carpet. The physical cause is the difference between cut-end luster and side luster of fibers.

shedding. Normal process of excess yarns coming to the surface in a freshly installed carpet.

skein dying. Undyed spun or filament yarns are plied and heat set.

solution dyed yarns. Pigment is added to the molten polymer from which the filaments are made. In synthetic fibers, the dye is part of the liquid chemical that forms the filament, resulting in a colorfast fiber.

sprouting. Protrusion of individual tuft or yarn ends above pile surface. May be clipped with scissors.

spun. Action of drawing out and twisting of numerous staple fibers into yarn.

staple fiber. Short lengths of fiber that may be converted into spun yarns by textile yarn spinning processes.

static electricity. Shoe friction against carpet fiber causes production of electrostatic charge that is discharged from carpet to person to conductive ground (e.g., a doorknob).

tack. Partially set.

tackless. Installation using narrow lengths of wood or metal containing either two or three rows of angled pins on which carpet is stretched and secured in a stretch-in installation.

velvet. Woven carpet made on a loom similar to a Wilton loom but lacking the Jacquard mechanism. These carpets are generally level loop, level cut/loop, or plush, in solid or tweed colors.

walk-off. Mats on which most of the exterior soil is deposited.

Wilton. Carpet woven on a loom with a Jacquard mechanism, which utilizes a series of punched cards to select pile height and yarn color.

wires. Stitches per inch.

yarns. A continuous strand composed of fibers or filaments and used in the production of carpet and other fabrics.

Yellowing. A discoloration sometimes occurring on light-colored carpets.

yellowing. An unwanted change of color.

NOTES

[1]*Brief History of the Pazryk Carpet.* Chicago, IL: Peerless Imported Rugs.

[2]Adapted from Wool Bureau Library, Volume 6, *Rugs and Carpets.*

[3]Carpet and Rug Institute. *Specifier's Handbook*, 5th ed. Dalton, GA: Carpet and Rug Institute, 1992, pp. 17–18. All quotes from *Specifier's Handbook* reproduced with permission.

[4]Carpet and Rug Institute website, www.carpet-rug.org, "Carpet Construction."

[5]Ibid, "Specifying Commercial Carpet—Modular Carpet Tiles and Six Foot Carpet."

[6]Ibid.

[7]*Carpet Specification and Appearance Guide.* DuPont Flooring Systems, p. 7.

[8]"Carpet Selection: Construction and Texture." Adapted by Shirley M. Niemeyer, Extension Specialist, Interior Design/Home Furnishings, website www.ianrpubs.unl.edu.

[9]Website, www.brintonsusa.com.

[10]DyeNamix™ Color System Solutia.

[11]Website, www.carpet-rug.org, "Carpet Maintenance," p. 3.

[12]Ibid, p. 51

[13]Ibid, p. 49.

[14]Ibid, p. 51.

[15]Ibid, p. 51.

[16]Website, www.indiaparenting/homedecor.com.

[17]Website, www.afceebrooks.af.

[18]Website, www.carpetbuyershandbook.com.

[19]Website, www.antrun.net.

[20]Website, www.dataspec.ultron.com/dataspec.

[21]Website, http://dataspec.ultron.com. MonsantoFiber and Intermediates Co. *Concepts, Ideas for Specifiers*, p. 11.

[22]Bridgepoint Corporation. *Protector Course.* Salt Lake City, UT: Bridgepoint Corporation, 1999.

[23]"Antimicrobial Issues Relating to Carpet." E.I. DuPont deMemours and Company, 2000.

[24]Carpet and Rug Institute website, www.carpet-rug.org, "Selecting Carpet & Rugs, Selecting Cushion/Pad."

[25]Carpet and Rug Institute website, www.cri.org.

[26]Website, www.carpetcushion.org/types.

[27]Website, www.floorfacts.com.

[28]Website, www.carpetcushion.org.

[29]Ibid.

[30]Carpet Cushion Council, *Commercial Carpet Cushion Guidelines*. Riverside, CT: Carpet Cushion Council, January 1997.

[31]Website, www.carpetcushion.org.

[32]Website, www.carpet-rug.org, "Carpet Specification."

[33]Ibid.

[34]Ibid.

[35]Website, www.carpet-rug.org, "Design Trends."

[36]Carpet and Rug Institute, *Specifier's Handbook*, pp. 61–62.

[37]Website, www.carpet-rug.org, "Maintenance and Troubleshooting."

[38]Carpet Cushion Council, Fact Sheet, 1994.

[39]Website, www.jwcarpet@earthlink.net.

[40]Website, www.carpet-rug.org, "Maintenance and Troubleshooting."

[41]Website, www.tactastsystems.com.

[42]Website, www.leescarpets.com.

[43]Website, www.carpet-rug.com, "Installation Method."

[44]Website, www.interfaceinc.com.

[45]Website, www.carpet-rug.org.

[46]Website, www.mannington.com.

[47]Carpet and Rug Institute, *Specifier's Handbook*, p. 56.

[48]Ibid, p. 64.

[49]Ibid.

[50]Ibid.

Floors

4

WOOD

Wood was used in ancient times for flooring. According to the Bible, Solomon's Temple had a floor of fir, whereas the Romans used wood on only the upper floors of their buildings and used stone on the main floor. These stone floors persisted throughout the Dark Ages. In peasant homes, of course, a dirt floor was spread with straw; however, heavy, wide oak planks predominated in larger domestic structures.

The first wood floors were called puncheon floors, made of split logs, flat side up, fitted edge to edge, and smoothed with an ax or an adz. When saws became available to cut the wood into planks, white pine plank flooring of great widths was used in the Colonial period in the United States and was pegged in place.

In 18th- and early-19th-century America, sand was frequently spread over the wood floor to absorb dirt and moisture. Later, these floors were stained and then covered by oriental rugs in wealthy homes; in more modest homes, they were left either bare or covered by homemade rugs. When renovating an old pine plank floor, the knots, which are much harder than the surrounding wood, have a tendency to protrude above the level of the worn floor and must be sanded to give a smoother surface. In some early floors that have not been renovated, it is possible to trip over these knots because they extend so far above the level of the floors. In the early 19th century, **stenciling** was done directly on the floor in imitation of rugs, parquet floors, marble, and tile. Painted floors and **floorcloths** came to be highly regarded until the carpet industry spelled the decline of floorcloths in the 1830s and 1840s. These floorcloths are now making a comeback.

Parquetry and **marquetry** were used in France from the early 1700s, with one of the most famous examples of this period being the beautiful parquet floor at the Palace of Versailles. In 1885, the invention of a machine capable of making a **tongue-and-groove** (often written as t & g) in the edge of the wood and the use of **kilns** combined to produce a draft-proof hardwood floor.

In the Victorian era, inlaid border patterns using contrasting light and dark wood were put together in an intricate manner. End-grain wood was even used to pave streets at the beginning of the 20th century. In the early 1920s, unit block flooring was introduced, which made parquet floors more reasonably priced because each piece did not have to be laid down individually, but more easily in one block.

As milling machinery became more refined, parquet became "the" floor of choice. These patterns or custom laid planks formed an important element in "Art Nouveau" interiors. These features gained much prominence in conjunction with their carpet counterparts. As parquet grew in popularity, these wood floor pieces were laid over the existing floor board, with many intricate borders and styles to accent carpets. Herringbone pattern of oak became the most popular with custom borders being introduced into the design. Some installations were being made over cement. As parquet styles and designs grew they were more commonplace in dining rooms, libraries and drawing rooms. Border motif parquets, using exotics such as mahogany and cherry, were not uncommon. Today inlays are used for logos and other symbols. [See Figure 4.1.]

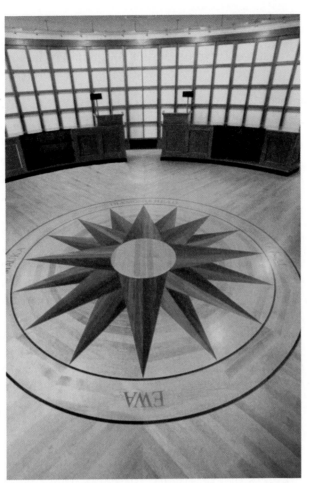

FIGURE 4.1
The compass was made of maple (the lighter wood that surrounds it) and Brazilian cherry (the darker reddish/brown wood). All of it came from Forest Stewardship Council (FSC)–certified forests. (Photo courtesy of Eco-Timber)

In colonial Revival houses, standard strips of oak became the norm, with planks being used. This would become the standard wood floor for years to come. Typically inlaid borders around the perimeter of main rooms were used. Minor rooms received oak plank strip flooring with pine upstairs. The lighter woods being more popular in the 20's and 30's, some variations of stained borders gained some acceptance in less smart houses. Throughout the 30's and 40's, strip oak was the main staple in the flooring industry. With an increase of parquet use in many patterns and species mixes, strip oak flooring outsold all wood flooring in the country. As the sizes changed, the various widths, oak strip in the late 30's was made into larger parquet or "unit blocks," at the same time a small amount of "factory finished" flooring began to appear. Following WWII, oak was the number-one floor of choice in homes built during the boom years of the 50's. As oak strip flooring peaked in 1956, major change was soon on the horizon including more **prefinished** products, on-slab construction, and the use of "**sleepers**" for the installation of oak floors. Even new methods of installation would not help the wood flooring regain its hey-day it no longer enjoyed.

With the approval of carpet as an accepted floor covering by the FHA in new home construction, major change for the wood flooring industry was soon to be reckoned with. As this tidal wave of carpet (being included in mortgage loans) hit the U.S. market, wood flooring would never be the same. A complete turnaround of some 10 years earlier had occurred. Now hardwood floors became a special surface of choice, and were only placed in special, formal areas and rooms. From this came the combination of parquet used with borders. As technology helped advance new products, such as elastomeric adhesives, wood floors now could be applied directly to concrete substrates. This could not have been at a better time, as on-grade (slab/concrete) construction increased more than 40%, wood was back in. As wood floors found their way back into our homes, in the 70's carpet was still king, (hardwood) was for the well-to-do and higher priced custom market. It has continued its growth more and more each year. With advanced technologies, adhesives, finishes, prefinishing techniques (factory finished), and a campaign to educate the public, wood flooring is on the rebound. As the market grows in addition to all the new products (engineered/laminates and impregnated) factory finished, the consumer now has many new products, wood species, sizes, and styles to choose from. There will be an increased demand for custom, one-of-a-kind wood floors, use of "mixed-media" and painted wood floors. With all the products and choices, prefinished wood floors will be the one to watch, as growth and consumer sales continue to rise. [emphasis added][1]

Also contributing to the popularity of wood floors are manufacturers' warranties, which vary from 5 to 25 years.

Wood is divided into two broad categories: hardwoods from deciduous trees, which lose their leaves in winter, and the softwoods, from conifers or evergreens. In reality, there is an overlapping of hardness because some woods from evergreens are harder than those from broad-leafed trees. The harder woods will, of course, be more durable. This durability, together with color and texture, must be considered in both flooring and furniture construction. Ease of finish should also be considered when the wood will have an applied finish.

According to the National Oak Flooring Manufacturers Association (NOFMA):

There are two types of oak used in flooring, white oak and red oak. White oak flooring typically presents more variations in color than its consistently pinkish cousin, red oak, thus adding more depth to the decorator's palette. Less porous than red oak, white oak flooring produces a smoother, more open **grain** appearance. Longer rays are accented by occasional swirls and **burls,** giving the floor a rich look. When stains are used to complement a color scheme, the select grade is often preferred for consistency of appearance in the finished floor. . . . White oak is also a very dense wood, making it an excellent choice for high traffic applications where its hardness provides greater resistance to heel dents and wear. Because it is plentiful, white oak strip flooring may cost from 5% to 20% less than the comparable grade in red oak. [emphasis added][2]

Weight is usually a good indicator of the relative strength of wood. Because wood is a natural material, it absorbs or eliminates moisture depending on the humidity to which it is exposed. Most shrinkage or swelling occurs in the width of the wood; the amount depends on the manner of the cut. **Quarter-sawn** woods are the least troublesome.

Warping is the tendency of wood to twist or bend when drying. Warping may occur as a **bow, crook, twist,** or **cup** (Figure 4.2). The moisture problem can be reduced to a minimum by using kiln-dried lumber. In the kiln-drying process, wood is stacked in an oven so heated air can circulate around each plank and thus render a uniform moisture content. Seven to 8 percent moisture content is acceptable in wood used for making floors and furniture, and 12 to 19 percent is acceptable for construction grades of wood. According to the Hardwood Information Center:

> Solid hardwood's natural response to extremely dry air is to lose moisture and contract a bit. Conversely, under high humidity conditions, the wood may absorb excess moisture from the air and expand. A humidifier in the winter and an air conditioner in the summer will stabilize the relative humidity at 25 to 35 percent. . . . Before a floor is installed, the hardwood should adjust to the new environment. It should be stored in the same room where it will be installed to reach a balance with the surroundings.[3]

Wood is composed of many cells that run vertically, thus giving wood its straight grain. At frequent intervals, **medullary rays** thread their way between and at right angles to the vertical cells. These rays are most noticeable in plain oak and beech.

We have all seen pictures or drawings of the circular rings of trees. Some of the giant sequoias of California and the ancient oaks of Great Britain have been dated by rings showing hundreds of years of growth. These rings show the seasonal growth and comprise springwood (formed early in the growing season) and summerwood or late wood. In some trees, such as ash and oak, the different times of growth are very obvious, whereas in others, such as birch and maple, the seasonal growth is more

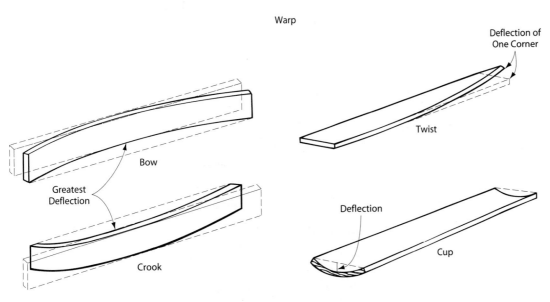

FIGURE 4.2
Warp.

blended. When there is an obvious difference in growth times, there is also a difference in weight and hardness. The faster-growing trees, usually those in more moderate climates, are softer than the same trees grown in northern areas, where the growing season is shorter. Next to the bark is the sapwood, which contains the food cells and is usually lighter in color. Heartwood contains the currently inactive cells and is slightly darker because of chemical substances that are part of the cell walls.

Figure is the pattern of the wood fibers, and the wood grain is determined by the arrangement of the cells and fibers. Some grains are straight and others are patterned; this characteristic is enhanced by the method of cutting the boards.

There are two principal methods of cutting lumber. One is called plain sawn for hardwoods and flat grained for softwoods. The second is quarter sawn for hardwoods or edge grained for softwoods. When referring to maple as a flooring material, the words *edge grained* are used, although maple is a hardwood. Oak is quarter sawn, but fir cut in the same manner is called vertical grain. Interior designers will probably be dealing mainly with hardwoods, so the terms *plain sawn* and *quarter sawn* will be used henceforth, with the exceptions just mentioned. Each method has its own advantages: Plain sawn is the cheapest, easiest, and most economical use of wood, whereas quarter sawn gives less distortion of wood from shrinkage or warping.

Each method of cutting gives a different appearance to wood. Plain sawing gives a cathedral or pointed-arch effect, whereas quarter sawing gives more of a straight-line appearance. Saw mills cut logs into boards producing 80 percent plain to 20 percent quartered lumber. Quartered oak flooring, therefore, is extremely hard to find and is expensive. Most production is mixed cuts (See Figure 4.3).

Veneer is a very thin sheet of wood varying in thickness from 1/8 inch to 1/100 inch. Wood more than 1/4 inch thick is no longer considered veneer. The manner in which the veneer is cut also gives different patterns. The three methods are rotary sliced, flat sliced, and quarter sliced. (These are discussed in more detail in Chapter 5.) **Laminated or engineered wood** is used for some floors and is a sandwich with an uneven number of sheets of veneer, layered at right angles to prevent warping, with the

FIGURE 4.3
Method of sawing.

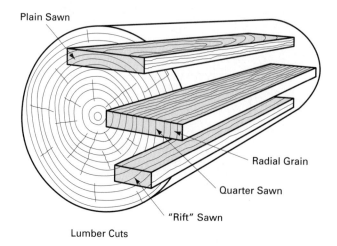

Plain Sawn

Radial Grain

Quarter Sawn

"Rift" Sawn

Lumber Cuts

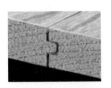

Solid Wood
Milled from one piece of wood into boards that are three-quarters of an inch thick.

• Should not install below grade, as moisture makes it expand and contract.

Engineered Wood
Constructed of multiple layers of crossgrain wood that are bonded together.

• Designed for installation at any house level including below grade.

FIGURE 4.4
Solid wood and engineered wood. This illustration not only shows the difference between solid wood and engineered wood but also shows a tongue-in-groove joint. (Drawing courtesy of Armstrong World Industries)

better veneers on the face. Water-resistant glue should be used for bonding the layers together, and the sandwich is placed in a hot press in which pressure of 150 to 300 pounds per square inch (**psi**) is applied. Heat around 250°F permanently sets the adhesive and bonds the layers together into a single strong panel. (See Figure 4.4.)

Laminated prefinished floors are less affected by humidity and are therefore considered more stable. Only laminated wood floors may be installed below grade, but the manufacturer's installation procedures must be followed exactly. Laminated products expand little, so they may be fitted close to a vertical surface. It is predicted that laminated wood flooring sales will more than double in the next five years, because strong environmental trends are leading consumers to these products.

Grades of oak are determined by appearance alone. Flooring generally free of defects is known as *clear* although it may contain burls, streaks, and pinworm holes. *Select* is almost clear, but this grade contains more of the natural characteristics including knots and other marks. The common grades have more marking than either of the other two grades and are often specified because of these natural features and the character they bring to the flooring. Although oak is the predominant wood used for flooring, maple, walnut, teak, and cherry are also used. Any wood can be used for any floor.

Three new products on the market are:

Handscraped Wood Floors—distinctive markings etched into face of wood and along edges, all done by hand (not machine scraped). Each plank has a very unique look. Also called hand sculptured.

Distressed Hardwood Floors—also have distinctive etched markings in the face of wood but it is done by machine.[4]

Durapalm® flooring is made from multiple layers of palm, creating both a stable and durable flooring product of great beauty. These tongue and groove planks come in lengths from two to six feet in length and are provided as unfinished or prefinished flooring. Durapalm® can be installed by either a nail-down or glue-down method following procedures laid out by NOFMA, the National Oak Floor Manufacturer's Association, and NWFA, the National Wood Flooring Association.[5] (See Figure 4.5.)

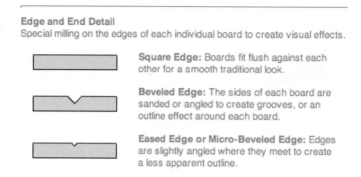

Edge and End Detail
Special milling on the edges of each individual board to create visual effects.

Square Edge: Boards fit flush against each other for a smooth traditional look.

Beveled Edge: The sides of each board are sanded or angled to create grooves, or an outline effect around each board.

Eased Edge or Micro-Beveled Edge: Edges are slightly angled where they meet to create a less apparent outline.

TYPES OF WOOD FLOORING

The three different types of wood flooring are strip, random plank, and parquet.

Strip

Usually 2 1/4″ wide, strip flooring is tongue and grooved on both sides and ends. This type of flooring is most commonly made of oak, although other woods may be used, such as teak and maple. Strip flooring may be laid parallel to the wall, or diagonally. Gymnasium floors are always constructed of maple but require a special type of installation that provides a slight "give" to the floor. Strip flooring is used for above-grade levels only, and is not recommended for concrete slabs.

Harris Tarkett's exclusive Alumide® is an advanced formulation of acrylic polyurethane that is enhanced by the addition of aluminum oxide granules. Invisible to the naked eye, these granules make Alumide® more resistant to wear than other wood finishes. They also protect the color, grain, and beauty of the wood, and are guaranteed to do so for up to 25 years.

Another variation of plank, strip, and parquet flooring is acrylic impregnated flooring. Liquid acrylic is evenly forced into the pore structure of select hardwood, and then is permanently hardened. The finish, therefore, is as deep as the wood itself, is highly resistant to abrasion and impact, never requires refinishing, and is easy to repair and maintain. Dyes and fire retardants may be added to the acrylic, if required. The stain penetrates throughout the wood so worn areas need only be retouched with a topcoat. The floor never needs sanding, staining, or refinishing. Acrylic impregnated hardwood is over 50% more crush proof than unimpregnated flooring. With impregnated woods, it must be remembered that the color cannot be changed because it has penetrated the whole depth of the wood. This can be an asset or a liability, depending on the purchaser's requirements.

Regular strip flooring is sold by the board foot and a 5 percent waste allowance is added to the total ordered. (See a strip floor with custom accents, Figure 4.6.)

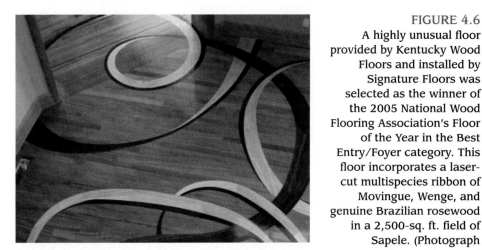

FIGURE 4.6
A highly unusual floor provided by Kentucky Wood Floors and installed by Signature Floors was selected as the winner of the 2005 National Wood Flooring Association's Floor of the Year in the Best Entry/Foyer category. This floor incorporates a laser-cut multispecies ribbon of Movingue, Wenge, and genuine Brazilian rosewood in a 2,500-sq. ft. field of Sapele. (Photograph courtesy of Kentucky Wood Floors)

Plank

Plank flooring is 3 to 8 inches wide, and most installations comprise three different sizes. The widths selected should correspond to the dimensions of the room to keep the flooring in proper scale: narrower ones for small rooms and wider ones for larger rooms. Random plank comes with a **square** or **beveled** edge and may be factory finished or finished after installation.

Plank floors also have a tongue-and-groove side. The prefinished tongue and groove disguises any shrinkage, because the V-joint becomes a fraction wider, whereas with a square edge, the crack caused by shrinkage is more obvious. This is why it is important that all wood be stored in the climatic conditions that will prevail at the installation site. Proper storage conditions will allow the wood to absorb or dissipate moisture and reach a stable moisture content. A white finish will also emphasize any shrinkage. In the past, some plank floors were installed using wooden pegs or plugs. A hole (or several holes for a wide plank) was drilled about 1 1/2 to 2 inches from the end of the plank. A **dowel** was pounded into the floor joist and glued into place. Any excess dowel was cut and sanded flush with the floor. Often, these plugs were constructed of a contrasting wood and became a decorative feature of plank flooring. Today it is recommended that, because of its width, plank flooring be screwed to the floor, then the screws should be countersunk and short dowels of walnut, other contrasting woods, or even brass are glued in to cover the screw for decorative purposes only.

Unfortunately, some prefinished floors may have plugs made of plastic, which seems incongruous in a wood floor. Another decorative joining procedure used in the past was the butterfly or key, where a dovetail-shaped piece of wood was used at the end joint of two boards. Plank flooring can also be of different species, which creates an interesting color combination.

By using the Pattern Guide for Pattern Plus, from Hartco, many patterns can be created. The guide computes the quantity needed. Planks range from 9 inches to 36 inches long. Another new line for Hartco is the Exotic Treasures, a "**floating floor**" design with new species including kempas, merbau, cherry, maple, and oak. Especially beneficial in remodeling installations, the floor may be installed over concrete, ceramic tile, vinyl, resilient tile, and hardwood.

For those desiring the authentic look of an old floor, Aged Woods® has recycled antique planks with varying amounts of character (e.g., knots and knot holes, nail holes, flat and vertical grain pattern, cracks and occasional insect marks, and **patina,** a dark, rich coloring). Aged Woods® supplies oak, chestnut, pine, hemlock, and poplar in various finishes for the old appearance. These are made from reclaimed wood from buildings that are going to be torn down. Plank flooring is sold by the square foot, and a 5 percent waste allowance is generally added to the total square footage. (See Figure 1.5 for Aged Wood floor.)

Parquet

Parquet is comprised of individual pieces of wood called **billets.** These are generally made of oak, from 3/8 to 3/4 inch thick, joined together to form a variety of patterns. These small pieces are held together by various methods, such as a **metal spline,** gluing to a mesh of paper, or gluing to a form of cheesecloth. Sizes vary from 9 to 19 inches square. There are many parquet patterns and most manufacturers make a similar variety of patterns, but the names may vary. For example, one company will name a pattern Jeffersonian; another will call it Monticello or Mt. Vernon, but they are variations of the same pattern. The Jeffersonian design is made with a central block surrounded by **pickets** on all four sides. The center may be made of solid wood, a laminated block, five or six strips all in the same direction, or a standard unit of four **sets.**

Designers need a word of warning about using some parquet patterns. Some parquets have direction (e.g., the herringbone pattern).

Hardwood Flooring Brand	Solid Strips and Planks	Prefinished Engineered Planks	Longstrip Engineered Planks	Exotic Species	Handscraped Floors	Glueless Installation
Anderson Hardwood Floors	Yes	Yes	Yes	Yes	Yes	–
Award Hardwood Floors	Yes	Yes	Yes	Yes	–	Yes
BR-111	Yes	Yes	–	Yes	–	–
Bruce Hardwood Floors	Yes	Yes	Yes	Yes	–	Yes
Capella Wood Floors	–	Yes	–	–	–	–
Columbia Flooring	Yes	Yes	Yes	Yes	Yes	Yes
Hartco Wood Flooring	Yes	Yes	–	Yes	–	–
HomerWood Hardwood Floors	Yes	–	–	–	Yes	–
Kahrs Wood Flooring	–	Yes	Yes	Yes	–	Yes
Kentucky Wood Floors	Yes	Yes	–	Yes	–	–
Lauzon Hardwood Flooring	Yes	Yes	Yes	Yes	–	–
Mannington Wood Floors	–	Yes	–	Yes	Yes	–
Mercier Wood Flooring	Yes	Yes	–	Yes	–	–
Mirage Wood Floors	Yes	Yes	–	Yes	–	–
Mohawk Hardwood Flooring	Yes	Yes	Yes	Yes	Yes	Yes
Mullican Flooring	Yes	–	–	Yes	Yes	–
Muskoka Hardwood Flooring	Yes	Yes	–	Yes	–	–
Robbins Hardwood Flooring	Yes	Yes	–	Yes	–	–
Shaw Hardwood Floors	Yes	Yes	Yes	Yes	Yes	Yes
Somerset Hardwood Flooring	Yes	–	–	Yes	Yes	–
Tarkett Wood Floors	Yes	Yes	Yes	Yes	–	–

Source: From Floor Facts website, www.floorfacts.com/hardwood-flooring-comparison.asp. Used with permission.

TABLE 4.1

Hardwood Flooring Brand Comparison

Depending on whether the pieces are laid parallel to the wall or at an angle, a client may see L's, zigzags, or arrows. The important thing is the client's expectations.

To reduce expansion problems caused by moisture, the oak flooring industry has developed several types of parquets. The laminated or engineered block is a product that displays far less expansion and contraction with moisture changes, and therefore can be successfully installed below grade in basements and in humid climates. It can even fit tight to vertical obstructions. Blocks can be glued directly to the concrete with several types of adhesive, which the industry is making VOC compliant. One concern in the past has been the ability of a laminated block to be sanded and refinished. Because the face layer is oak, with proper maintenance the initial service life can be expected to be 20 to 30 years. Any of the laminated products on the market today can be sanded and refinished (at least twice) using proper techniques and equipment, so the expected life of a laminated block floor is 60 to 90 years.

Parquet flooring comes packed in cartons with a specific number of square feet. When ordering parquet flooring, only whole cartons are shipped, so the allowance for cutting may be taken care of with the balance of the carton.

All the parquet woods mentioned in this subsection are quarter sawn or plain sawn, but some species are cut across the growth rings (end grained). End-grain patterns are formed by small cross-cut pieces attached into blocks or strips with the end grain exposed. The thickness may vary from 1 inch to 4 inches, depending on the manufacturer. A block with 1 1/2 inches of end-grain has insulating qualities equal to 23 inches of concrete. Some end-grain block floors are still in place after more than 40 years of heavy industrial use. These blocks absorb noise and vibration and have been installed in museums and libraries.

Grade Levels

Figure 4.7 illustrates the differences among on grade, above grade, and below grade. Above grade is not a problem for installation of wood floors, because no moisture is present. As mentioned earlier, moisture is the major cause of problems with wood. On grade means that the concrete floor is in contact with the ground. The floor usually has a

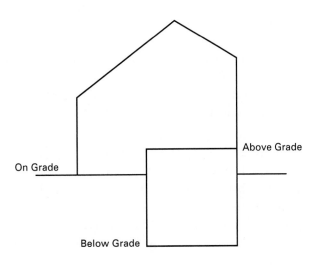

FIGURE 4.7
Grade levels.

drainage gravel as a base, covered by a polyethylene film to prevent moisture from migrating to the surface. The concrete is then poured on top of this polyethylene sheet. Below grade means a basement floor in which the presence of moisture is an even greater problem. All freshly poured concrete should be allowed to **cure** for 30 to 60 days.

The National Oak Flooring Manufacturers Association (NOFMA) provides the following information on testing for excessive moisture: Make tests in several areas of each room on both old and new slabs. When tests show too much moisture in the slab, do not install hardwood floors. For a moist slab, wait until it dries naturally, or accelerate drying with heat and ventilation; then test again. If moisture is still present, consult a specialist in this field to avoid flooring problems.

There are four tests for moisture: rubber mat, polyethylene film, calcium chloride, and phenothalein.

1. *The rubber mat test.* Lay a smooth, noncorrugated rubber mat on the slab, place a weight on top to prevent moisture from escaping, and allow the mat to remain 24 hours. If the covered area shows water marks when the mat is removed, too much moisture is present. This test is worthless if the slab surface originally is other than light in color.

2. *The polyethylene film test.* Tape a 1-foot square of 6-mil clear polyethylene film to the slab, sealing all edges with plastic moisture-resistant tape. If, after 24 hours, there is no "clouding" or drops of moisture on the underside of the film, the slab can be considered dry enough to install wood floors.

3. *The calcium chloride test.* Place a quarter teaspoonful of dry (anhydrous) calcium chloride crystals inside a 3-inch diameter putty ring on the slab. Cover this with a glass so the crystals are totally sealed off from the air. If the crystals dissolve within 12 hours the slab is too wet.

4. *The phenothalein test.* Put several drops of a 3 percent phenolphthalein solution in grain alcohol at various spots on the slab. If a red color develops in a few minutes, too much moisture is present.[6]

Particleboard underlayment is a product used widely as a substrate for floors in residential construction. Flooring manufacturers always specify the type of underlayment to be used with their products.

Particleboard is a composite panel product consisting of cellulosic particles of various sizes that are bonded together with a synthetic resin or binder under heat and pressure. Particle geometry, resin levels, board density, and manufacturing processes may be modified to produce products suitable for specific end uses. At the time of manufacture, additives can be incorporated to provide greater dimensional stability, better fire and moisture resistance, or to impart additional characteristics.[7]

Substrates must be clean (free of dust, grease, or oil stains), dry, and level. As stressed in Chapter 3 and repeated throughout this book, **surface preparation is extremely important.** The completed floor is only as good as the substrate. Any high spots should be ground down and low spots filled using the correct leveling compound. One floor installer related a story about a client who complained of a loose wood floor installed over a slab. When the loose wood was removed, not only did the wood come up, but attached to it was the material used as a filler for the low spots. The person who leveled the floor had used the wrong leveling compound.

Two types of patching compounds are available for use under flooring: gypsum and portland cement. Whichever type is used, antimicrobial agents must be added to prevent mold and mildew growth.

> Solid strip products are nailed down, and parquet products are glued down.
>
> Laminated planks are the only product that can be either nailed or glued.

The National Oak Flooring Manufacturers Association suggests that several factors may contribute to an unsatisfactory installation. First, the wood floor should be scheduled at the end of construction. Because most other work is completed, the floors will not be abused. The building should now be dry, with any moisture introduced during construction now gone. Second, a substrate of 5/8-inch or thicker plywood or $1'' \times 6''$ edge boards is preferred. A thicker, well-fastened substrate provides better installation. Third, the wood flooring should be well nailed; there should be no skimping on the number of nails per strip, plank, etc.

Walls are never used as a starting point for installation because they are never truly square. Wood parquet must always be installed in a pyramid or stair-step sequence, rather than in rows, to avoid a misaligned pattern. (See Figure 4.8.) Parquet may also be laid either parallel or at a 45-degree angle to the wall.

Reducer strips may be used at the doorway if there is a difference in level between two areas, and they are manufactured to match the wood floor. Most wood floor **mastics** take about 24 hours to dry, so no one must walk on the floor or place furniture in the room during that period. Laminated planks must be rolled with a 150-pound roller before the adhesive sets. An unfinished wood floor is sanded with the grain using progressively finer grits until the floor is smooth and has an almost shiny appearance. After vacuuming to eliminate any dust particles, finishing materials specifically manufactured for use on wood floors are applied.

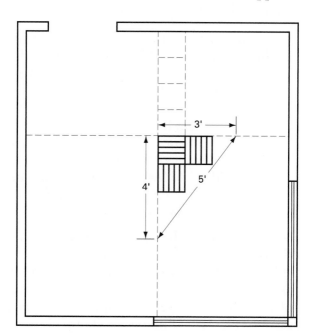

FIGURE 4.8
Method of laying parquet.

For open-grained wood such as oak, a filler with or without stain may be used after sanding to provide a more highly reflective surface. Often there is a preference for natural-color hardwood floors, but stain may be used to bring out the grain or produce a darker tone. When a very light finish is desired, the wood may be bleached or pickled. If a white floor is needed, a laminated wood floor is better because such floors are less likely to expand and contract (problems that show up as dark lines).

There are two main types of finish applied to wood floors: polyurethane and Swedish finish. Polyurethane finish will normally yellow with time, whereas the Swedish finish will not. Basic Coatings' Street Shoe XL® Commercial Wood Floor Finish system is a water-based finish that contains a special UV-blocker designed to reduce the sun's damaging effects. This finish is used for both commercial and residential applications. Several companies have introduced a low-gloss finish on their prefinished floors, which complements a more historic decor and is reminiscent of the original style of hardwood floors.

The latest material to be used in the finish of wood floors is aluminum oxide, with each company having its own brand name. This finish increases the durability of the wood floor.

Maintenance

A floor surface requires eight steps to remove sand or dirt from the bottom of shoes. Walk-off or tracking mats should be used at all exterior doors. (See Figure 3.9.) General housekeeping prolongs the life of a wood floor. The main problem with maintenance of any floor is *grit,* which can be removed by dust mop, broom, or vacuum. Another problem is indentations caused by heels, especially women's high heels. A 125-pound woman wearing high heels exerts as much pressure as an elephant, and therefore indentations should be expected. Round-headed chair glides and narrow wheels on furniture legs are also damaging. They can scratch or permanently dent the floor. Congoleum's® *Consumer Flooring Guide* has the following information on how to protect against indentations and furniture damage:

> Always make sure furniture legs have large-surface, nonstaining floor protectors. [They recommend that] the homeowner replace small, narrow metal or dome-shaped glides.
>
> Use hard, plastic casters and cups because some types of rubber casters and cups may permanently stain the floor.
>
> Use wide, flat casters and cups for heavy furniture.
>
> Use nonstaining rubber-surfaced wheels that are a minimum 3/4″ wide instead of metal casters.
>
> Glides and furniture cups should be covered with felt pads. The pads should be checked periodically for grit and wear and replaced when necessary.[8]

If the floor is the type that may be waxed (very few are), a thin coat of wax should be allowed to dry and harden. When dry, an electric bristle brush buffer is used. Because old wax holds dirt and grease and a buildup of "scuffs," it should be removed periodically by means of a solvent type of wax remover specifically designed for wood floors. Food spills may be wiped up with a damp cloth.

Certain chemicals in wood oxidize in strong light, causing the wood to change color; therefore, rugs or area rugs should be moved periodically.

Wood and water do not mix. No matter what claims the manufacturer makes for the wood finish, water must never be poured onto the floor intentionally. A damp mop is fine for nonwaxed polyurethane and other surface finishes in good condition. Wax-coated finishes should **never** be cleaned with water, not even with a damp mop. (The *Wood Floor Care Guide* is available from the Oak Flooring Institute, an affiliate of NOFMA.)

Many manufacturers sell a line of maintenance products specially prepared for their own products. Custom finishes, such as polyurethane and Swedish, should **not** be waxed. Manufacturers of acrylic wood provide special cleaning materials for their products.

If cracks appear in the wood floor, they are probably caused by lack of humidity and can be reduced by installing a humidifier.

Wood floors can be refinished. The old method was to sand the floor with a power sander, which created dust throughout the area. Now Basic Coatings has introduced the TyKote® Dustless Recoating System, which is simply a thorough cleaning with IFT and Squeaky, followed by the application of TyKote and then coating the floor with StreetShoe XL®.

BAMBOO AND PALM

Bamboo is actually in the "grass" family and is the latest product for use on floors. It is manufactured from timber bamboo that grows to a height of 40 feet and matures in less than five years. The bamboo is split into strips, kiln-dried, and laminated together to produce a multiple bamboo plywood. Boric acid, a benign pest repellent, is applied during the process to protect the bamboo.

> Plyboo® flooring is twice as stable and nearly as hard as standard red oak flooring. It has performed exceptionally well on both residential and commercial projects and can be installed, finished and maintained like other hardwood floors. Plyboo flooring is distinguished by its long continuous grain interspersed with characteristic nodes, or knuckles. Plyboo flooring comes both finished and unfinished in two colors, natural and amber.[9]
>
> Teragren's bamboo is harvested at 5 1/2 to 6 years (at maturity, for a more durable finished product), leaving behind a thriving plant and new shoots. Harvesting sooner than 5 1/2 years results in softer fiber and a less stable finished product.[10]

The hardness of bamboo does vary from species to species.

> Palm is harvested from coconut plantations at the end of their coconut bearing years and is then cut down and replanted with new coconut palms with the old palms made into . . . palm flooring.
>
> Bamtex Palm provides its own unique graining and is offered in either medium or soft brown shades.[11]

The finish is either a UV-applied polyurethane or aluminum oxide and resists 20,000 revolutions on the **taber test.** PVA-C formaldehyde-free glue is used and the finish is also formaldehyde free. Plyboo is available in horizontal and vertical grains.

Installation

Bamboo hardwood floors can be floated, nailed, or glued. They may also be floated over slab or radiant heat systems. Bamboo flooring should be allowed to acclimatize on site for at least three days. Each plank should be laid out separately during the acclimatizing process. The method of installation is similar to other wood tongue-and-groove planks.

LAMINATE

In 1977 Pergo®, Inc., originated the idea for **laminate floor** and the product was introduced to the European market in 1984. Wilsonart International manufactured the first laminate flooring in the United States. This type of floor is not to be confused with a laminated wood floor (also called engineered wood).

Laminate flooring is actually a composite that's designed to endure more-than-average wear and tear. A direct-pressure manufacturing process fuses four layers into one extremely hard surface. The four layers are:

> **back layer**—the back is reinforced with melamine for structural stability and moisture resistance.
>
> **fiberboard core**—Shaw Laminate's ultra-dense core board provides impact resistance and stability. It also features an edge-sealing treatment that provides even further structural stability.
>
> **decorative layer**—providing the floor's beauty, the decorative layer is actually a highly detailed photograph that gives the laminate the appearance of wood or tile.
>
> **wear layer**—the melamine wear layer is a tough, clear finish reinforced with aluminum oxide, one of the hardest mineral compounds known to man, to resist staining, fading, surface moisture, and wear.[12]

Wilsonart® Commercial Flooring has introduced a new premium commercial flooring line called Contact™, which features the company's award-winning Tap-N-Lock™ installation system. . . . The new value-priced line is designed specifically to fit the needs of smaller, more mainline commercial installations on a fixed technical improvement budget.

> A new high performance commercial overlay that's wear, stain and fade resistant, adds increased durability in high traffic areas. The crystalline surface promotes design clarity and definition, increasing the realistic look of the 19 wood grain planks and 7 tile patterns available in the design line.[13]

Other laminate floors may vary in core and surface.

> iCore® is Advanced Composite Flooring, an entirely new category of hard surface flooring that's ideal for commercial installations in retail/restaurants, healthcare, education and hospitality spaces. Featuring new technology, exclusive to Mannington Commercial, iCore® has an extruded synthetic core that is impervious to moisture and incorporates unique sound-dampening chambers for a quieter sound underfoot than other floors.[14]

Many laminate floor products are available. Because these products carry a lower warranty, it is probably best to stay with a nationally known brand.

Installation

According to Wilsonart International:

> Laminate flooring is installed using the "floating floor" system: Planks or tiles are glued together using a tongue and groove system, and are installed over a padding which increases sound absorption and provides some flexibility to the floor. Laminate flooring is not nailed or glued to the substrate; a small gap is left at walls allowing for expansion and contraction without damage to the floor. It can be installed over most existing floors, making it ideal for retrofit situations.
>
> Reduced prep time prior to installation (e.g., tear out is often unnecessary), and the simple installation process provides both time and cost savings. Wilsonart Flooring features an exclusive, patented tongue and groove system that makes installation simple and ensures proper bonding and seal.[15]

Some laminate floors may be glued.

Maintenance

Wilsonart suggests the following:

> For everyday cleaning, simply vacuum the floor to remove loose dirt and debris. Mop occasionally, using a minimal amount of water (a cotton string mop is recommended). For more thorough cleaning, mop using a solution of two ounces of Wilsonart Flooring Cleaner or a mixture of soap-free household cleaner and water (vinegar and ammonia both work well).
>
> Wipe stains away with a damp cloth. For difficult stains caused by ink, paint, etc., a cloth moistened with acetone (nail polish remover) or a household solvent is usually all that's needed. To remove chewing gum, tar, etc., let the spot harden completely, then gently scrape away. Apply felt protectors to the bottom of furniture and use floor mats at entryways to preserve the appearance of the floor. A few Notes of Caution: Abrasive cleansers and scouring pads can scratch and damage the surface of Wilsonart flooring. Please do not use them. Important! Never wax, sand or apply lacquer to Wilsonart Flooring.[16]

GROUT

As most of the hard-surface materials that follow require the use of **grout** to finish the floor, it is mentioned before those materials. Grout is the material used to fill the joints between hard-surface materials. The type of grout employed, if any, depends on which variety of tile is being used (see Table 4.2). Therefore, not only is the type of grout important,

W = Wall Use F = Floor Use	Jobsite Mix (Sanded)	Grouts Containing Portland Cement		
		Standard Unsanded Cement Grout A118.6 (4)	Standard Sanded Cement Grout A118.6 (4)	Polymer Modified Unsanded Tile Grout A118.7 (4, 9)
Tile Type				
Glazed Wall Tile (7)		W	W	W
Glazed Floor Tile (7)	W, F	W, F	W, F	W, F
Ceramic Mosaics	W, F	W, F	W, F	W, F
Quarry, Paver, and Packing House Tile (8)	W, F		W, F	
Large Unit Porcelain or Vitreous Tile (8)	W, F	W, F	W, F	W, F
Dimension Stone (7, 8) (including Agglomerates)	W, F	W, F	W, F	W, F
Use				
Dry/Limited Water Exposure	W, F	W, F	W, F	W, F
Wet Areas (10)	W, F	W, F	W, F	W, F
Exteriors (8, 9, 10)	W, F	W, F	W, F	W, F
Performance	(Note: There are five performance ratings, from Best [A] to Minimal [E])			
Suggested Joint Widths (5)	1/8″ to 5/8″	1/16″ to 1/8″	1/8″ to 5/8″	1/16″ to 1/8″
Stain Resistance	E	D	D	C
Crack Resistance	E	D	D	C
Color Availability	D	B	B	B

Notes:
(1) Mainly used for chemical resistant properties.
(2) Special tools needed for proper application. Silicone, urethane, and modified polyvinylchloride used in pregrouted ceramic tile sheets. Silicone grout should not be used on kitchen countertops or other food preparation surfaces unless it meets the requirements of FDA Regulation No. 21, CFE 177.2600.
(3) Special cleaning procedures and materials recommended.
(4) Follow manufacturer's directions.
(5) Joint widths are only guidelines. Individual grout manufacturer's products may vary. Consult manufacturers' instructions.
(6) Epoxies are recommended for prolonged temperatures up to 140°F, high-temperature-resistant epoxies and furans up to 350°F.
(7) Some types of glazed ceramic tiles, polished marble, marble agglomerates, and granite can be permanently scratched or damaged when grouted with sanded grout formulas. DO NOT use sanded grout or add sand to grout when grouting polished marble, marbled agglomerates, and ceramic wall tiles with soft glazes. Check the tile or marble manufacturer's literature and test grout on a separate sample area prior to grouting.
(8) Some types of ceramic tiles and dimension stone may be permanently stained when grouted with pigmented grout of a contrasting color. WHITE GROUP IS BEST SUITED FOR GROUTING WHITE OR LIGHT-COLORED MARBLE OR GRANITE.
(9) Latex modification may be required in areas subject to freezing temperatures. Consult grout manufacturer for recommended products and methods.
(10) Colored cementitious grouts may darken when wet.

Source: 2006 Handbook for Ceramic Tile Installation. Copyright© Tile Council of America, Inc. Reprinted with permission.

TABLE 4.2
Grout Guide
These guidelines cannot address every installation. The type and size of tile, service level, climatic conditions, tile spacing, and individual manufacturer's recommendations are all factors that should be considered when selecting the proper grout.

Polymer Modified Sanded Tile Grout A118.7 (4, 9)	Modified Epoxy Emulsion A118.8 (4)	100% Solid Epoxy A118.3 (1, 3, 4, 6)	Furan A118.5 (1, 3, 4, 6)	Silicone Urethane (2, 4)	Mastic Grout (3, 4)
W		W		W	W
W, F	W, F	W, F			W, F
W, F	W, F	W, F		W	W, F
W, F	W, F	W, F	W,		
W, F	W, F	W, F	F	W	W, F
W, F	W, F				
W, F	W, F	W, F	W, F	W, F	W, F
W, F	W, F	W, F	W, F	W, F	
W, F	W, F	W, F (4)	W, F (4)	W, F	
1/8″ to	1/16″ to	1/16″ to	3/8″ to	1/16″ to	1/16″ to
5/8″	5/8″	5/8″	5/8″	1/4″	1/4″
C	C	A	A	A	B
C	C	B	C	A	C
B	B	B	Black only	B	B

but also the spacing of the tile. Proper joint placement is crucial so that both sides of the room have equal-size pieces. The use of crack isolation membranes in thin-bed installations is necessary to prevent cracks in the substrate from cracking marble or ceramic tiles installed over them.

The Tile Council of America states that:

> Grouting materials for ceramic tile are available in many forms to meet the requirements of the different kinds of tile and types of exposure. Portland cement is the base of most grouts and is modified to provide specific qualities such as whiteness, mildew resistance, uniformity, hardness, flexibility, and water retentivity. Complete installation and material specifications are contained in **ANSI** A108.10, A118.6 and A118.7. Non-cement based grouts such as epoxies, furans, and silicone rubber offer properties not possible with cement grouts. However, special skills on the part of the tile setter are required. *These materials can be appreciably greater in cost than* cement-based grouts. [emphasis added][17]

Commercial portland cement grout for floors is usually gray (but colors are available) and is designed for use with ceramic **mosaics,** quarry, and paver tile. Damp curing is required, which is the process of keeping the grout moist and covered for several days and results in a much stronger grout. For areas that must be opened for traffic as quickly as possible, quick-set grout additives are available (see Table 4.2).

Grouts with sand are not used with highly reflective tiles, because the roughness of the grout is not compatible with the high gloss. For glazed tiles, unsanded grout or mastic grout is used. Special grouts that are chemical resistant, fungus and mildew resistant, or of a latex composition are used when movement is anticipated. Grout sealers form an invisible barrier that is resistant to moisture and stains while allowing vapor to escape.

MARBLE

Marble is a **metamorphic** rock derived from limestone. Pressure and/or heat created the metamorphic change that turned limestone debris into marble. Today all rocks that can take a polish come under the heading of marble. Dolomitic limestone ("hard" limestone), although technically limestone, is known commercially as marble. Travertine and onyx are related stones; travertine is the more important for flooring purposes because it is easier to work with. Onyx is brittle and is mostly relegated to decorative uses. Serpentine is of a different chemical makeup, but because it can be polished, it is classified as marble. All of the aforementioned stones are calcareous.

The minerals that result from impurities give marble a wide variety of colors. The colored veins of marble are as varied and numerous as the areas from which it is quarried. One famous type, Carrara marble, is pure white. Michelangelo used this marble for many of his sculptures. Other Carrara marble may have black, gray, or brownish veining. The name *verd antique* is applied to marbles of prevailing green color, which consists chiefly of serpentine, a hydrous magnesium silicate.

Verd antiques are highly decorative stones; at times the green is interspersed with streaks or veins of red and white. The pinks, reds, yellows, and browns are caused by the presence of iron oxides, whereas the blacks, grays, and blue-grays result from bituminous deposits. Silicate, chlorite, and mica provide the green colors.

Marble is the most ancient of all finished materials currently in use today. Some authorities believe that the onyx marble of Algeria was employed by the Egyptians as early as 475 B.C. Biblical references show that marble was used in King Solomon's Temple at Jerusalem, and in the palace of Sushun more than one thousand years before Christ. Parian marble from the Aegean Sea was found in the ruins of ancient Troy.

Pentelic marble was used in the Parthenon in Athens and is still available today. Phidias used this marble for the frieze of the Parthenon, and portions of this frieze known as the **Elgin Marbles** are intact today and are on display at the British Museum. Makrana marble, a white marble, was used in the Taj Mahal in India. Inside the Taj Mahal, sunlight filters through marble screens as delicate as lace and the white marble walls are richly decorated with floral designs in onyx, jasper, carnelian, and other semiprecious stones.

Knoxville, Tennessee, was known at the turn of the 20th century as the marble capital of the United States. Marble is found in many eastern states, from Vermont to Georgia, and in some western states. The Georgia Marble Company ranks as the world's largest producer of marble products. Dolomitic marble is quarried in Tennessee and Idaho. The famous Yule Quarry in Marble, Colorado (from which came the columns of the Lincoln Memorial and the massive block forming the Tomb of the Unknown Soldier), has been reopened. The white marble from this quarry may be the purest marble in the world.

Marble floors were used in the Baroque and Rococo periods in Europe. During the French empire, black and white marble squares were used, and they remain a popular pattern for marble floors today. In the formal halls of Georgian homes, the marble floors were appropriate for mahogany tables and chairs. In his Barcelona Pavilion, Mies Van der Rohe used great slabs of marble as freestanding partitions. Today, marble is used for furniture, floors, and interior and exterior walls.

Marble does not come in sheets (slabs) and must be quarried. There are three principal quarrying methods utilized today. The first is by drilling holes and thus outlining the block. Then wedges are driven into the holes and the blocks are split from the surrounding rock. The second method uses wire saws. A long steel cable with diamond teeth is passed over the stone with downward pressure, cutting the block of stone free from the deposit. The third method employs a large chain-saw-type machine to saw the stone free from the deposit. Marble chips are used in the production of **terrazzo, agglomerated** marble tiles, and cast polymer products.

Marble is a relatively heavy and expensive material for use on floors because of the necessity of using the conventional thick-bed installation method. Fiberglass and epoxy resins employed as a backing hold delicate stones together during fabrication, shipment, and installation. This mass-produced method allows expensive decorative stone to be furnished more economically than with conventional methods (i.e., permanent stone liners also known as backer slabs).

The following properties need to be considered for marble floors:

Density. Averages 0.1 pound per cubic inch. This figure may be used to calculate the weight of the marble.

Water absorption. Measured by total immersion of a 2-inch cube for 48 hours and varies from 0.1 to 0.2 percent, which is less than that for other natural stones. The maximum absorption as established by ASTM C503 is 0.20 percent.

Abrasion resistance. Measured by a scuffing method that removes surface particles similar to the action of foot traffic, abrasion resistance for commercial flooring should be at least a hardness value of 10, as measured by ASTM C241. The Marble Institute of America (MIA) recommends a hardness value of 12. This value is not necessary for single-family homes.

Marble is also classified as A through C, according to the fabrication methods considered necessary and acceptable in each instance, as based on standard trade practice.

A polished finish reflects light and emphasizes the color and marking of the material. The polished finish may be used in residential installations, but not for commercial installations. The biggest problem with a polished floor is that the shine is removed in the traffic area but the edges retain the shine, emphasizing the difference in the two areas. A honed surface is satin smooth with little light reflection. A honed finish is preferred for floors, stair treads, thresholds, and other locations where heavy traffic will wear off the polished finish.

When using marble or any other natural stone, the weight of these materials must be calculated to ensure that the substrate is strong enough to support the extra weight. This is where 3/8-inch-thick marbles come into use; especially in remodeling, the floor was probably not constructed to bear heavy stones. Substrates must meet a maximum deflection of 1/180 of span. The stiffer the substrate, the longer lasting the finished floor. Substrates that have measurable deflection will fail.

Two of the materials used to help provide rigidity to a stable substrate are a cementitious backer unit (CBU) and glass water-resistant gypsum backer board.

CBU is a backing and underlayment deigned for use on floors, walls, and ceilings in wet or dry areas. This board is applied directly to wood or metal wall studs or over wood substrates. Ceramic tile can be bonded to it with dry-set, latex/portland cement **mortar** or epoxy by following the backer board manufacturer's instruction. Complete interior installation and material specifications are contained in ANSI (American National Standards Institute) A108.11 and ANSI A118.9 or ASTM C. 1325.

Coated Glass Mat Water-Resistant Gypsum Backer Board is a backer board conforming to ASTM C-1178. Designed for use on floors, walls, and ceilings in wet or dry areas, this board is applied directly to wood or metal studs or over wood substrates. Ceramic tile can be bonded to it with dry-set, latex/polymer modified portland cement mortar, organic adhesive of epoxy by following the backer board manufacturer's instructions.[18]

A crack-suppression membrane allows the stone setting bed to span cracks and narrow expansion joints without the fear of the stone floor following the crack. There are, of course, limits to which crack-suppression membranes can work.

Large stone medallions have been a popular decorative element used in grand residences for thousands of years. Reserved for princes and prelates in the past, these incredible pieces are now available to those working within a more modest budget.

> Walker Zanger offers medallions handcrafted in Italy and the United States to the industry's highest standards. All medallions are fully assembled for ease of installation.[19]

Mosaic medallions are crafted from thousands of different chips of stone, painstakingly combined to form a brilliant pattern, and mounted on sheets for easy installation. Medallions are created by hand-cutting pieces of stone and terra cotta, and carefully fitting them together to form the design. This process is a rare art, practiced only by a few workshops in Italy. Water-jet medallions take advantage of modern technology. The stone is cut by a super-pressurized stream of water that is controlled by a computer programmed with the shapes that comprise the design. This process allows for incredible precision. Installed, water-jet cut medallions create a seamless design.

Installation

Several associations are responsible for installation codes and standards based on the consensus of their membership. The natural stones, such as marble, travertine, and slate, use the specifications and test methods contained in the ASTM manual, Section 4, Construction, Volume 04.08, Soil and Rock; Building Stones. The ceramic tile industry uses ANSI A108 for installation specifications.

Because marble is the first hard-surface material covered in this book, installation methods will be discussed in detail. The same methods are used for all natural stones, ceramic tile, quarry tile, and other types of hard-surface materials.

Setting materials account for only 10 percent of installation costs, but account for 90 percent of problems, so proper specification and professional installation are crucial and will eliminate most problems. Skinning, a film that forms on the surface of the setting materials and causes improper bonding, is a common cause of installation failure for all setting materials. To cure this problem, the application tool should be used again to break up the skin.

According to the Tile Council of North America:

> Portland cement mortar is a mixture of portland cement and sand, roughly in proportions of 1:5 on floors and of portland cement, sand and lime in proportions of 1:5:1/2 to 1:7:1 for walls.

Performance-Level Requirement Guide and Selection Table

Based on results from ASTM Test Method C-627 "Standard Test Method for Evaluating Ceramic Floor Tile Installation Systems Using the Robinson Type Floor Tester." All methods are material dependent performance rating should not exceed rating of weakest component consult each material manufacturer for individual component rating.

SERVICE REQUIREMENTS
Find required performance level and choose installation method that meets or exceeds it. Performance results are based on ceramic tile meeting ANSI A137.1, or tile designated by tile manufacturer.

FLOOR TYPE—Numbers refer to Handbook Method numbers

Service Requirements	Concrete	Page	Wood	Page
EXTRA HEAVY: Extra heavy and high-impact use in food plants, dairies, breweries, and kitchens. Requires quarry tile, packing house tile, or tile designated by tile manufacturer. (Passes ASTMC 627 cycles 1 through 14.)	F101, F102, F111 F112, F113, F114 F115, F116, F121 F125[i], F125A[i] F131, F132 F133, F134, F205	17, 17, 18 19, 19, 20 20, 20, 22 23, 23 24, 24 25, 25, 21		
HEAVY: Shopping malls, stores, commercial kitchens, work areas, laboratories, auto showrooms and service areas, shipping/receiving, and exterior decks. (Passes ASTM C627 cycles 1 through 12.)	F103, F111, F112 F113, F121	17, 18, 19 19, 22	F143[a, g]	33
MODERATE: Normal commercial and light institutional use in public space of restaurants and hospitals. (Passes ASTM C627 cycles 1 through 10.)	F112, F115 F122[c], F200 RH110, RH111 RH115, RH116	19, 20 22, 21 26, 27 27, 28	F121, F141, F145	22, 32, 32
LIGHT: Light commercial use in office space, reception areas, kitchens, and bathrooms. (Passes ASTM C627 cycles 1 through 6.)	F122[c]	22	F143[a], F144[b, e&f] F146, F150[h] F160, F175, F180 RH122 RH130[h], RH135[e&f]	33, 34 35, 33 34, 36, 39 29 29, 30

RESIDENTIAL:
Kitchens, bathrooms, and foyers. (Passes ASTM C627 cycles 1 through 3.)

F116[j]	20	F142, F144	32, 34
TR711[d]	61	F147, F170	36, 35
F135	26	F148, F149	37, 37
		F150[h], F151, F152	33, 37, 38
		F155, F180, F185	38, 39, 40
		RH130[h], RH135	29, 30
		RH140	31

Notes:

Consideration must also be given to (1) wear properties of surface of tile selected, (2) tile size, (3) coefficient of friction. Unglazed Standard Grade tile will give satisfactory wear or abrasion resistance in installations listed. Glazed tile or soft body decorative unglazed tile should have the manufacturer's approval for intended use. Color, pattern, surface texture, and glaze hardness must be considered in determining tile acceptability on a particular floor.

Selection Table Notes:

Tests to determine Performance-Levels utilized representative products meeting recognized industry standards:

a. ANSI A118.3 epoxy mortar and grout.
b. Data in Selection Table based on tests conducted by Tile Council of North America, except data for F144 Method, which is based on test results from an independent laboratory.
c. ANSI A118.4 latex-portland cement mortar and grout.
d. Tile bonded to existing resilient flooring with epoxy adhesive.
e. 7/16"-minimum-thick cementitious backer unit or minimum 1/4"-thick fiber-cement underlayment tested.
f. Minimum 1/4" thick cementitious backer unit can be used for residential applications over 19/32" minimum thick subfloor; minimum 1/4" thick cementitious backer unit can be used for light commercial applications over minimum 23/32" thick subfloor.
g. Requires tile designated by tile manufacturers as suitable for the rating.
h. Requires minimum 19/32" exterior glue plywood underlayment for light rating; 15/32" exterior glue plywood underlayment may be used for residential rating.
i. Requires membrane designated by membrane manufacturer as suitable for the rating.
j. F116 with epoxy is extra heavy while F116 with organic adhesive is rated residential.

Source: Courtesy of the Tile Council of North America.

TABLE 4.3
Floor Tiling Installation Guide

Portland cement mortar is suitable for most surfaces and ordinary types of installation. A mortar bed, up to 2″ in thickness, facilitates accurate slopes or planes in the finished tile work on floors and walls.

The mortar bed can be modified with the inclusion of a latex/redispersable polymer per the manufacturer's directions as part or all of the liquid portion of the mixture to enhance certain performance properties.

There are two equivalent methods recognized for installing ceramic tiles with a portland cement mortar bed on walls, ceilings and floors. They are: (1) the method covered by ANSI A108.1A, which requires the tile be set on a mortar bed that is still workable, and (2) the method covered by ANSI A108.1B, which requires the tile to be set on a cured mortar bed with dry-set or latex-portland polymer modified cement mortar. Absorptive ceramic tiles must be soaked before setting on a mortar bed that is still workable when using a neat portland cement bond coat.

Portland cement mortars can be bonded to concrete floors; backed with membranes and reinforced with wire mesh or metal lath; or applied on metal lath over open studding on walls. They are structurally strong, are not affected by prolonged contact with water, and can be used to **plumb** and square surfaces installed by others.

Suitable backings, when properly prepared, are: brick or cement masonry, concrete, wood or steel stud frame, rough wood floors, plywood floors, foam insulation board, gypsum board, and gypsum plaster. The one-coat method may be used over masonry, plaster, or other solid backing that provides firm anchorage for metal lath.

Complete installation and material specifications are contained in ANSI A108.1A, A108.1B, and A108.1C. [emphasis added][20]

Thick-set or thick-bed *must* be used for setting materials of uneven thickness such as natural flagstone and slate. It may also be used for hard-surfaced materials of uniform thickness. Tiles are placed on the mortar and tapped into place until the surface is level. The mortar used on floors is a mixture of portland cement and sand, roughly in proportions of 1:6.

According to the Tile Council of North America:

Dry-set mortar is a mixture of portland cement with sand and additives imparting water retentivity which is used as a bond coat for setting tile.

Dry-set mortar is suitable for **thin-set** installations of ceramic tile over a variety of surfaces. It is used in one layer, as thin as 3/32″, after tiles are embedded, has excellent water and impact resistance, is water-cleanable, nonflammable, good for exterior work, and does not require soaking of the tile.

Dry-set mortar is available as a factory-sanded mortar to which only water need be added. Cured dry-set mortar is not affected by prolonged contact with water but does not form a water barrier. It is not a setting bed and is not intended to be used in truing or leveling the work of others.

Suitable backings, when properly prepared, include plumb and true masonry, concrete, gypsum board, cementitious backer units fiber-cement underlayment, coated glass mat water-resistant gypsum backer board, cementitious coated foam backer board, cured portland mortar beds, brick, ceramic tile and dimension stone.

Complete specifications and material specifications are contained in ANSI A108.5 and ANSI A118.1. For conductive dry set mortar see ANSI A108.7 and ANSI 118.2.[21]

Another thin-set method is to use an adhesive that is spread with a trowel. The trowel is used not only for spreading, by using the flat edge for continuous coverage, but is also a metering device for determining the proper amount of adhesive. Oil-based adhesives should be avoided when installing marble because they stain the marble. Again, it must be repeated that thin-bed should be used only where the substrate is solid and level.

Almost all marble and granite tile produced today is manufactured for use with a joint, and is furnished with a slight **chamfer** (bevel) at the junction of the face and edge.

Maintenance

The following information is condensed from the booklet *Care & Cleaning for Natural Stone Surfaces,* available from the Marble Institute of America, Inc. This institute serves the dimension stone industry. This information covers all natural stones, including marble, granite, limestone, onyx, and slate.

Blot the spill with a paper towel immediately. Do not wipe the area; it will spread the spill. Flush the area with plain water and mild soap and rinse several times. Dry the area with a soft cloth. Repeat as necessary. Identifying the type of stain on the stone surface is the key to removing it. Sometimes the location and color of the stain in proximity to possible culprits will make identification easier (i.e., plants, food service area, cosmetics, etc.). Surface stains can often be removed by cleaning with an appropriate cleaning product or household chemical. Deep-seated or stubborn stains may require using a poultice or calling in a professional.[22]

TERRAZZO

Terrazzo was developed by the Venetians in the 16th century and is still widely used. Terrazzo as we know it today, however, was not produced until after the development of portland cement in the 18th century.

Terrazzo is a composite material poured in place or precast, which is used for floor and wall treatments. It consists of marble, quartz, granite, glass or other suitable chips, sprinkled or unsprinkled, and poured with a binder that is cementitious, chemical or a combination of both. Terrazzo is cured, ground and polished to a smooth surface or otherwise finished to produce a uniformly textured surface.[23]

Terrazzo encompasses the following types:

Standard Terrazzo: Most common type of Terrazzo using relatively small chip sizes.

Venetian Terrazzo: Terrazzo in which larger chips are used.

Palladiana: Utilization of thin, random fractured slabs of marble, sometimes with Terrazzo joints between each slab.

Structural Terrazzo: Terrazzo Contractor places 4 inches of 4,000 psi concrete plus cementitious Terrazzo topping.

Rustic Terrazzo: A uniformly textured form of Terrazzo in which the **matrix** is depressed to expose the chips.

Resinous Matrices: A Terrazzo system usually applied in a thin cross-section in which small chip sizes are used. The matrix is composed of resinous or chemical materials or, in some cases, resinous additives to Portland cement, which are often highly resistant to acids, alkalis and other normally harmful materials.[24]

According to the National Terrazzo and Mosaic Association (NTMA), three types of binders are used to anchor marble chips or other aggregate in a terrazzo floor. One is a portland cement product; the second is a polyacrylic modified portland cement that includes an acrylic additive. The third is an epoxy or polyester system, often referred to as a resinous thin-set system. Although each system has the role of anchoring the aggregate into the topping, the treatment of each does vary.

Divider strips of brass, zinc, or plastic are attached to the substrate and are used for several purposes: as expansion joints to take care of any minor movement; as dividers when different colors are poured in adjacent areas; and as enhancements of a design motif, logo, or trademark. Because of the labor involved in a monolithic installation, terrazzo tiles consisting of portland cement with an aggregate of marble chips may be used. Wausau Tile is the only domestic manufacturer of cementitious precast terrazzo tile, available in 12, 16, and 24 inches square by 5/8 inch thick, in both square and chamfered edges. With the tile set method, chamfered-edge tiles are set with 1/16″ to 3/16″ joints, then grouted. With the new tight-joint method, square-edge tiles are set with a 1/16″ minus joint, then grouted flush and ground and polished on the job for a monolithic look. The size of the chips may be large or small, or a mixture of sizes. The finish may be polished or slip-resistant.

Agglomerated marble tiles consist of 90 to 95 percent marble chips, combined with 5 to 10 percent resins and formed into blocks in a vacuum chamber. They are available as floor tile or marble wall veneers. Agglomerated marble sometimes is classified as cast marble, but the term *cast* is also used to describe a polyester product containing ground marble.

Installation

When cementitious terrazzo tiles are used, they may be installed using the thin-set method or other cement mortar methods. The installation of poured-in-place (monolithic) terrazzo was described previously.

Maintenance

Moisture is added to the Terrazzo products in the composition, curing, grinding, grouting and polishing stages. Structurally, with this much moisture, you can be assured of a quality installation; however, you can also expect the water to dissipate and escape through the finished surface. Here again, however, it is necessary to retard this moisture evaporation. Therefore, the Terrazzo must be sealed with a penetrating-type sealer. This further increases the time that it takes for the system to cure. Each passing day, with normal maintenance the aesthetics of your Terrazzo floor will increase. Obviously, this requires your patience, but you can be assured that the results will be rewarding.

Because there are three types of binders used to anchor marble chips or other aggregate in the terrazzo floor, it is necessary to know which type has been used in order to decide the correct maintenance procedure. The National terrazzo and Mosaic Association specifically warns that soaps and scrubbing powders containing water-soluble inorganic salts or crystallizing salts should never be used in the maintenance of terrazzo. Alkaline solutions will sink into the pores and, as they dry, will expand and break the cells of the marble chips and matrix, causing **spalling**. [emphasis added][25]

This is similar to the problem that occurs with cement floors. The NTMA has an excellent booklet, "The Care of Terrazzo."

After the initial cleaning, the terrazzo floor should be allowed to dry and then sealed with a water-based sealer in the acrylic family especially designed for terrazzo use. The Underwriters Laboratories classification of this sealer should include slip resistance with a coefficient of friction rating at a minimum of 0.5.

The NTMA recommends the following maintenance plan for terrazzo floors:

1. Daily sweeping with yarn-wick brush treated with sweeping compound.
2. Weekly damp mop lightly soiled floors with a neutral cleaner.
3. Heavily soiled floors should be scrubbed with a mechanical buffing machine and neutral cleaner. Mop up residue with clean water before it dries. Allow to dry and buff with a dry brush.
4. Semi-annually strip all old sealer and any finish coats. Reseal clean floors.

Stain removal for terrazzo is the same as for marble.

TRAVERTINE

Travertine is a dense, closely compacted form of limestone found mostly in banded layers. It is formed from the **precipitation** of mineral springs, has holes in it because of escaping gas, and is a calcareous stone. When it is to be used as a floor, travertine is filled with a cement fill. Epoxy-filled travertine is available only on special order and is much more expensive than cement filled. Epoxy is subject to color change and strength loss (failure) when subjected to sunlight (ultraviolet rays).

The Sedimentaria line is a replica of a stone from a region of Tuscany called "Alta Maremma" (the region of Grosseto). It belongs to the same family as limestones, but has a very high percentage of ferrite that gives the stone its peculiar "cloudy" movements and creates the typical blossomy designs (also called loins—if you check the tiles you can find some of them). There are very few quarries of this stone so it is not widely exported.[26]

Maintenance

The maintenance of travertine is the same as for marble.

GRANITE

Granite is technically an igneous rock having crystals or grains of visible size. These grains are classified as fine, medium, or coarse.[27]

The *World Book Encyclopedia* states that "geologists conclude that most granite is formed by the slow cooling and crystallization of molten material called magma. This magma has the same chemical composition as granite."[28]

Granite consists of chiefly three minerals—quartz, alkali feldspar, and plagioclase feldspar, which make granite white, pink, and light gray. Granite also contains other minerals that account for buff, beige, red, blue, green, and black tones; however, within these colors, the variegations run from light to dark. The color gray, for example, may be light, medium, or dark, or vary between dark and purplish gray or dark and greenish gray. It is important to see an actual sample of the type of granite to be used.

The National Building Granite Quarries Association (NBGQA) recommends submitting duplicate 12″ × 12″ samples to show the full range of color, texture, and finish. The designer retains one set and the other is returned to the granite supplier for reference.

Granite is the latest material used for kitchen counters (see Chapter 9).

In addition to color, finish is important. The NBGQA has established the following definitions:

Polished: Mirror gloss, with sharp reflections.
Honed: Dull sheen, without reflections.
Fine rubbed: Smooth and free from scratches; no sheen.
Rubbed: Plane surface with occasional slight "trails" or scratches.
Shot ground: Plane surface with pronounced circular markings or trails having no regular pattern.
Thermal: Finish produced by application of high-temperature flame to the surface. Large surfaces may have shadow lines caused by overlapping of the torch.
Sand blasted, coarse stippled: Coarse plane surface produced by blasting with an abrasive; coarseness varies with type of preparatory finish and grain structure of the granite.
Sand blasted, fine stippled: Plane surface, slightly pebbled, with occasional slight trails or scratches.

As with other stones, polished granite should not be used for floors because the mirror gloss and color will eventually be dulled by the abrasion of feet. Where water may be present, flamed or thermal textures are used to create a nonslip surface.

The method of veneered construction used to make thinner and lighter-weight marble squares is also used with granite, and for the same reasons. When a feeling of permanence and stability is needed, granite is a good choice; therefore, granite is often used in banking institutions.

Installation

Honed granite is installed using the same methods as for marble. When more textured finishes are specified and when the granite has not been cut to a definite size, a mortar joint is used.

Maintenance

Granite floors, particularly those with rougher surfaces, require ordinary maintenance by means of a brush or vacuum cleaner. The more highly finished granite surfaces should be maintained in the same manner as marble.

FLAGSTONE

Flagstones were used on the floors in Tudor England (1485–1603). Flagstone is defined as thin slabs of stone used for paving walks, driveways, patios, etc. It is generally fine-grained **sandstone, bluestone, quartzite,** or slate, but thin slabs of other stones may be used. One-inch-thick bluestone flagging in a random multiple pattern compares favorably in price to premium vinyl tiles. Flagstones are siliceous and very durable because they are composed mainly of silica or quartzlike particles.

Flagstone may be irregularly shaped, the way it was when quarried, varying in size from 1 to 4 square feet, or the edges may be sawn to give a more formal appearance. Thickness may vary from 1/2 inch to 4 inches; therefore, the flagstone *must* be set in a thick mortar base to produce a level surface.

The extra thickness of the flagstone must be considered when positioning floor joists. One client had flagstones drawn and specified on her blueprints. The carpenter misread the plans, however, and assumed that it was to be a flagstone-patterned floor and not the real thing. The client arrived at the house one day to discover that the entryway did not have the lowered floor necessary to fit the extra thickness of the stone. The contractor had to cut all the floor joists for the hall area, lower them 4 inches, and then put in additional bracing and supports in the basement—a costly error.

Another point to remember with flagstones is that the surface is usually uneven because it comes from naturally cleaved rock; therefore, flagstones are not suitable for use under tables and chairs. In addition, an entrance hall of flagstones is very durable but the stone needs to be protected from grease, which can be absorbed into the stones.

The grout used in setting flagstones is a sand portland cement type and fills all areas where flagstones adjoin.

Maintenance

Flagstones are relatively easy to clean with mild acidic cleaning solutions. Sealing compounds are available that make flagstones **impervious** to any staining and wear. These compounds are available in gloss and matte finishes and protect the treated surface from the deteriorating effects of weathering, salts, acids, alkalis, oil, and grease. The gloss finish does seem to give an unnatural shiny appearance to the stone, but where the impervious quality rather than the aesthetic quality is important, these sealers may be used. Vacuuming will remove dust and siliceous material from the surface and a damp mop will remove any other soil from the sealed surface.

SLATE

Slate was also used as a flooring material in Tudor England (1585–1603). In 17th-century France, slate was combined with bands of wood. Slate is a very fine-grained metamorphic rock cleaved from sedimentary rock shale. One characteristic of slate is that this cleavage allows the rock to be split easily into thin slabs. The most common colors for slate range from gray to black, but green, brown, and red are also available. In areas of heavy traffic, honed black slate tends to show the natural scuffing of shoes, and the scratches give the black slate a slightly grayish appearance. All stones will eventually show this scuffing, and therefore highly polished stones should be avoided as a flooring material. Although slate used to come mainly from Vermont, most of the slate used in this country is now imported from India and China. The current trend seems to be the Chinese slate called China Lotus, a light greenish-brown stone with strong gold influences.

Different finishes are available in slate, as in other stones. The Structural Slate Company describes the following finishes:

Natural cleft: The natural split or cleaved face. This finish is moderately rough, with some textural variations. Thickness will have a plus or minus tolerance of 1/8 inches.
Sand rubbed: This finish has a slight grain or stipple in an even plane. No natural cleft texture remains. Finish is equivalent to **60-grit** and is obtained by wet sand on a rubbing bed.
Honed: This finish is equivalent to approximately **120-grit** in smoothness. It is semi-polished, without excessive sheen.[29]

The standard thickness of sawed flooring slate is 1/2 inch. Also available are 3/4-inch and 1-inch thicknesses, which are suitable for both interior and exterior use. One-half-inch slate weighs 7 1/2 pounds per square foot, 3/4-inch weighs 11 1/4 pounds, and 1-inch weighs 15 pounds. The absorption rate of slate is 0.23 percent. One-quarter-inch slate is used for interior foyers in homes and commercial buildings using the thin-set method. This thickness is an excellent remodeling item over wood or slab and gives a rug-level effect when it adjoins carpet. One-quarter-inch slate weighs only 3 3/4 pounds per square foot.

Installation

As can be seen from the preceding types, slate is available for both thin-set and thick-set applications. When thin-set mastic or adhesive is used, a 1/4″ × 1/4″ notched trowel held at a 45-degree angle is suggested.

Several points need to be remembered with both types of installations. If grout is used with slate (the spacing should be 3/8″ minimum), it is important that any excess be cleaned off immediately, because grout that has dried on the slate surface will probably never come off. If grout is not used, the slate tiles are butted against each other. Joint lines are staggered so no lines are more than 2 to 3 feet long in a straight line.

Thick-bed installation is similar to that for flagstones. All joints should be 3/8-inch-wide flush joints and should be **pointed** with 1:2 cement mix the same day the floor is laid to make the joints and setting bed **monolithic.**

Maintenance

The Structural Slate Company has the following information on its website:

> Although slate needs no sealer or other treatment, the joints are susceptible to minor cracks and separations. Use of a sealer/impregnator is useful in protecting water infiltration through these cracks into the setting bed. Sealers usually darken the slate and give a glossy appearance. Natural cleft finish and Sand Rubbed finish may be sealed suitably; however, sealers may not adhere nor give a desirable appearance to Machine gauged or Honed finish. . . .
> **Note:** Care should be taken in selecting a treatment that is slip resistant.[30]

CERAMIC TILE

Because ceramic tile was one of the most durable materials used by ancient civilizations, archaeologists have discovered that thin slabs of fired clay, decorated and glazed, originated in Egypt about 4700 B.C. Tile was, and currently is, used in Spanish architecture to such a degree that a Spanish expression for poverty is "to have a house without tiles." The Spanish also use decorative ceramic tiles on the **risers** of stairs. The Romans used fired clay pipes to carry water and sewage and used terra cotta to construct and decorate their public and private buildings.

In England, many abbeys had mosaic tile floors and the European cathedrals of the 12th century also had tile floors. In ancient times, tiles were used to make pictures on the walls, and these patterns were spread over many tiles. A good example is the bulls and dragons design in the Ishtar Gate from Babylon, which is now in the Pergamon Museum in Berlin. Later, each tile was decorated with intricate patterns, or four tiles were used to form a complete pattern. Eighteenth- and 19th-century tiles used a combination of these two design types.

Tiles were named after the city where they originated: Faience, with its striking opaque glazes, from Faenza in Italy; Majolica, with bright decorations, from Majorca, Spain; and Delft tiles, from the town of Delft in Holland. Delft tiles, with their blue and white designs, are known worldwide. Production tiles are made by two methods, dust press and extruded. Floor and wall tiles for interior use are produced by the dust-press method. The clay mixture is forced into steel dies under heavy pressure and is fired at very high temperatures to form a **bisque,** a tile ready to be glazed. These tiles are then sprayed with a surface glaze and fired at a lower temperature than before. This second firing fuses the glaze to the tile. The dust-press method produces distinct shapes and sizes. The second production method is an extruded or ram process in which the clay is mixed to form a thick mud and is then forced through a die. This process forms a slightly rougher-looking and larger tile, which is glazed in the same manner as the dust-process tiles. The temperature and proportions of the ingredients dictate the tile use: walls, floors, interior or exterior, and residential or commercial. Seneca Tiles, Inc. has a new line called Seneca Handmold®.

This line uses a special blend of local clays, wooden molds, and techniques developed hundreds of years ago. While soft, moldable clay, individually batched glazes, and natural oxides are the ingredients of the tiles, the "magic" that is Seneca Handmold is in the human hand. Skilled craftsmen vigorously beat handfuls of plastic clay into shallow wooden molds. Excess clay is then scraped from the top of the mold. A wooden drying board is placed over the mold; together they are carefully inverted; the mold is lifted, and a tile falls free. "Handmade". . . . This age-old process is completed by drying the tile, applying one of many glazes and, finally, firing under carefully controlled conditions.

Handmold Series 3-D creates a whole new dimension in tile installations. By using geometric shapes combined with high relief, you can add character that interacts with light and creates a natural three-dimensional depth to your installation.[31]

Water absorption tests can also be used as a good indicator to predict the stain resistance of unglazed tile. The lower the water absorption, the greater the stain resistance. (See Table 4.4.)

Porcelain tiles are inherently impervious and are used frequently in heavy-use commercial and retail areas. Porcelain tiles are made with ball clays, feldspar and kaolin. According to one tile manufacturer, its porcelain tiles are fired at a temperature that exceeds 2200°F, at which point they have a viscous liquid phase in which crystallization occurs. During the cooling stage, the materials fuse together and solidify again to gain strength and hardness. These tiles can be used in light colors that give an airy and spacious feeling to the installation. The

TABLE 4.4
Porosity Variances

Type	Water Absorption Rate
Impervious	0.5% or less
Vitreous	More than 0.5% but less than 3%
Semivitreous	More than 3% but less than 7%
Nonvitreous	More than 7%

color of the ceramic tile results from the addition of body stains, which consist of inert crystalline metals in oxides or salts. The breaking strength of porcelain tile is approximately three times stronger than that of a glazed tile. Additionally, the low absorption of porcelain tile yields a tile that is frost-proof, unlike a glazed product, which when exposed to freezing and thawing may have the glazing separate from the body of the tile.[32] (See Figure 4.9.)

Because of the low absorption rate of porcelain tiles, bond-promoting additives are added to the mortars and grouts.

Many types of finishes and patterns are available in ceramic tiles, ranging from a very shiny, highly reflective glaze to a dull matte finish and even an unglazed impervious tile. Tiles may be solid color or hand painted with designs.

The surface texture of the ceramic tile relates to the reflectance qualities. For example, a perfectly smooth tile will have a much higher reflectance rate than a rough-surface tile, although both tiles have identical glazes. Ceramic tiles are available in many different shapes and sizes. Instead of the traditional 4 1/4″ × 4 1/4″ tile, 8″, 12″, and even 18″ square tiles are widely used.

Highly glazed tiles are not recommended for floor use for two reasons: First, the surface can become extremely slippery when wet; second, some wearing and scratching can occur over time, depending on type of use. Of course, if moisture and wear are not a problem, then glazed tiles may be used.

ASTM C-1028-89 is the standard test method for determining the static coefficient of friction of ceramic tile and other like surfaces by the dynamometer pull meter method. Static coefficient of friction is a term used in physics to describe the amount of force required to cause an object (shoe sole material) to start moving across a surface (flooring material). A higher coefficient indicates increased resistance of shoe sole material to start moving across a flooring material. The ASTM procedure states that "the measurement made by this apparatus is believed to be one important factor relative to slip resistance. Other factors can affect slip resistance, such as the degree of wear on the shoe and flooring material; presence of foreign material, such as water, oil and dirt; the length of the human stride at the time of slip; type of floor finish, and the physical and mental condition of humans. Therefore, this test method should be used for the purpose of developing a property of the flooring surface under laboratory conditions, and should not be used to determine slip resistance under field conditions unless those conditions are fully described.

Although ANSI has not established a standard value for coefficient of friction, OSHA (Occupational Safety and Health Administration) has established a recognized industry of 0.5 (wet and dry) for slip-resistant surfaces. The Americans with Disabilities Act (ADA) recommends but does not require "a Static Coefficient of Friction of 0.60 for accessible routes and 0.80 for ramps." ADA does not specifically state that 0.60 is both a dry and a wet requirement.[33]

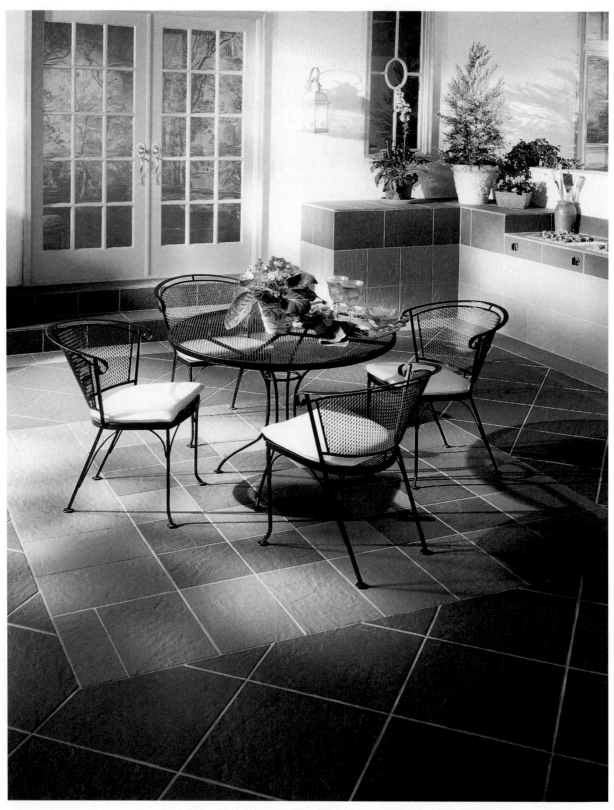

FIGURE 4.9
Made of porcelain stone for strength and durability, each color coordinates with at least two or three other colors, and all are designed to coordinate with Bentley Prince Street carpet. (Photo courtesy of Crossville Tile)

Stone/USA is a nonslip porcelain stone tile developed to reduce "slip and falls" in restaurants. Cross-Grip is part of Crossvile's Cross-Tech series, and comes in 8 × 8-inch formats.[34]

Most ceramic tile companies produce a raised-dome surface tile that can be detected under foot and by cane contact (which meets the guidelines set by the ADA). Its yellow color serves as a caution for platform and curb edges.

When ceramic or quarry tiles are used on a floor, the floor is usually finished with a **base** or combination trim tile having a **bullnose** at the top and a **cove** at the bottom in the same material as the floor tiles. If ceramic tiles are to be continued onto the wall surface, a cove base is used (see Figure 4.10).

Questech® Metals Floor Borders from Crossville come in bronze, copper, and nickel-silver. Borders are either 2 or 4 inches wide with tiles 4 inches square and a 2 × 2-inch border corner rosette. These tiles are installed in the same manner as ceramic tile. Questech Metals borders are ideal for trim, surrounds, feature walls, edging, and backsplashes. Walker Zanger also has a collection of handmade copper tiles.

CERAMIC MOSAIC TILE

According to *Compton's Interactive Encyclopedia™*,

> The earliest Greek patterned mosaics are made with small, naturally rounded pebbles set into fine cement. Early examples from the 8th century B.C. have been found at Fordion in Phrygia (Asia Minor). The technique may have been invented in Greece, where unpatterned pebble floors have been found to date from the Bronze Age. . . . In the Americas the Pueblo Indians of the Southwestern United States use turquoise to make mosaic plaques. Mexican mosaic made before Christopher Columbus includes examples of mosaic masks. There are references in surviving documents to architectural decoration in mosaic. Mosaic also reached a high level of excellence in ancient Peru . . . . By the 15th century mosaic was executed exclusively by craftsmen without the participation of the artist who supplied the design.[35]

Today, mosaic tile is used for intricate designs for floors, walls, and ceilings, copying the ancient art. Ceramic mosaic tile is usually formed by the dust-press method and is 1/4 to 3/8 inch thick, with a facial area of less than 6 square inches. Pigments and, if required, abrasives, are added to the porcelain or clay mixture, and therefore the color is dispersed throughout the tile. Ceramic mosaic tiles are fired in kilns with temperatures reaching 2150°F. Ceramic tile is impervious, stain proof, dent proof, and frost proof. Because of a mosaic tile's small size, the individual tiles are mounted on a sheet to simplify setting.

The Tile Council of North America, Inc. (TCNA) notes the following types of tile:

Mounted tile: Tile assembled into units or sheets by suitable material to facilitate handling and installation. . . . Tile may be back-mounted, edge-mounted, or face-mounted tile (refer to ANSI A137.1).

FIGURE 4.10
Crossville line drawings.

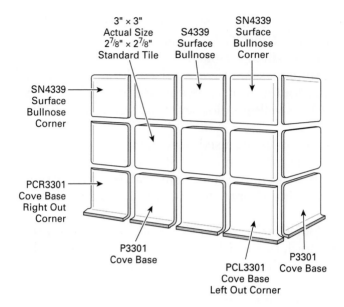

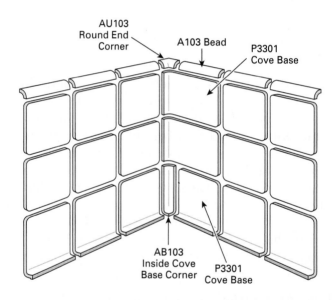

Back- and edge-mounted tile assemblies may have perforated paper, fiber mesh, resin, polyurethane, or other bonding material on the back or edges of each tile, which becomes an integral part of the tile installation.

Clear film-faced tile is assembled with clear plastic adhesive film on the face, which is removed after final set has occurred.

Paper-faced has paper applied to the face of the tile with water-soluble adhesives which should be removed during the installation process by wetting and removing the paper, followed by adjusting the tile prior to its final set.

Mounted tile assemblies shall have sufficient exposure to bonding surfaces of the tile body to allow for 80% coverage of the bond mortar in dry areas and 95% in wet areas.

Tile manufacturers must specify whether their assemblies are suitable for installation in swimming pools, on exteriors, and other wet areas. Paper back-mounted mosaics are not recommended in wet areas.[36]

A paver tile has the same composition and physical properties as a mosaic tile, but it is thicker and has a facial area of more than 6 square inches.

Installation

The Handbook for Ceramic Tile Installation is published by the TCNA each year. Table 4.2 comes from this publication. The designer can choose the correct tile installation for every type of floor use and specify a *Handbook* method number, grout, and setting method. The *Handbook* is also a guide in developing job specifications. As can be seen from Table 4.2, ceramic tile for floor use may be installed by both thick- and thin-set methods. When ordering any tile, 2 percent extra of each color and size should be added for the owner's use. This will allow immediate replacement of damaged tiles, and the color will match exactly.

OTHER TYPES OF TILE

Fiberoptic floors combine the beauty of a fine tile floor with the practical functionality of an embedded fiberoptic display. Logos, decorative patterns, text and other graphic images can be combined to achieve almost any desired effect. Images can range from simple to highly complex patterns.[37]

Conductive tile is made from a special body composition by adding carbon black or by methods resulting in specific properties of electrical conductivity while retaining other normal physical properties of a tile. Conductive tiles are used in hospital operating rooms, certain laboratories, or wherever the presence of oxygen and sparks from static electricity could cause an explosion. Conductive tiles should be installed using a conductive dry-set mortar with an epoxy grout.

Pregrouted tiles usually come in sheets of up to 2.14 square feet that have already been grouted with an elastomeric material such as silicone, urethane, or polyvinyl chloride (**PVC**) rubber, each of which is engineered for its intended use. The perimeter of these factory pregrouted sheets may include all or part of the grout between sheets, or no grout. Field-applied perimeter grouting should be of the same elastomeric materials used in the factory-pregrouted sheets or as recommended by the manufacturer. Pregrouted tiles save on labor costs because the only grouting necessary is between the sheets, rather than between individual tiles.

Slip-resistant tiles contain abrasive particles that are part of the tile. Other methods of slip-resistance may be achieved by grooves or patterns on the face of the tile.

Some tiles are self-spacing because they are molded with **lugs.** Other means of spacing are achieved by using plastic spacers to ensure alignment of tiles and an even grout area.

QUARRY TILE

A quarry tile is a strong, hard-body tile made from carefully graded shale and fine clays, with the color throughout the body. Depending on the geographic area where the clays are mined, the colors will vary from warm brown-red to warm beige. The face of a quarry tile may be solid colored, variegated with light and dark shades within the same tile, or flashed, in which the edges of the tile are a darker color than the center. A quarry tile is extruded in a 1/2-inch-thick ribbon and then cut to size. The qualities of the clays and temperatures at which they are fired (up to 2000°F) provide a variety of finished products. Quarry tiles are generally considered stain resistant but not stain proof. The rugged, unglazed surface of quarry tiles develops an attractive patina with wear. An abrasive grit surface is available for installations in which slip resistance is important. Most quarry tiles are manufactured unglazed to retain the natural quality of the tile, but some quarry tile is available glazed.

> Seneca Tile has chosen to resurrect the more traditional methods, providing handcrafted, intrinsically interesting tiles . . . tiles that express the warmth of the human hand. Instead of masking the natural variations of the tiles with highly refined ingredients made under laboratory-like conditions, the Seneca Tiles philosophy celebrates the inherent characteristics of naturally made tiles. It is this difference that inspires architects and designers to include Seneca Tile in some of their finest creations as well as in their own homes. . . . Their kilns, as big as houses, were made of brick and shaped like beehives. These early methods are used today by Seneca Tile to produce this series of natural paver tiles. . . . The practice of "flashing" these kilns creates a rich and varied coloration that cannot be duplicated in modern kilns. The unique "heart" shadings and natural ironspots are the result of soaking in this long, slow process.[38] (See Figure 4.11.)

Installation

Quarry tiles may be installed by either thick- or thin-set methods. The grout is either a sanded portland cement mix or an epoxy grout with a silica filler. It is the responsibility of the tile installer to remove all excess grout as part of the contract.

Maintenance

Ceramic or quarry tiles may be cleaned with a damp mop if the soil is light, or with water and a detergent if the soil is heavier. Tile and grout are two different materials, with grout being the more porous. Any soil that is likely to stain the grout should be removed as soon as possible.

MEXICAN OR SALTILLO TILE

In Mexican or saltillo tile, clay, taken directly from the ground, is shaped by hand into forms. Saltillo tile differs from ceramic and quarry tile in

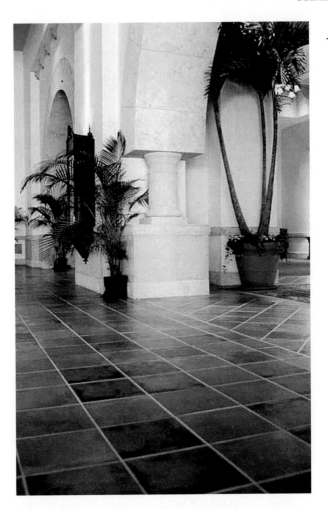

FIGURE 4.11
The lobby sets the ambience
of this restaurant. (Photo by
Ceramic Matrix, distributor
for Seneca Tiles, Inc.)

that the proportion of ingredients in the clay is not measured. The clay form is allowed to dry in the sun until it is firm enough to be transported to the kiln. Because Mexican tile is a product of families working together, it is common to find a child's handprint or a dog or cat paw imprinted in the surface of the tile. Leaf prints may also be noticed, in which a leaf drifted down when the tile was drying. These slight imperfections are part of the charm of using saltillo tile. Mexican tile is often named for the town in which it is made, thus the name *Saltillo*, the capital of Coahuila, Mexico. Today, Mexican factories are producing tiles of more consistent quality.

Because of the uneven thickness of Mexican tile, it should be installed using the thick-set method. If it is being used in a greenhouse or similar area where drainage is possible, Mexican tile may be laid in a bed of sand, which will adapt to any unevenness of the tile. All cracks or joints are then filled with sand.

Saltillo tile is extremely porous—the most porous of all tile—because of its natural qualities. If the tile is not sealed in the factory (and most are not), a "grout release" *must* be sponged, sprayed, or rolled on. Another method of preventing the grout from staining the tile is to use a sealer before grouting. It is recommended that one of the many new sealer/finish products, which allow the combination of linseed oil and wax into one process application, be used. Additional coats can be applied to provide a matte or gloss finish—the more coats applied, the higher the gloss will appear. The benefits are cost, labor, and an environmentally friendly finish.

Maintenance

A Mexican tile floor should be kept free of dust and dirt by sweeping or vacuuming, and when the floor shows signs of wear, another coat of wax or sealer/finish should be applied and buffed. Traffic areas may need to be frequently touched up with wax or sealer.

GLASS BLOCK

The glass block used for floors may be VISTABRIK® from Pittsburgh Corning. The blocks come in 6-, 8-, and 12-inch squares 3 inches thick, with either a clear or stippled finish. These units provide excellent light transmission and good visibility, with high-impact strength. These blocks may also be used as covers for light fixtures recessed in floors. Glass block material is also used where special lighting effects are required.

GLASS TILE

Crossville's new Water Crystal Mosaics, designed by Boyce & Bean, are made of cast, translucent glass that captures, reflects and refracts light like no other mosaics on the market. Providing a shimmering, ever-changing light show on floors, walls and countertops, Water Crystal Mosaics are available in nine water-inspired colors in three finishes: clear, frosted or iridescent. . . . Face-mounted on paper sheets of approximately 1 sq. ft in size, for quick and simple installation.[39] (See Chapter 10, Figure 10.3.)

Maintenance

Simple cleaning with clean water and a sponge or mop should suffice. Any oily deposits should be removed by using soap and water and then rinsing with clean water.

CONCRETE

Concrete is a mixture of two materials: **aggregates** and paste. The paste, comprised of portland cement and water, binds the aggregates (sand and gravel or crushed stone) into a rocklike mass as the paste hardens because of the chemical reaction of the cement and water.

According to the Portland Cement Association:

Aggregates are generally divided into two groups: fine and coarse. . . . Since aggregates make up about 60 percent to

75 percent of the concrete, their selection is important. Aggregates should consist of particles with adequate strength and resistance to exposure conditions. They should not contain materials that will cause deterioration of the concrete. . . . In properly made concrete, each particle of aggregate is completely coated with paste (portland cement and water), and all the space between aggregate particles is completely filled with paste.[40]

A good rule of thumb is as follows: the denser the better.

The following was condensed from information supplied by R. Godfrey Consulting, Forensic Floor Covering Specialists: Irrespective of what may be claimed or in print, *all* concrete will allow the passage of water vapor. Concrete will always absorb and evaporate moisture until it is restricted. The source may be one or more of the following: subterranean moisture, lateral moisture absorbed through the edges of the slab, internal moisture from a leaking pipe, or topical moisture caused by excessive application of adhesive/wet installation. Moisture indicators include color (darker is generally wetter), smell, effervescence (alkali and salts from concrete), and by touch (this is the worst way). Moisture will discolor most flooring materials. The following should be used as a guide for the basic evaluation of vapor emissions and associated problems:

1. *All* concrete is permeable.
2. One volume unit of water in a liquid form is capable of producing as much as 1,700 volume units of water in a vapor form.
3. Vapor emissions *can only be measured*, not calculated.
4. Water, whether it is in a liquid or vapor form, will *always* seek the path of least resistance.
5. Irrigation or landscaping surrounding irrigation can contribute to vapor emission conditions.

A concrete floor is low in cost as compared with other materials and is very durable. Maintenance for interiors is difficult, however, unless the surface has been treated with a floor sealer specially manufactured to produce a dust-free floor. Color may be added when the concrete is mixed, or it may be dusted on the surface during the finishing operation. A concrete floor looks less like an unfinished floor or substrate if it is stamped and/or colored into squares. In addition, any cracking is more likely to occur in these stamped grooves and be less visible. Several pattern products are available to mark the surface of the **plastic** concrete, so that it imitates the shapes and patterns of brick or natural stone.

Dark-colored concrete floors are used in passive solar homes because the large mass absorbs the rays of the sun during the day and radiates the heat back at night.

Concrete floors may be painted with an epoxy, polyurethane, or acrylic paint. Generally, epoxy paints are the best for adhesion.

A custom aggregate mix can be made from Syndecrete, a precast lightweight concrete. For a description of Syndecrete, see Chapter 1.

Maintenance

Because cured concrete can sometimes absorb harmful chemicals, prewetting must be done before using any cleaning solution. Synthetic detergent should be used because soap will react with the lime and cause a scum.

EXPOSED AGGREGATE

When an exposed aggregate floor is specified, the type of aggregate used is extremely important because it is visible on the finished floor. River stone gives a smooth, rounded texture. Today, the river stone effect may be achieved by tumbling stones in a drum to remove sharp edges.

Installation

While the concrete is still plastic, the selected aggregate is pressed or rolled into the surface. Removal of the cement paste by means of water from a hose when the concrete is partially hardened will expose the aggregate and display the decorative surface. For interior use, most of the aggregate should be approximately the same size and color, but other values within that hue may also be used, with a scattering of white and black stones.

One drawback to the use of exposed aggregate is that, like any other hard-surfaced material, exposed aggregate is not sound absorbent and is hard on the feet during prolonged standing. A clear polyurethane finish specially formulated for masonry surfaces can be applied. This finish brings out the natural color of the stone—similar to the way a wet stone has more color than a dry one. Coated exposed aggregate seldom seems to become soiled. A vacuum brush used for wood floors will pick up any loose dirt from between the stones.

BRICK

Prehistoric men made brick from dried mud, but they soon discovered that when mixed with straw, the shaped brick could withstand the elements. Kiln-burned brick made by the Babylonians 6,000 years ago still exists. Sun-dried brick, or **adobe,** dates from around 5000 B.C. and is still used in some areas of the southwestern United States, but with some modern-day materials added. Fired bricks and kilns first appeared between 2500 and 2000 B.C. in Mesopotamia and India, but the art was lost around 1700 B.C. and fired brick was not used again until 300 B.C.

The earliest recorded use of brick is in the Bible: The Egyptians made the Israelites work "in mortar and in brick" (Exodus 1:14). There was a limitless supply of clay from the bed of the Nile River. Sun-baked brick was used in the Tower of Babel and in the wall surrounding the city of Babylon.

The Chinese used brick in the 3rd century B.C. for building part of the Great Wall. The Romans used sun-dried bricks until about A.D. 14, when they started using bricks burnt in kilns. The Romans took this knowledge of brick making to Europe and Britain, but after they left in A.D. 410, the art died out and was not restored until the 11th and 13th centuries. The first brick buildings in the United States were built in Jamestown, Virginia, by British settlers, and on Manhattan Island by the Dutch. Bricks used in Virginia were probably made locally because there are records of brick being exported in 1621. Of course, the Aztecs of Mexico and Central America also used adobe bricks for building purposes.

Until about the mid-1850s, brick was molded by hand, but from then on it was made using mechanical means. Bricks are made by mixing clays and shales with water and are formed, while plastic, into rectangular shapes with either solid or hollow cores.

During the process of heating the bricks, the clay loses its water content and becomes rigid but it is not chemically changed. During the higher temperatures used in burning, the brick undergoes a molecular change: The grains fuse, closing all pores, and the brick becomes vitrified or impervious.

The color of brick depends on three factors: chemical composition of the clay, method of firing control, and temperature of the kiln. A red color comes from the oxidation of iron to form iron oxide. Lighter colors (the salmon colors) are the result of underburning. The higher the temperature, the harder the brick. Harder bricks have lower absorption potential and higher compressive strength than softer ones. Generally, the denser the brick and the lower the absorption, the easier it is to clean and maintain. Flooring brick, used in such places as factories, where floors receive heavy use, is hard and dense.

Installation

For areas in which spilled liquids are likely, such as in a kitchen or bathroom, a mortared installation is appropriate. When installing over a wood-frame floor, a thin brick paver may be selected to reduce the additional dead weight of the floor assembly. Brick pavers weigh approximately 10 pounds per square foot (psf) per inch of thickness. Installation methods are shown in Figure 4.12. Pavers are laid in a conventional manner in a 1/2-inch wet mortar bed with mortar joints. When the joints are thumbprint hard, they are **tooled,** compacting the mortar into a tight, water-resistant joint. Where moisture is not a problem, a mortarless method may be used. Patterns used should be interlocking to ensure a secure floor.

Maintenance

Brick may be vacuumed, swept, damp mopped, or spray buffed.

LINOLEUM

Linoleum is derived from two Latin words: *Linum*, "linen," and *Oleum*, "oil." Linoleum was invented in 1860 by English rubber manufacturer Sir Frederick Walton. Linoleum is extremely durable, resistant to acid, grease, oil, solvents, and cigarette burns. It is only sensitive to alkaline solutions that dissolve the linseed oil and dry out the material.

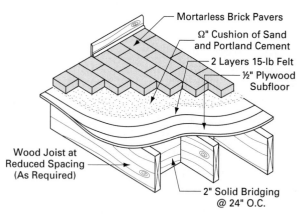

Mortarless Brick Pavers
Ω" Cushion of Sand and Portland Cement
2 Layers 15-lb Felt
½" Plywood Subfloor
Wood Joist at Reduced Spacing (As Required)
2" Solid Bridging @ 24" O.C.

Brick Paving Over Wood Joists

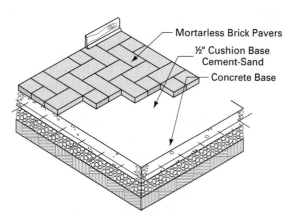

Mortarless Brick Pavers
½" Cushion Base Cement-Sand
Concrete Base

Brick Paving Over Concrete Slab

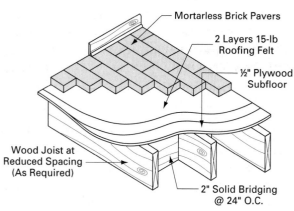

Mortarless Brick Pavers
2 Layers 15-lb Roofing Felt
½" Plywood Subfloor
Wood Joist at Reduced Spacing (As Required)
2" Solid Bridging @ 24" O.C.

Brick Paving Over Wood Joists

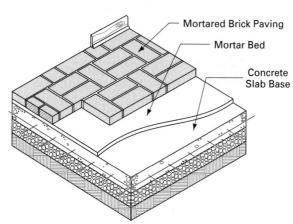

Mortared Brick Paving
Mortar Bed
Concrete Slab Base

Brick Paving Over Concrete Slab

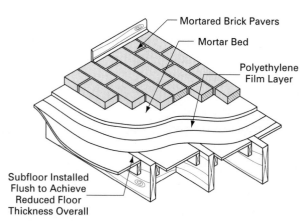

Mortared Brick Pavers
Mortar Bed
Polyethylene Film Layer
Subfloor Installed Flush to Achieve Reduced Floor Thickness Overall

Brick Paving Over Wood Joists

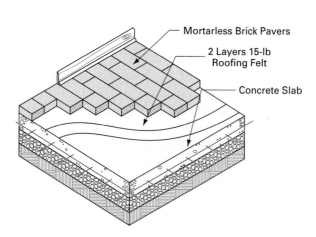

Mortarless Brick Pavers
2 Layers 15-lb Roofing Felt
Concrete Slab

Brick Paving Over Concrete Slab

FIGURE 4.12
Methods of installing brick.

Linoleum has been a mainstay floor covering for over 100 years because it is one of the few products made from primarily natural raw materials. It is made up of linseed oil, rosins, and wood flour, calendered into a natural jute backing (backing for tile is polyester). It is a tough yet visually striking floor covering, highly resistant to heavy rolling loads and foot traffic. Because linoleum is a natural organic product, its performance is enhanced by time, as exposure to air serves to harden and increase its durability. Although linoleum continues to harden over time, the floor remains quiet and comfortable under foot.[41]

Another ingredient in linoleum is wood powder, which is salvaged from sawdust. Forbo imports linoleum, Marmoleum®, from Europe (Scotland and Holland) for the environmentally conscious user. The manufacture of linoleum requires less energy than the manufacture of most popular floor coverings. Beneficial bactericidal properties halt the spreading of many microorganisms, and the natural static resistance provides a safe environment for data-processing facilities. There are no harmful VOC emissions, and natural antistatic properties repel dust and dirt. Because linoleum is made from natural materials, it is biodegradable. Forbo recycles 100 percent of its postproduction waste. Marmoleum Dual-13 (DIY), in this case standing for "design-it-yourself," is now available and should be of interest to interior designers. The solid-color tiles are 13 × 13 inches and borders are 4 3/8″ × 39 3/8″ long with corners 4 3/8″ square. These borders and corners are made to order, with the designs having from two to six colors.

Forbo has just introduced Marmoleum Global 2 with Topshield™, which consists of a durable primer and top layer to resist scuffing and dirt. This top coat can be renovated.

Installation

One hundred percent solvent-free adhesive is used to install linoleum. Seams for linoleum sheet, vinyl sheet, and specialty sheet floors are sealed by means of weld rods. Each material has its own type of weld rods. Heat-welding blocks the penetration of dirt and moisture.

Maintenance

Forbo Industries recommends the following maintenance procedures: "For initial cleanup and daily maintenance remove all surface soil, debris, sand, and grit by sweeping or dust mopping. Damp mop with a neutral pH detergent, such as Butcher Sundance®, TASKI R-50, Johnson Stride™, or an equivalent. . . . For a matte-satin shine, apply one or two thin coats of floor finish such as TASKI Ombra or equivalent, or for a high-gloss shine apply two or three thin coats of floor finish such as Butcher Mainstay®, TASKI Brilliant, or an equivalent." These finishes are applied with a clean-finish mop or finish applicator, with 30 minutes dry time between each coat. For further maintenance instructions, see *Linoleum Maintenance* from Forbo Industries.

ASPHALT TILE

Dark-colored asphalt flooring was developed in the United States in the 1920s. Like linoleum, however, asphalt tile is a flooring material that has been gradually phased out because of advanced technology. Asphalt tile was very inexpensive, but it was not resistant to stains and could be softened by mineral oils or animal fats. The individual tiles were brittle and had poor recovery from indentation. Asphalt tile may still be found in some older homes.

VINYL COMPOSITION

Vinyl composition tile (VCT) is a commonly used floor tile for less expensive installations. VCT is composed of binder (organic), fillers (inorganic), and pigments. The organic binder portion contains vinyl resins; plasticizer; additives; and in the case of Mannington, 5 percent or greater recycled vinyl content. Armstrong vinyl composition tile is composed of 85 percent limestone filler, which is a common material available in great supply. Color and pattern are commonly distributed evenly throughout the thickness of the tile. The mixture is formed into thin sheets under heat and pressure and is then cut into 12″ × 12″ tiles with a **gauge** of 3/32 inch or 1/8 inch. Inspirations™ and Essentials® are vinyl composition tiles from Mannington Commercial (see Chapter 1).

> Brand new from Mannington, SafeWalks™ is an attractive, slip retardant vinyl composition tile that is recommended for areas where slip/fall is a concern. SafeWalks meets the requirements of the Americans with Disabilities Act for static coefficient of friction as manufactured.[42]

Patterns in VCT may include a simulated brick paver, ceramic tile, and wood parquet. Accent strips are typically solid colors.

Vinyl composition tiles were once made with asbestos. In recent years, however, asbestos has been proven to have adverse health effects, so VCTs are no longer made with asbestos fibers. Therefore, there are no health hazards now associated with VCTs. **Note:** The Occupational Safety and Health Administration has provided rigid rules for safely removing old vinyl asbestos floors.

The thickness, or gauge, as it is sometimes called, of VCTs is 3/32 inch, or 1/8 inch. For commercial and better residential installations, the 1/8-inch gauge should be used.

The advantages of vinyl composition tile are that it (1) is inexpensive, (2) is easy to install and maintain, (3) may be installed on any grade, (4) resists acids and alkalis, and (5) withstands strong cleaning compounds. The disadvantages are that it (1) has low impact resistance, (2) has poor noise absorption, and (3) is semiporous as compared with solid vinyls and solid rubber. Armstrong has added new colors to its Standard EXCELON® Imperial Texture & MultiColor, including blue dreams, animal crackers, mint masquerade, and bubblegum.

Installation

Vinyl composition, vinyl, and some other tiles are all installed using the thin-set method. The most important step in this installation procedure is to be sure the substrate is smooth and level. With thinner tile, any discrepancies in the substrate will be visible on the surface of the tile. In a residential installation of thinner tile, a newly installed floor developed a wavy and bumpy appearance after only several weeks, because the wood substrate had not been sanded.

Materials and the installation site should be at a minimum temperature of 65°F for 48 hours before, during, and after installation. The substrate is troweled with the manufacturer's suggested adhesive and, as with the installation of parquet floors, the walls should not be used as a starting point.

Maintenance

Mannington Commercial suggests the following maintenance procedures for a VCT tile:

Initial Maintenance

Do not wash or scrub the floor for at least 4–5 days. Keep heavy furniture and equipment off the floor for 48 hours.

Apply multiple (3–5) coats of a high-quality cross-linked acrylic floor finish to the thoroughly clean, dry floor to protect the surface.

Regular Care and Maintenance
(after initial cleaning and polishing)

Clean frequently with a treated dust mop or clean, soft push broom.

Remove stains and spills promptly. Damp mop as needed with a dilute, neutral detergent solution. In heavily soiled areas, scrub lightly with an automatic floor machine.

Rinse the floor with clean water and allow to dry completely. Restrict traffic when cleaning to prevent slipping.

Spray buff or perform high-speed burnishing to protect the surface and restore gloss.[43]

Many of the same maintenance procedures may apply for commercial installations of other types of vinyl floors. See the manufacturer's specifications.

SOLID VINYL

Solid vinyl tile is really not all vinyl. It has a lower percentage of fillers and a higher percentage of PVC than vinyl composition tiles. It usually consists of a fiberglass-reinforced backing on which the pattern is printed. The final coat may be either clear vinyl or vinyl with urethane. The latter is tougher and wears longer. Sizes are 12 inch, 18 inch, and 24 inches square.

Maintenance

Maintenance is the same as for vinyl composition tile.

PURE VINYL TILE

Pure vinyl tiles are homogeneous or, in other words, pure vinyl with few, if any, fillers, with the color throughout the tile. Vinyl tiles have a higher resistance to abrasive wear than VCT. They are available in faux-stone finishes, marble, travertine, brick, and slate. Pure vinyl tiles are also used as feature strips or for borders. Borders should be of approximately the same width at all walls. Mannington Assurance™ II is a slip-retardant sheet vinyl, also available in modular form. A conductive tile is required in environments where static electricity poses a danger to sensitive electronic devices, and in areas where flammable gases or explosives may be present. If high voltages are used in the working environment, then a static dissipative vinyl tile should be used. A vinyl wall base effectively trims off a floor installation and helps hide minor wall and floor irregularities. Its distinctive profile consists of a reclining curvature at the top and a descending thin-toe line that conforms snugly with the wall and floor. Some vinyl cove bases can be hand-formed to make the corners, whereas others come with both inside and outside corners preformed. The cove wall base comes either in 20-foot rolls or 48-inch strips in 2 1/4-inch or 4-inch heights.

Installation

Pure vinyl tiles are installed with a specified adhesive and are laid in a pyramid shape as seen in Figure 4.8.

Maintenance

A new vinyl tile floor should not be washed, only damp mopped for a week to allow the adhesive to set. Spots of adhesive can be removed with a clean white cloth dampened with paste wax or lighter fluid. Periodically sweeping with a soft broom or vacuum will prevent the buildup of dust and dirt. Spills should be cleaned immediately. Damp mopping with a mild detergent is sufficient for slightly soiled floors, or scrubbing with a brush or machine for heavy soil. Soap-based cleaners should not be used because they can leave a dulling film. The floor should be rinsed with clean water after cleaning. The floor should never be flooded, and excess dirty water should be removed with a mop or wet vacuum. No-wax floors can be damaged by intense heat, lighted cigarettes, and rubber or foam-backed mats or rugs. If stubborn stains persist, they should be rubbed with alcohol or lighter fluid.

RUBBER

Rubber flooring is now made of 100 percent synthetic rubber. Rolls of rubber flooring are 4 feet wide and rubber tiles are 9-, 12-, 18-, 20-, 36-, and 39-inch squares, depending on manufacturer. Thickness varies from 3/32 to 3/16 inch. The tiles are usually marble or travertine patterned and are laid at right angles to each other. They may be laid below grade and are extremely sound absorbent. Stair treads are being made of rubber to comply with the California building code, which calls for a clearly contrasting color on the stair tread in public buildings.

Although available with a smooth surface, multilevel rubber flooring (raised discs or pastilles, solid or dual-colored squares, or even rhythmic curves) has become increasingly popular where excessive dirt or excessive moisture is likely to be tracked inside. Raised portions have beveled edges, causing the dirt to drop down below the surface, which reduces abrasion on the wear surface. The same thing happens with water; most of it flows below the wear surface. Although the original purpose of this type of rubber tile was to reduce wear from moisture or dirt, rubber floors are now used to meet the minimum requirements of the American with Disabilities Act (ADA). Rubber flooring is considered an ideal product for public areas because it offers excellent traction.

Johnsonite® produces Tactile Warning Surface to address accessibility requirements where detectable warnings on walking surfaces are specified. Manufactured in strips, it is designed to extend across the full width of the hazardous area for a continuous depth of 3 feet. This product has an undulated surface to alert individuals to potentially dangerous areas, such as the top of open stairwells, in front of doors leading to loading platforms, and on theatrical stages and other similar areas. Tactile Warning Surface meets all relevant ANSI requirements. Several other manufacturers have similar warning surfaces for the visually impaired.

Many large office buildings have no source of daylight in stairwells or hallways. When an emergency evacuation of the building is necessary, many times the electricity is not working and exit signs and stairwells are in the dark. As a result of the first World Trade Building bombing, Johnsonite® pioneered the SAFE-T-FIRST™ System, which integrates color with Permalight® self-illuminating technology in vinyl or rubber flooring products and accessories, such as exit signs and directional arrows. Johnsonite has received many awards for this extensive product offering, which includes rubber cove base, vinyl handrail tape, and even disc inserts for raised-disc flooring. (See Figure 4.13.) The SAFE-T-FIRST System has won many design awards.

Roppe uses Alpha Base™, which combines a wall base with an innovative "signage" capacity, and uses such wording as "In Case of Fire Use Stairs," "Fire Exit," etc. In case of fire, the first thing building occupants are often instructed to do is to "get close to the floor" in order to avoid dangerous, impeding smoke. When this happens, standard signs are often invisible. It is ideal for schools, hospitals, dormitories, public buildings—anywhere you need to show exits and escape routes.

The two products just described may have saved many lives in the attacks on the World Trade Center and the Pentagon. The author heard one story from the Pentagon attack in which 12 people held hands and crawled along the floor, and they were all saved.

> SafeTcork Slip-Resistant Tile & Tread, from Roppe, is a special rubber compound formulated for toughness and added traction where there is a threat of moisture on the walking surface. Roppe can add any of the following to the rubber tile, antifungal, flame-retardant and oil/grease resistant.[44]

Dodge-Regupol has several ECO® surfaces made from a combination of recycled tire rubber and postindustrial colored rubber, with the durability of the original tire rubber and resilience and comfort of carpeting.

FIGURE 4.13
The Safe-T-First System from Johnsonite has won many design awards. It is visible in light and sudden darkness, as can be seen in these two photographs. (Photos courtesy of Johnsonite)

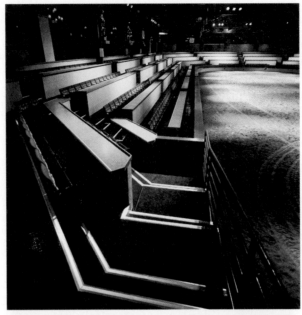

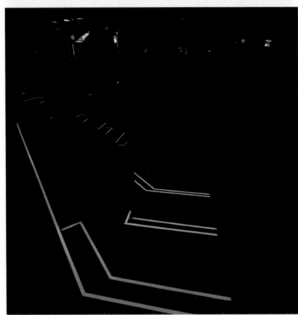

Maintenance

Proper maintenance is essential to the appearance and wear life of rubber tiles. The tile should be swept and mopped daily with a neutral pH detergent.

New rubber floor should not be cleaned for a minimum period of 72 hours after installation to ensure proper adhesive curing. Stripping of a new rubber floor may not be required unless the end user intends to apply an acrylic floor finish. If buffing is the user-preferred method of maintenance, stripping will remove the internal waxes that continuously bloom to the surface of the tile. Typically, a wax containing detergent is used to clean the tile for a period of 90 days to allow the waxes to uniformly bloom prior to routine buffing of the tile. The equipment used to buff rubber floor tiles should never exceed 350 rpm.

SHEET VINYL

Sheet vinyl manufacturers have greatly improved not only the quality but also the designs of their products. Precise information regarding construction is a trade secret, but the following information is generic to the industry.

Sheet vinyl comes in widths of 6 feet, 6 feet 6 inches, 9 feet, and 12 feet and is manufactured by two methods—inlaid or rotogravure. Most inlaid sheet vinyls are made of thousands of tiny vinyl granules built up layer by layer, and then fused with heat and pressure. The result is a resilient, hefty flooring with a noticeable depth of color and a crafted look. Some sheet vinyls have extra layers of foam cushioning to provide comfort underfoot and muffle footsteps and other noises. Color chips are distributed throughout the depth of the wear surface. A fibrous backing will produce a light, flexible flooring that virtually eliminates tearing and creasing and the telegraphing of irregularities from the old flooring to the new.

Armstrong defines the three categories of vinyl sheet flooring:

Heterogeneous—A layered structure with beautiful designs protected by a high-performance, easy-to-maintain wear layer. A flexible floor that is easy to install.

Homogeneous—Floor surfacing in sheet form that is of uniform structure and composition throughout, usually consisting of vinyl plastic resins, plasticizers, fillers, pigments, and stabilizers (sometimes called unbacked vinyl sheet flooring). The flooring meets requirements of ASTM F 1913, Standard Specification for Sheet Vinyl Floor Covering without Backing.

Inlaid Sheet Flooring—Floor surfacing material in which the decorative pattern or design is formed by color areas set into the surface. The design may or may not extend through to a backing.[45] (See Figure 4.14.)

Rotovinyls are made by a rotogravure process that combines photography and printing. Almost anything that can be photographed can be reproduced on a rotovinyl floor. The printed layer is protected by a topping (called the wear layer) of vinyl resin (PVC) either alone or in combination with urethane. Vinyl resin composition often produces a gloss surface, whereas urethane creates a high-sheen result. A mechanical buffer with a lambswool pad will bring back the satin gloss of the vinyl resin composition wear layers. Urethane wearlayer flooring should not be buffed. All rotovinyls are made with an inner core of foamed or expanded vinyl, which means they are cushioned to some extent. At the lower end of the price scale, cushioning may be thin. Most sheet vinyls are flexible enough to be coved up the **toe space** to form their own base (check manufacturer's specifications).

The wear layer is the final, protective topcoat on sheet vinyl or vinyl tile flooring products. Usually consisting of clear vinyl or urethane, wear layers enable the flooring to resist scuffs, stains, and other evidence of wear. The thicker the wear layer, the better the protection

FIGURE 4.14
The waiting room of a health facility has a four-color design that leads the eye to the desk. (Photo courtesy of Armstrong World Industries)

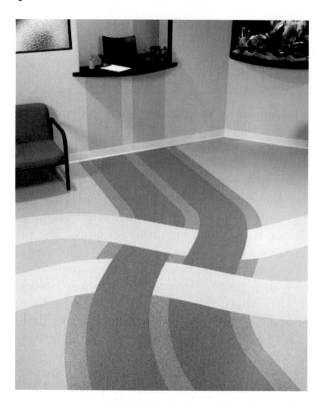

FIGURE 4.14
The waiting room of a health facility has a four-color design that leads the eye to the desk. (Photo courtesy of Armstrong World Industries)

against the effects of foot traffic, dirt, and overall daily use. Generally, for residential rotogravure products, those with the thickest wear layers often have long-term warranties. There is a definite distinction, however, between residential and commercial flooring. Product characteristics, maintenance, and warranties vary considerably.

For residential installations, high-gloss finishes are still available, but the trend seems to be patterns that copy natural materials, such as stone, wood, marble, and slate. The warranties, ranging from 5 to 11 years and more, cover manufacturing defects and wear.

Multilevel embossed sheet vinyl flooring has become increasingly popular where excessive dirt or excessive moisture is likely to be tracked inside. Lonseal® has many different configurations including large or small raised discs, squares, cobblestone effect, and even a deeply grooved "sound wave" pattern. Raised portions have beveled edges, causing the dirt to drop down below the wear surface, which reduces the abrasion on the wear surface. The same thing happens with water; most of it flows below the wear surface and makes the floor more slip resistant. For a transitional flooring between indoors and outdoors, Londeck® can be heat-welded to achieve a watertight, weatherproof surface. All Lonseal floors exceed requirements of the Americans with Disabilities Act (ADA).

Tarkett Inc. offers 12-feet-wide sheet vinyl flooring, featuring a wearlayer with silicone, for seamless installation in most residential rooms. All manufacturers make a polish that will renew the shine. Some even recommend wax (again, follow the manufacturer's directions).

Armstrong produces Clean Sweep® which is a new, patented, stain-resistant surface engineered to keep the floor looking like new without waxing.

Mannington Commercial BioSpec™ homogeneous sheet vinyl was developed specifically for health-care and clean room environments, where added protection against germs and moisture penetration is important. BioSpec features superior stain and chemical resistance and a rugged 80-mil wear layer for durability and resistance against indentations and rolling-load damage. Six of the patterns feature low-contrast colors, which makes it easier to see materials dropped on the floor and facilitates faster cleanup, especially in operating rooms. These six colors were developed with the input of health-care designers and hospital staff, who requested warm, neutral colors to help reduce eye fatigue during long surgical procedures. BioSpec is also ideally suited for heavy-traffic areas such as classrooms and auditoriums, and it meets the ADA specification for static coefficient of friction. Armstrong manufactures Step Master®, a slip-resistant floor covering.

Installation

Seaming methods vary from manufacturer to manufacturer, depending on the product and its application. Installation may be a perimeter-bond system stretched over the floor and secured only at the edges. The other option—a full-adhered system—is set in a full bed of mastic. The correct trowel notch size is important with resilient floors. The latter type should be rolled with a weighted roller to eliminate air pockets and form a good bond between the backing and the adhesive. Installing new flooring over an existing floor is preferable to removal, particularly if it is known that the existing floor contains asbestos. As noted in Chapter 1 and previously in the vinyl asbestos section of this chapter, removal of old floor coverings or adhesives that might contain asbestos requires, in some states, a trained asbestos abatement contractor, whether or not the asbestos is friable.

The old floor must be fully adhered. A perimeter-bonded system must not be covered. When covering a textured or embossed surface, a manufacturer-recommended embossing leveler must be used. Asphalt tiles or asphalt adhesive must not be covered, because asphalt eats through vinyl. Furniture should be equipped with the proper load-bearing devices; otherwise, indentations will mar the vinyl surface. Static load limitations vary for each product. Refer to each manufacturer's information. (See Figure 4.15.)

Heavy refrigerators and kitchen or office equipment should not be dragged across the floor, because this will damage and tear the surface. These items should be "walked" across the floor on a piece of wood or on Masonite® runways. Runways must be used even if using an appliance dolly or if the heavy objects are equipped with wheels or rollers.

Discoloration has been a problem with some light-colored resilient floors. There are several ways the vinyl flooring may discolor. Bottom-up discoloration may result from the following conditions: Use of the wrong adhesives can cause discoloration. Follow the manufacturer's recommendations, and use the appropriate adhesives. These are specially formulated for that particular product. Failure to remove existing adhesives or staining agents may discolor the vinyl surface.

TYPE OF LOAD	KENTILE FLOORS INC. RECOMMENDS	KENTILE FLOORS INC. DOES NOT RECOMMEND	TYPE
HEAVY FURNITURE, more or less permanently located, should have composition furniture cups under the legs to prevent them from cutting the floor.	Right 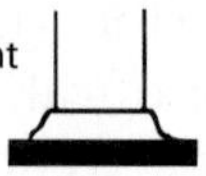 Wide Bearing Surfaces Save Floors	Wrong 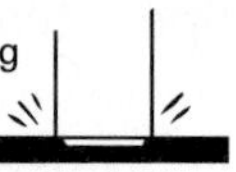 Small Bearing Surfaces Dent Floors	Composition Furniture Cups 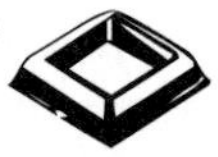
FREQUENTLY MOVED FURNITURE requires casters. Desk chairs are a good example. Casters should be 2" in diameter with soft rubber treads at least ¾" wide and with easy swiveling ball bearing action. For heavier items that must be moved frequently, consult the caster manufacturers as to the suitable size of equipment that should be used.	Right 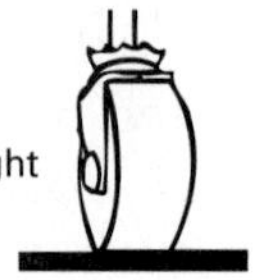 Rubber Rollers Save Floors	Wrong 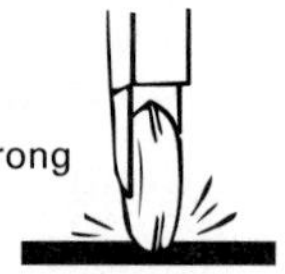 Hard Rollers Mark Floors	Rubber Wheel Casters 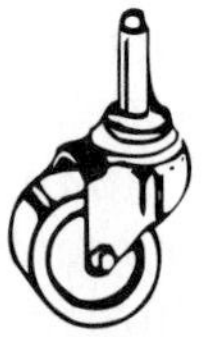
LIGHT FURNITURE should be equipped with glides having a smooth, flat base with rounded edges and a flexible pin to maintain flat contact with the floor. They should be from 1¼" to 1½" dia., depending upon weight of load they must carry. For furniture with slanted legs apply glides parallel to the floor rather than slanted ends of legs.	Right 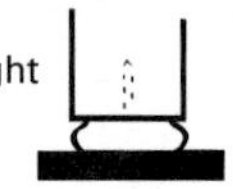 Use Flat Bearing Surfaces	Wrong 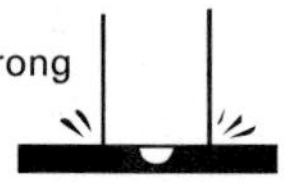 Remove Small Metal Domes	Flat Glides With Flexible Shank 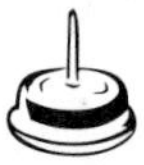

FIGURE 4.15
Static load.

Sometimes gypsum products, when combined with the slightest amount of moisture, can create an environment for fungus growth, causing discoloration. To eliminate this problem, use only portland-cement-based patching compounds for *all* underfloor patching needs. A synthetic polyurethane patch sometimes used for filling voids on the surface of wood panels will also cause discoloration in the shape of the patch. This problem can also be avoided by using an underlayment grade of plywood.

If there are dark pieces of wood or bark in wafer board and oriented strand board (OSB), they will cause staining. The use of construction adhesives to cement underlayments of substrates is another major cause of discoloration. Rubber-backed mats may cause staining, and coco fiber mats may cause scratches.

Maintenance

Remember that no-wax does not mean *no maintenance*. Congoleum has the following information on resilient sheet flooring, which is probably generic to most similar types of flooring:

Protect and do not disturb the sealed seams for at least 16 hours after seam sealer application to ensure a proper seam bond. Permanent damage may result if seam sealer is stepped on or disturbed before it is dry.

Keep traffic to a minimum during the first 48 hours on all resilient sheet and tile floors to allow the adhesive to harden.

Furniture should not be placed on the floor until the adhesive has had adequate time to dry (at least 24 hours).[46]

CORK

Cork is the name given to the bark of the cork oak, a tree from the beech family, characteristic of western Mediterranean countries. The bark acts as a protective shell to the harsh climate changes and numerous fires affecting the region. Cork trees are stripped of their bark every 9 to 14 years; the tree is never cut and the habitat remains undisturbed. The properties of cork are derived naturally from the structure and chemical composition of the inner cells. Each cubic centimeter of cork's honeycomb structure contains between 30 to 50 million cells.

Hence, cork provides:

Insulation. Because 90% of the tissue consists of gaseous matter, the density of cork is extremely low, giving the material wonderful insulating properties, thermal as well as acoustical.

Resiliency. When cork is subjected to pressure, the gas in the cells is compressed and volume reduces considerably. When released from pressure, cork recovers very rapidly to its original shape.

Impermeability. The presence of Suberin, an inherent waxy substance, renders cork impervious to both liquid and gases. As a result, it does not rot and may therefore be considered the best seal available.

Hypoallergenic. Cork does not absorb dust and consequently does not cause allergies.

Durability. Cork is remarkably resistant to wear, as it is less affected by impact and friction than other hard surfaces because of its cellular composition. [Author's note: A church in Chicago had cork installed in its entire area in 1890 and is still in use.]

Fire Retardant. A natural fire retardant, cork does not spread flames and does not release toxic gases during combustion.

Cork waste from the stopper industry (wine corks) and low-quality bark is used to produce cork granules. These are classified according to density and grain size.

Flooring tiles are produced from cork granules bound with resins and molded to obtain the desired density under pressure and heat. Cork wear layers can be waxed, varnished, urethane or acrylic coated.

This past decade the floating floor technology has been successfully adapted to cork flooring to produce one of the highest-quality floor coverings.[47]

Cork today can be found in many products and applications, from the wine bottle stopper to the insulation panels of the NASA space shuttle. Frank Lloyd Wright, in 1937, used cork as a decorative durable flooring material in his renowned Falling Waters house in Pennsylvania, and he was one of the first American architects to do so.

Natural CORK™ has prefinished parquet tile suited for installation over smooth and level underlayment-grade plywood, and above-grade and on-grade concrete. Natural Cork Floating Floor™ is 1-foot by 3-foot interlocking planks that are supplied with their own underlayment. They fit together to make a floor that floats on the slab. Humidity should be controlled (between 50 and 70 percent) because cork is a natural material and will react to extremes in humidity, shrinking in low humidity and peaking in high humidity, just like wood.

Unfinished tile and plank must be finished with a hardwood floor protective coating of either water-based or oil-based polyurethane or paste wax. Unfinished cork products may be stained a color before the protective coating is applied.

A unique blend of rubber and cork used in Natural CORK® is extremely durable and wear resistant. The color and pattern run throughout the entire thickness of the tile. This product has been used throughout Europe and Asia in public transportation as well as in airports and train stations.

Installation

Because cork is a wood product, the floor tiles should be acclimatized to the installation site for 72 hours before installation. Because of cork's natural qualities, no two tiles are identical in pattern or color. Pieces may vary slightly in color, tone, and grain configuration. It is the installer's or client's responsibility to mix colors and patterns in an acceptable manner. The cork tiles should be shuffled to get the desired aesthetic mix. Only those substrate materials and adhesives specified by the manufacturer of the cork flooring should be used. Expansion and contraction, resulting from climatic conditions, will occur, so an approximate 1/8- to 1/4-inch space around the perimeter of the room must be allowed for. This space is covered by a base. Natural CORK Planks Plus do not require an underlayment, only a moisture barrier of 6-mil polyethylene film over the substrate.

Natural CORK provided the following information on installation on a concrete substrate: "Check concrete slab for moisture by chipping quarter size sections 1/8″ deep in several places and applying two drops of 3% phenophalen in alcohol solution (readily available at drug stores) with a dropper in each section. If solution turns red, too much moisture is present for safe installation of Cork Parquet."[48] A calcium chloride test is also acceptable.

Maintenance

Walk-off mats should be used, provided they do not have a rubber back, which may cause permanent discoloration. Furniture guards should also be used. (See Figure 4.15.) Spills should be picked up immediately; wet spills or water should not be allowed to stand on the cork floor. With factory-refinished cork parquet tiles and Planks Plus™, a high-quality hardwood floor polyurethane cleaner should be used in accordance with the manufacturer's instructions. When the finish begins to show wear, the floor should be cleaned and one of Natural CORK's recommended topcoat finishes should be used.

FORMED-IN-PLACE OR POURED FLOORS

Formed-in-place floors come in cans and are applied at the site in a seamless installation. The basis of the "canned floors" may be urethane, epoxy, polyester, or vinyl, but they are all applied the same way. First, as with all other floor installations, the surface must be clean, dry, and level. Second, a base coat of any of the aforementioned materials is applied to the substrate according to manufacturer's directions. Third, colored plastic chips are sprinkled or sprayed on the base and several coats of the base material are applied for the wearlayer.

Formed-in-place poured floors seems popular in veterinary offices, where a nonskid and easily cleaned surface is desirable. Such floors can also be coved up a base in the same manner as sheet vinyl, which eliminates cracks between floor and base. Of course, this type of flooring may be used in any area where cleanliness is paramount.

Maintenance

Maintenance is the same as that for sheet vinyl.

BIBLIOGRAPHY

Berendsen, Anne. *Tiles: A General History*. New York: Viking Press, 1967.

Byrne, Michael. *Setting Tile*. Newton, CT: Taunton Press, 1996.

Oak Flooring Institute. *Hardwood Flooring Finishing/Refinishing Manual*. Memphis, TN: Oak Flooring Institute, 1986.

Oak Flooring Institute. *Wood Floor Care Guide*. Memphis, TN: Oak Flooring Institute, 2004.

Tile Council of America. *2006 North America Handbook for Ceramic Tile Installation*. Anderson, SC: Author, 2006.

GLOSSARY

adobe.   Unburnt, sun-dried brick.

agglomerate.   Marble chips and spalls of various sizes, bonded together with a resin.

aggregate.   The solid material in concrete, mortar, or grout.

ANSI.   American National Standards Institute.

ASTM.   American Society for Testing and Materials.

base.   A board or moulding at the base of a wall that comes in contact with the floor; protects the wall from damage.

beveled.   In wood flooring, the top edge is cut at a 45-degree angle.

billets.   Small pieces of wood making up a parquet pattern.

bisque.   Once-fired clay.

bluestone.   A hard sandstone of characteristic blue, gray, and buff colors, quarried in New York and Pennsylvania.

bow.   Longitudinal curvature of lumber.

bullnose.   A convex rounded edge on tile.

burl.   An abnormal growth or protuberance on a tree, resulting in a very patterned area.

chamfer.   Tile with a slight beveled edge.

cove.   A concave rounded edge on tile.

crook.   The warp of a board edge from the straight line drawn between the two ends.

cup.   Deviation of the face of a board from a plane.

cure.   Maintaining the humidity and temperature of freshly poured concrete for a period of time to keep water present so the concrete hydrates or hardens properly.

dowel.   Round wooden rod to join two pieces of wood.

Elgin Marbles.   (Pronounced with a hard "g.") Lord Elgin, the British Ambassador to Turkey from 1799 to 1802, persuaded the Turkish government in Athens to allow him to remove the frieze of the Parthenon to the British Museum in London to prevent further damage.

figure.   The pattern of wood fibers.

floating floor.   A wood floor that is not attached to the substrate, merely laid on top.

floorcloth.   Painted canvas used in the early 1800s.

gauge.   Thickness of tile.

grain.   Arrangement of the fibers of the wood.

grout.   Material used to fill in the spaces between tiles.

impervious.   Less than 0.5 percent absorption rate.

kiln.   An oven for controlled drying of lumber or firing of tile.

laminate floor.   Same construction as a decorative laminate, only specially made for flooring.

laminated or engineered wood.   Bonding of two or more layers of material.

lug.   A projection attached to the edges of a ceramic tile to provide equal spacing of the tiles.

marquetry.   Veneered inlaid material in wood flooring that has been fitted in various patterns and glued to a common background.

mastic.   An adhesive compound.

matrix.   The mortar part of the mix.

medullary rays.   Ribbons of tissue extending from the pitch to the bark of a tree, particularly noticeable in oak.

metal spline.   Thin metal wire holding strips of parquet together.

metamorphic.   Changes occurring in appearance and structure of rock caused by heat and/or pressure.

monolithic.   Grout and mortar base become one mass.

mortar.   A plastic mixture of cementitious materials, with water and fine aggregates.

mosaic.   A small size tile, ceramic or marble, usually 1-inch or 2-inch square, used to form patterns.

nonvitreous.   Tile that absorbs more than 7 percent moisture.

120-grit.   A medium-fine grade of sandpaper.

parquetry.   Inlaid solid wood flooring, usually set in simple geometric patterns.

patina.   Soft sheen achieved by continuous use.

pickets.   Wood strips pointed at both ends, used in parquet floors in patterns such as Monticello.

plastic.   Still pliable and soft, not hardened.

plumb.   Exactly vertical.

pointed.   Act of filling joints with mortar.

precipitation.   Action of solids settling out of the mineral springs.

prefinished.   Factory finished, referring to wood floors.

psi.   Pounds per square inch.

PVC.   Polyvinyl chloride. A water-insoluble thermoplastic resin used as a coating on sheet vinyl floors.

quarter sawn.   Wood sliced in quarters lengthwise that shows the grain of the wood to best advantage.

quartzite.   A compact granular rock, composed of quartzite crystals usually so firmly cemented as to make the mass homogeneous. Color range is wide.

reducer strip.   A tapered piece of wood used at the joining of two dissimilar materials to compensate for difference of thickness.

riser.   The vertical part of a stair.

sandstone.   Sedimentary rock composed of sand-sized grains naturally cemented from mineral materials.

semivitreous.   Three percent but not more than 7 percent moisture absorption.

sets.   Groups of parquet set at right angles to each other, usually four in a set.

60-grit.   A medium grade of sandpaper.

sleepers.   Horizontal timbers laid on a concrete slab to which the wood floor is nailed.

spall.   A fragment or chip, in this case of marble.

spalling.   Flaking of floor because of expansion of components.

square.   Edges cut at right angles to each other.

stenciling.   Method of decorating or printing a design by painting through a cut-out pattern.

taber test.   Scientific method to measure the amount of wear a surface can take before it is worn out.

terrazzo.   Marble chips of similar size combined with a binder that holds the marble chips together. This binder may be cementitious or noncementitious (epoxy resin).

thin-set.   The method of installing tile with a bonding material usually 3/32 to 1/8 inch in thickness. In certain geographical areas, the term *thin-set* may be used interchangeably for dry-set portland cement mortar.

toe space.   Area at base of furniture or cabinets that is inset to accommodate the toes.

tongue and groove. A wood joint providing a positive alignment.

tooled. A mortar joint that has been finished by a shaped tool while the mortar is plastic.

twist. A spiral distortion of lumber.

veneer. A very thin sheet of wood varying in thickness from 1/8 to 1/100 inch.

vitreous. Moisture absorption of 0.5 percent to less than 3 percent.

NOTES

[1]Wood Floors International, Inc. "Wood Floors—A History," www.woodfloosonline.com.

[2]The National Oak Flooring Manufacturers Association, *Oak Flooring Advocate*, Volume 4, Number 2.

[3]Hardwood Information Center, *Managing Natural Expansion and Construction of Hardwood Floors*, www.hardwood.org/flooring.

[4]Website, www.woodfacts.com.

[5]Smith & Fong website, www.durapalm.com.

[6]Website, www.nofma.org.

[7]Website, www.pbmdf.com.

[8]Congoleum, "Maintenance & Warranty Information, Consumer Flooring Guide."

[9]"Bamboo Flooring . . . The Natural Choice." Brochure from Smith & Fong Company, San Francisco, CA 94080.

[10]Website, www.teragren.com.

[11]Website, www.bamtex.com.

[12]Shaw Industries website, www.shawfloors.com.

[13]Website, www.wilsonart.com.

[14]Website, www.mannington.com.

[15]Website, www.wilsonart.com.

[16]Ibid.

[17]Tile Council of America (TCA), *2005 Handbook for Ceramic Tile Installation*, Clemson, SC, 2005, p. 9 (italics in original).

[18]Ibid.

[19]Walker Zanger, Medallion Collection, www.walkerzanger.com.

[20]TCA, *Handbook for Ceramic Tile Installation*, p. 6.

[21]Ibid, p. 5.

[22]Marble Institute of America, *Care & Cleaning of Natural Stone Surfaces*, 1995.

[23]Website, www.ntma.com.

[24]The National Terrazzo and Mosaic Association, "The Care of Terrazzo," Leesburg, VA.

[25]Website, www.ntma.com.

[26]Ibid.

[27]Website, www.nbgqa.com.

[28]*Compton's Interactive Encylopedia*™, Version 2.01W, ©1994 Compton's New Media Inc., a Tribune New Media Company.

[29]Website, www.structuralslate.com.

[30]Ibid.

[31]Website, www.senecatiles.com.

[32]Letter from Crossville Tile, Crossville, TN.

[33]Website, www.floridatile.com.

[34]Crossville website, www.crossvilleinc.com.

[35]*Compton's Interactive Encyclopedia*.

[36]Tile Council of America, *Handbook for Ceramic Tile Installation*, p. 10.

[37]Website, www.fiberopticsfloors.com.

[38]Website, www.senecatile.com.

[39]Website, www.crossvilleinc.com.

[40]Portland Cement Association, *Design and Control of Concrete Mixtures*, Skokie, IL.

[41]Forbo Industries, "The Linoleum Story," brochure. Forbo Industries Hazelton, PA.

[42]Website, www.mannington.com.

[43]Ibid.

[44]Website, www.roppe.com.

[45]E-mail from Armstrong World Industries.

[46]Website, www.congoleum.com.

[47]Website, www.naturalcok.com.

[48]Ibid.

5

Walls

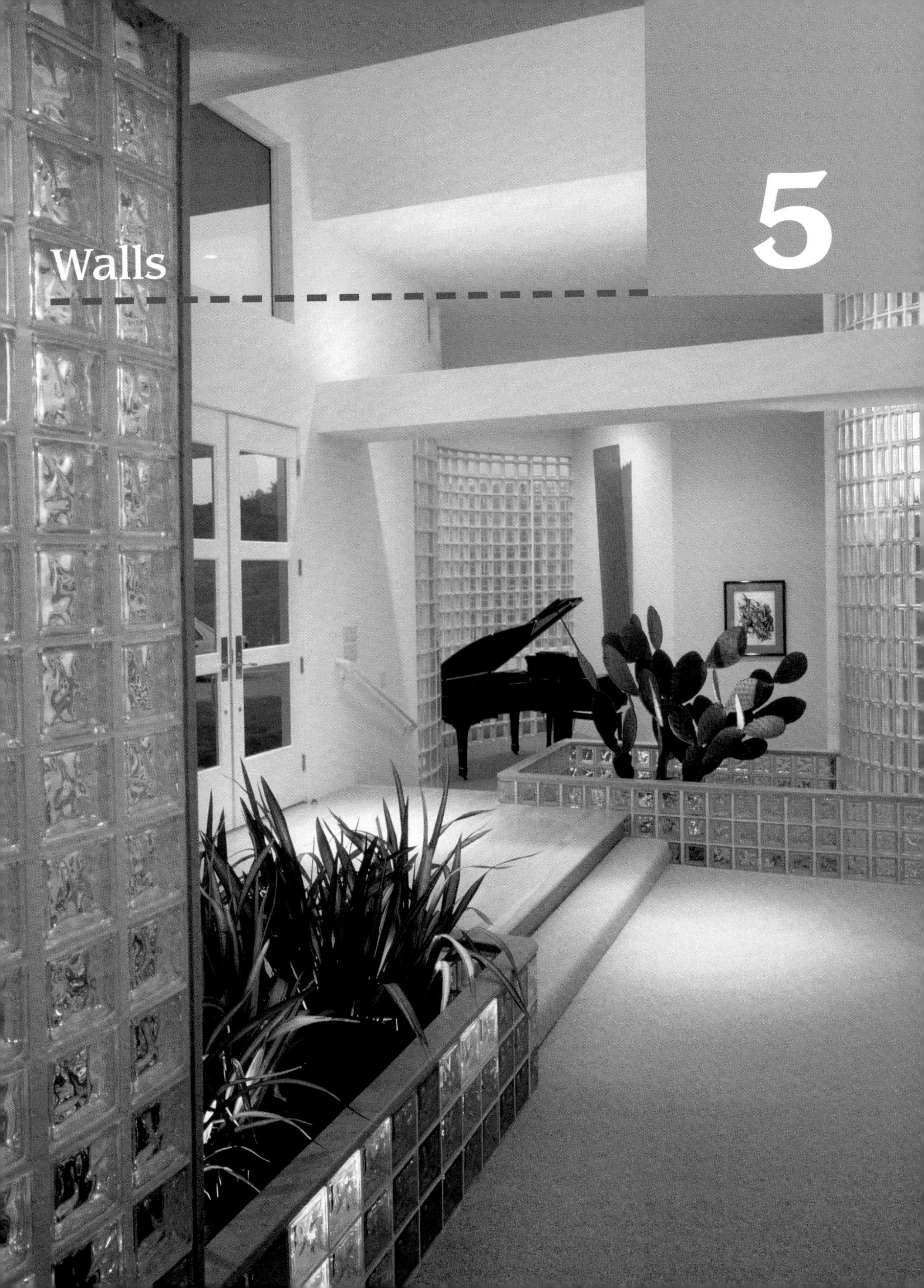

In floors, the weight of flooring material is spread over a large area; however, when these same materials are used on walls, they create a heavy dead load. Thus, walls—whether constructed or veneered with granite, stone, or brick—must have a foundation prepared to withstand this additional weight. **Compressive strength** is also important for wall installation materials.

There are two types of walls: load bearing and nonbearing. Interior designers need to know the difference between the two. **Load-bearing** walls are those that support an imposed load in addition to their own weight; a nonbearing wall is just for utilitarian or aesthetic purposes. The architect deals with both, but the interior designer probably deals more with nonbearing walls. A load-bearing wall should never be removed or altered without consulting an architect or engineer.

STONE

Most interior designers do not specify stone except maybe for fireplaces; however, it is important to understand the various patterns.

FIGURE 5.1
Types of stonework.

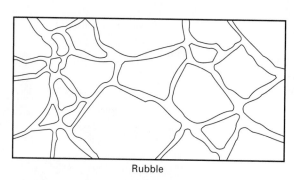

Rubble

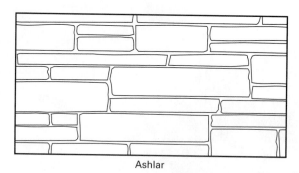

Ashlar

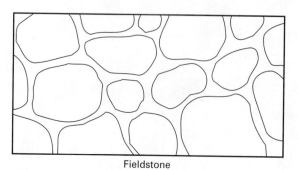

Fieldstone

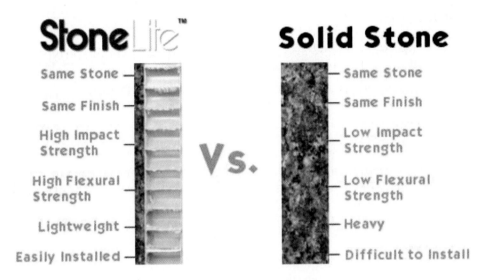

FIGURE 5.2
Drawing of Ultra-Lite Stone
Panels versus Solid Stone.
(Courtesy of Stone
Panels Inc.)

A stone wall, in a residence, is usually a veneer and may be constructed of any type of stone. **Rubble** is uncut stone or stone that has not been cut into a rectangular shape. **Ashlar** is stone that is precut to provide enough uniformity to allow some regularity in assembly. The rubble masonry is less formal, requires the use of more **mortar,** and is not as strong as the other types of **bonds** because of the irregular shapes. Uniform mortar joints are a mark of a skilled worker. **Fieldstone** or **cobble** has a more rounded feeling than does ashlar or rubble (Figure 5.1).

Maintenance

Stonework should be cleaned with a stiff brush and clean water. If stains are difficult to remove, soapy water may be used, followed by a clean-water rinse. Stonework should be cleaned by sponging during construction, which facilitates final cleaning. The acids used to clean brick should never be used on stone walls.

Regular maintenance consists of brushing or vacuuming to remove dust. It is important to remember that, generally, igneous types are impervious, but sedimentary and metamorphic stones are more susceptible to stains. Stone walls should not be installed where grease or any substance that may stain the stone is present. "Ultra-Lite Stone panels are composite wall panels made up of a thin natural stone veneer reinforced with an aluminum honeycomb backing. The stone veneer can be almost any stone including granite, marble, and limestone."[1] (See Figure 5.2.)

GRANITE

Granite is used wherever a feeling of stability and permanence is desired, which is probably why one sees so much granite in banks and similar institutions. The properties of granite were mentioned in Chapter 4. Granite for walls may be used polished, or honed, because abrasion is not a problem with walls.

Installation

Anchors, **cramps**, dowels, and other anchoring devices should be type 304 stainless steel or suitable nonferrous metal. A portland cement sand mortar is used and, where applicable, a sealant is used for pointing the joints.

Maintenance

If required, granite walls may be washed with a weak detergent solution and rinsed with clear water. The walls should be buffed with a lambswool pad to restore shine.

MARBLE

Marble has the same elegant and formal properties whether used for walls or for floors. According to the Marble Institute of America, interior marble wall facing may be installed by mechanical fastening devices utilizing nonstaining anchors, angles, dowels, pins, cramps, and plaster spots, or in a mortar setting bed to secure smaller units to interior vertical surfaces. The overall dimensions of the marble determine the setting method. Resilient cushions are used to maintain joint widths, which are then pointed with white cement or other approved material.

In addition to the traditional sizes, new thin marble veneers that are backed with lighter-weight materials have less weight per square foot and, depending on job conditions, may be set in either a conventional full mortar bed or by any of the several thin-bed systems.

Maintenance

Maintenance is the same as that for marble floors.

TRAVERTINE

When travertine is used in wall applications, it is not necessary to fill the voids. Unfilled travertine gives an interesting texture to the wall surface, but for a perfectly smooth installation, filling is required. Like flooring, wall applications of travertine may be filled with a translucent epoxy or an opaque epoxy matching the color of the travertine. Filled travertine does tend to have less sheen on the opaque-filled area than on the solid area. The surface of the travertine may be left in its rough state, providing texture, or it may be cut and sanded or ground smooth.

Installation

Installation methods of travertine are the same as for marble.

BRICK

Brick is used for both exterior and interior walls, and the surface of the brick may be smooth, rough, or grooved. Bricks with these surface textures create interesting wall designs with their varied shadows. Bricks are available in whites, yellows, grays, reds, and browns and may be ordered in special sizes or shapes. Firebrick is used for lining boilers and fireplaces and is made of special fire-resistant clays.

The standard brick size is 3 3/4 inches wide by 8 inches long and 2 1/4 inches high. Bricks laid to expose the long side in a horizontal position are called **stretchers;** vertically laid bricks are called soldiers. When the ends of the bricks show horizontally, the bricks are called **headers,** and vertically they are called **rowlocks** (Figure 5.3). A bond is the arrangement of bricks in rows or **courses.** A common bond is defined as bricks placed end to end in a stretcher course with vertical joints of one course centered on the bricks in the next course. Every sixth or seventh course is made up of headers and stretchers. These headers provide structural bonding as well as pattern. A bond without headers is called a running bond. It is interesting to note that in some historical digs of buildings dating from the 1880s, it is possible to discover the nationality of the builders of brick walls (e.g., English and Flemish, as well as several other European nationalities). See Figure 5.3 for types of brick bonds.

Masonry walls may be hollow masonry, where both sides of the wall are visible, or they may be veneered. When both sides are visible,

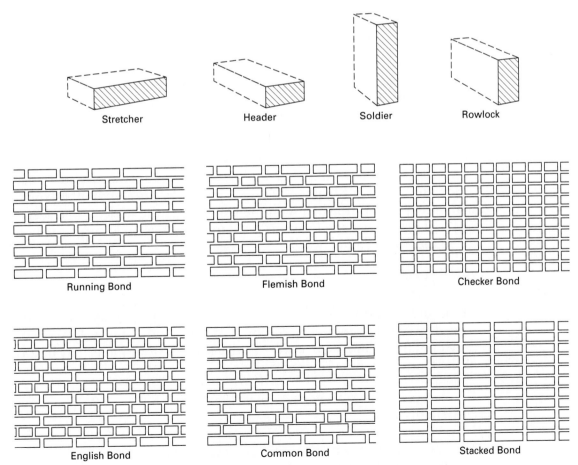

FIGURE 5.3
Stretchers, headers, and bonds.

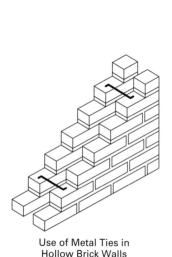

Use of Metal Ties in
Hollow Brick Walls

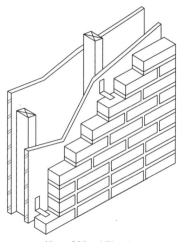

Use of Metal Ties in a
Brick Veneer Wall

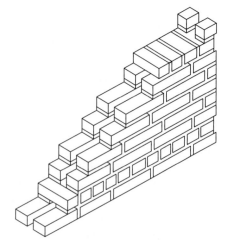

Use of Headers in a Hollow Brick
Wall Visible from Both Sides

FIGURE 5.4
Brick wall construction.

the **header course** ties the two sides together. A veneered wall is attached to the backing by means of metal ties (Figure 5.4).

The joints in a wall installation are extremely important because they create shadows and special design effects. The joints of a brick wall are normally 3/8 inch thick. The mortar for these joints consists of a mixture of portland cement, hydrated lime, and sand. The mortar serves four functions:

1. It bonds the brick units together and seals the spaces between them.
2. It compensates for dimensional variations in the units.
3. It bonds to reinforcing steel and therefore causes the steel to act as an integral part of the wall.
4. It provides a decorative effect on the wall surface by creating shadow or color lines.

Mortar joint finishes fall into two classes: troweled and tooled joints. In the troweled joint, the excess mortar is simply cut off (**struck**) with a trowel and finished with the trowel. For the tooled joint, a special tool other than the trowel is used to compress and shape the mortar in the joint (Figure 5.5).

Installation

Brick and concrete blocks are both installed by masons. Bricks are placed in a bed of mortar and mortar is laid on the top surface of the previous course, or row, to cover all edges. The mortar joints may be any of the types shown in Figure 5.5.

Maintenance

The major problem with finishing brick walls is the **mortar stain**, which occurs even if the mason is skilled and careful. To remove mortar stain, the walls are cleaned of surplus mortar and dirt; then scrubbed with a

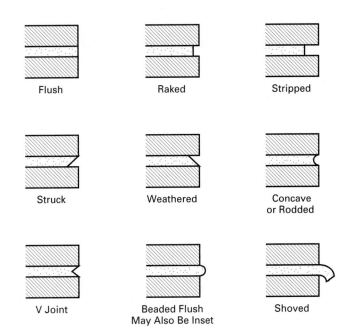

FIGURE 5.5
Mortar joints.

solution of trisodium phosphate, household detergent, and water; and then rinsed with water under pressure. If stains are not removed with this treatment, a solution of muriatic acid and water is used. The acid should be poured into the water, and not vice versa, to avoid a dangerous reaction. Just the bricks themselves should be scrubbed. The solution should not be allowed to dry but should be rinsed immediately with clean water. For cleaning light-colored bricks, a more diluted solution of muriatic acid and water should be used to prevent burning.

Regular maintenance for bricks includes brushing and vacuuming to remove dust that may have adhered to the rough surface. Masonry walls that may come in contact with grease, such as in kitchens, should be either impervious or sealed to prevent penetration of the grease.

CONCRETE

In a March 2004 article, Dr. Oliver Graydon, editor of Optics.org and *Opto & Laser Europe* magazine, notes that light-transmitting concrete is set to go on sale later this year.

> The days of dull, grey concrete could be about to end. A Hungarian architect has combined the world's most popular building material with optical fiber from Schott to create a new type of concrete that transmits light.
>
> A wall made of "LitraCon™" allegedly has the strength of traditional concrete but thanks to an embedded array of glass fibers can display a view of the outside world, such as the silhouette of a tree, for example.
>
> "Thousands of optical glass fibers form a matrix and run parallel to each other between the two main surfaces of every block," explained its inventor Áron Losonczi. "Shadows on the lighter side will appear with sharp outlines on the darker one. Even the colours remain the same. This special effect creates the general impression

that the thickness and weight of a concrete wall will disappear." The hope is that the new material will transform the interior appearance of concrete buildings by making them feel light and airy rather than dark and heavy.

Losonczi, a 27-year-old architect from Csongrád, recently came up with the idea while he was studying at the Royal University College of Fine Arts in Stockholm, Sweden. After demonstrating the material at design exhibitions all over Europe he has now formed a company to commercialize the concept.

His new company, also called LiTraCon, is now optimizing its manufacturing methods and hopes to start selling prefabricated blocks of the material later this year.

"In theory, a wall structure built out of the light-transmitting concrete can be a couple of meters thick as the fibers work without any loss in light up to 20 m," explained Losonczi. "Load-bearing structures can also be built from the blocks as glass fibers do not have a negative effect on the well-known high compressive strength of concrete. The blocks can be produced in various sizes with embedded heat isolation too."[2] (See Figure 5.6.)

Currently, many architects of contemporary buildings, particularly in the commercial, industrial, and educational fields, are leaving poured concrete walls exposed on the interior. The forms used for these walls may be patterned or smooth, and this texture is reflected on the interior surface. The ties that hold the forms together may leave holes that, if properly placed, may provide a grid design. From the interior designer's point of view, a poured concrete wall is a *fait accompli*. The surface may be left

FIGURE 5.6
Translucent concrete. (Photo courtesy of Optics.org)

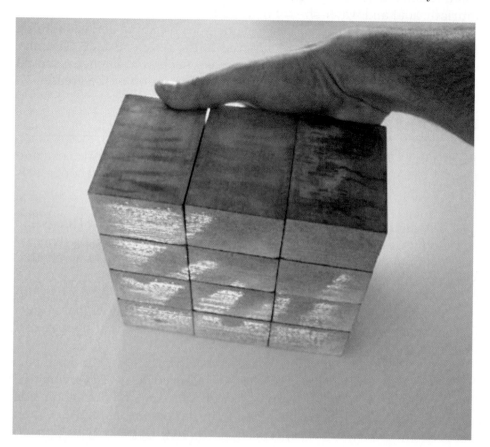

with the outline of the forms showing, patterned or plain, or it may be treated by the following methods to give a different surface appearance: bush hammering, acid etching, and sandblasting. Bush hammering is done with a power tool that provides an exposed aggregate face by removing the sand-cement matrix and exposing the aggregate. Sandblasting provides a textured surface. Bush hammering produces the heaviest texture, whereas the texture from sandblasting depends on the amount and coarseness of sand used. Acid etching just removes the surface.

If concrete is left in its natural poured state, the main problem facing the designer is using materials and accessories that will be compatible with cast concrete. Obviously, such materials need to imply weight and a substantial feeling, rather than delicacy or formality. The massive feeling can be overcome, however, by plastering over the concrete.

CONCRETE BLOCK

Concrete block is a hollow concrete masonry unit (CMU) composed of portland cement and suitable aggregates. Walls of this type are found in homes, but they are more frequently used in commercial and educational interiors. There are several problems with concrete block. It has extremely poor insulating qualities if used on an exterior wall; if used on an outside wall and moisture is present, **efflorescence** will form; and it has a fairly rough surface that is difficult to paint, although coverage may be accomplished by using a specially formulated paint and a long-nap roller.

Installation

The mason erects a concrete block wall in a similar manner to a brick one except that, whereas a brick wall is viewed only from one side, a concrete block wall is often visible from both sides; therefore, the joints need to be finished on both sides of the block. Concrete block may be erected in either a running bond pattern or stacked (running bond is stronger).

Maintenance

Acid is not used to remove mortar smears or droppings, as with brick. Excess mortar should be allowed to dry and then chipped off. Rubbing the wall with a small piece of concrete block will remove practically all the mortar. For painting instructions, see Chapter 3.

GLASS BLOCK

In the 1920s and 1930s, glass block seemed to be used only in bathrooms and on the sides of front doors, but today modern technology and the innovation of architects and designers have led to a revival and growth of its use in a variety of design environments. Glass block must only be used for non-load-bearing installations, but creative designers have nonetheless found many appealing uses for it.

Glass block, by definition, is composed of two halves of pressed glass fused together. The hollow in the center is partially **evacuated,** which provides a partial vacuum with good insulating qualities. The construction of the block is such that designs may be imprinted on both the inside and the outside of the glass surfaces. In all of their applications, glass blocks permit the control of light—natural or artificial, day or night—for function and drama. Thermal transmission, noise, dust, and drafts may also be controlled (Figure 5.7). For curved panel radius minimums, refer to Table 5.1.

Pittsburgh Corning Corporation, the only American manufacturer of glass block, produces a variety of styles that may be used for both exterior and interior purposes.

The IceScapes® pattern provides a high degree of privacy while maintaining maximum light transmission. Similar to other Pittsburgh Corning glass block, the 12-inch by 12-inch by 4-inch IceScapes® pattern glass block provides the benefits of security, noise control, durability and low maintenance.[3]

The range of privacy varies from the VUE® pattern, which is clear for the greatest combination of light transmission/maximum privacy, to

FIGURE 5.7
Glass block is used in multiple ways. For inside and outside walls and as a divider between rooms. (Photo courtesy of Pittsburgh Corning Glass Block)

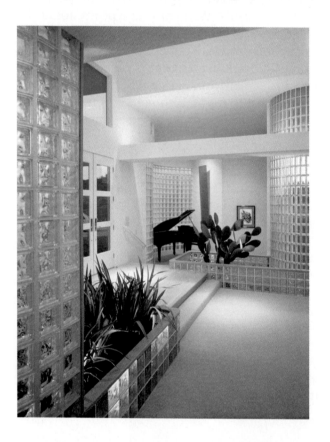

TABLE 5.1
Radius Minimums for Curved Panel Construction

Block Size	Outside Radius in Inches	Number Blocks in 90° Arc	Joint Thickness in Inches	
			Inside	Outside
6 × 6	52 1/2	13	1/8	5/8
4 × 8	36	13	1/8	5/8
8 × 8	69	13	1/8	5/8
12 × 12	102 1/2	13	1/8	5/8

Source: Courtesy of Pittsburgh Corning Corporation.

the ARGUS®, narrow flutes that provide moderate light transmission with maximum privacy. There are specialty blocks for finishing a free-standing glass block wall in offices and residences. The newest block from Pittsburgh Corning is a sandblasted VUE pattern that provides a frosted look for complete privacy. Another pattern is SPYRA®, a wave effect that provides many options for decorative designs.

Standard glass block is 3 7/8 inches thick; the Thinline Series units are 3 1/8 inches thick. Glass block is available in 6-, 8-, and 12-inch squares, and some styles come in 4″ × 8″ and 6″ × 8″ rectangular blocks. Thinline block has the additional advantage of 20 percent less weight.

Specialty blocks such as VISTABRIK® units are solid glass and provide maximum protection from vandalism and forcible entry.

Installation

The mortar-bearing surfaces of glass block have a coating that acts as a bond between the block and the mortar. Additionally, the coating acts as an expansion-contraction mechanism for each block. An optimum mortar mix is one part portland cement, one-half part lime, and four parts sand. Panel reinforcing strips are used in horizontal joints every 16 to 24 inches of height, depending on which thickness of block is used. Expansion strips are used adjacent to **jambs** and **heads.** Joints are struck whereas plastic and excess mortar are removed immediately. Mortar should be removed from the face of the block with a damp cloth before final set occurs. For easier cleaning of glass block showers, use a non-mildew-forming silicone or acrylic sealer to coat the mortar joints. Prefabricated panels with or without ventilation are also available.

Maintenance

Ease of maintenance is one of the attractive features of block. Mortar or dirt on the face of glass block may be removed by the use of water, but not with abrasives (steel wool, wire brush, or acid).

PLASTER

The Egyptians and ancient Greeks used plaster walls that they painted with murals. The frescoes of early times were painted on wet plaster, which absorbed the pigment so it dried as an integral part of the plaster. The frescoes of Michelangelo's Sistine Chapel still retain their original brilliant color after 400 years. Historically, plaster was also used for intricate mouldings and decorations. Today, plaster-covered walls are used only in commercial installations and expensive custom-built homes, because applications are expensive as compared to **drywall.** The plastering process is also extremely labor intensive, involving three coats of plaster over gypsum or metal lath.

Surface finishes called veneer plaster are on the market; they create the upscale look of solid plaster at a lower cost (about 25 percent more than gypsum board). Veneer plaster has high resistance to cracking, nail popping, and impact and abrasion failure, and is particularly suited to accommodate wall situations where light conditions require smooth, even expanses of wall.

> Terramed is a textured wall treatment made in France, to recreate the ambiance of Mediterranean interiors. It is all natural, authentic, affordable, and easy to use. Terramed is the right treatment to achieve a certain refined style. Adding straw, finely crushed shells, or small pebbles during the mixing stage will result in a more rural or nautical or rustic wall surface. Simply add a cup or two, but no more than 7% by volume, of your choice of additive to the mix and apply to your walls as usual. After waiting half-an-hour for Terramed to set, go over the surface with a damp sponge to reveal the added texture.[4] (See Figure 5.8.)

National Gypsum's Gold Bond® BRAND Uni-Kal® is a single-component veneer plaster for application over Gold Bond Kal-Kore® tapered-edge 1/2″ Regular or 5/8″ Kal-Kore Hi-Impact® or as a finish over Kal-Kote base. When applied in a thin coat 3/32″ thick and troweled to a smooth finish, it provides a durable, abrasion-resistant surface for further decoration. Uni-Kal may be worked to a variety of textured finishes.

Joints are reinforced with a fiberglass webbing; steel corners and **casing beads** protect corners. An alkali-resistant primer formulated for use over new plaster should be used if the surface will be painted.

If a gypsum board wall is already installed, a plaster bonding agent must be applied before using the veneer plaster, which is then applied in two coats.

Lath is the foundation of a plaster wall. In the pyramids of Egypt, the lath was made of intertwined reeds. The construction of the half-timbered homes of the English Tudor period is often referred to as daub and wattle (the daub being the plaster and the wattle the lath), this time a woven framework of saplings and reeds. When restoration work is

FIGURE 5.8
Terramed from Eco
by design.

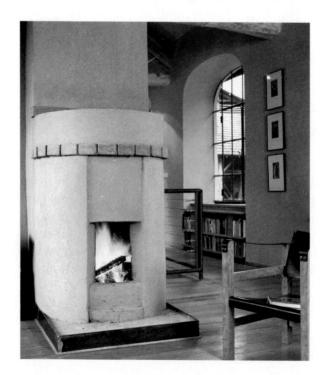

done on houses built in the United States prior to the 1930s, the lath will probably be thin wood strips nailed to the studs about 3/8 of an inch apart.

Modern lath is gypsum board, metal, or masonry block. The gypsum lath consists of a core of gypsum plaster between two layers of specially formulated, absorbent, 100 percent recycled paper. The gypsum lath is 3/8 or 1/2 inch thick, 16 inches wide by 48 inches long, and is applied horizontally with the joints staggered between courses. Other sizes are also available. Special types of gypsum lath may have holes drilled in them for extra adhesion or may have a sheet of aluminum foil on one side for insulating purposes.

Metal lath is expanded metal that is nailed to the studs and is used not only for flat areas but also for curved surfaces and forms. The **scratch coat** is troweled on and some plaster is squeezed through the mesh to form the mechanical bond, whereas the bond with gypsum board is formed by means of **suction.** Beads or formed pieces of metal are placed at exterior corners and around casings to provide a hard edge that will not be damaged by traffic.

Plaster used to be troweled on the lath in three different coats. The first coat bonded to the lath; the second was the brown coat; and the third, the finish coat, was very smooth. The first two coats were left with a texture to provide tooth. A three-coat plaster job is still done sometimes, but two coats or even one may be used to complete the finished surface.

As mentioned in Chapter 3, because of its extreme porosity, plaster must be sealed before proceeding with other finishes.

GYPSUM BOARD

Gypsum board has the same construction as gypsum board lath. Sheets are normally 4 feet wide and 8 feet long, but they may be obtained in lengths up to 16 feet. The long edges are usually tapered with a beveled edge; sometimes the short sides are also coated with the paper.

In some areas of the United States the term *drywall* is synonymous with *gypsum board*. The term *drywall* originated to differentiate between plaster or "wet wall" construction and any dry material, such as gypsum board, plywood, or other prefabricated materials, that does not require the use of plaster or mortar.

Another term mistakenly used as a synonym for *drywall* is Sheetrock®, a registered trademark of the U.S. Gypsum Company for its brand of gypsum board. The term *gypsum wallboard* implies use on walls only, whereas most gypsum board companies now produce a type of reinforced gypsum board specially for ceilings, which can withstand deflection. All gypsum board companies produce their product with 100 percent recycled paper on both the face and the back of the board.

Gold Bond® BRAND Sta-Smooth® Wallboard is a drywall system offering maximum joint strength and easy application. It can be used in any gypsum drywall system where conventional types of gypsum wallboard are recommended. This system features Gold Bond® BRAND Sta-Smooth® Gypsum Wallboard with a unique edge. The two edge configurations relieve joint deformity problems caused by twisted framing, damaged wallboard edges, poor alignment and extremes in humidity and temperature. Regular Sta-Smooth Panels are available in 1/2″ thicknesses, 4′ wide and in customary wallboard lengths. The Sta-Smooth System is also composed of Sta-Smooth® BRAND Joint Compounds, a hardening-type taping compound and regular Proform® BRAND Joint Tape and finishing compounds. The taper is scientifically designed to reduce crowned joints.[5]

Some edges are square; the square edge was designed to be a base for a fabric covering or wallpaper, paneling, or tile. The square edge also can be used where an exposed joint is desired for a paneled effect. Tapered, round-edge gypsum board can be used for walls and ceilings in both new construction and remodeling. It is designed to reduce the beading and ridging problems commonly associated with standard-type gypsum board.

There are several types of specialty gypsum wallboards available— for fire-resistant purposes, for abrasion resistance mold/mildew resistance, for use as a vapor retarder barrier on exterior walls, or for radius construction. National Gypsum Company's 1/4″ High Flex® Wallboard is specifically designed for radius construction such as curved walls, archways, and stairways. It can be used for both concave and convex surfaces, but not **compound curves.** High Flex is typically applied in double layers.

In new construction, 1/2-inch thickness is recommended for single-layer application; for laminated two-ply applications, two 3/8-inch-thick sheets are used. The horizontal method of application is best adapted to rooms in which full-length sheets can be used, because horizontal application minimizes the number of vertical joints. Today, screws are used rather than nails, because screws can be installed by automatic screw guns and will not pull loose or "pop." Screws are placed a maximum of 12 inches on center (o.c.) on ceilings and 16 inches o.c. on walls where framing members are 16 inches o.c. Screws should be spaced a maximum of 12 inches o.c. on walls and ceilings where framing members are 24 inches o.c. In both cases, the screw heads should be slightly below the surface. A very good drywall installation may also have an adhesive applied to the studs before installing the panels, in which case screws may be farther apart.

If nails are used, the spacing is slightly different. Nails should be spaced a maximum of 7 inches o.c. on ceilings and 8 inches o.c. on walls along framing supports. The ceilings are done first and then the walls.

A thorough inspection of the studs should be made before application of the gypsum board to ensure that all warped studs are replaced. If this is not done, the final appearance of the plaster board will be rippled. Of course, this problem is not present when metal studs are used (e.g., in commercial construction).

After all the sheets have been installed, outside corners are protected by a metal corner or bead. The beads are either right angled or curved. Trim strips are available for a **reveal** effect.

Joint cement, spackling compound, or, as it is called in the trade, "mud" is applied to all joints with a 5-inch-wide spackling knife. Tape is placed to cover the joint and is pressed into the mud. (*All* seams or joints must be taped regardless of length; otherwise, cracks will soon appear). The outside beads have joint cement feathered to meet the edge. Another layer of compound is applied, **feathering** the outer edges. After drying, the compound is sanded and a third coat is applied, the feathering extending beyond the previous coats. All screw holes are filled with joint cement and sanded smooth. Care must be taken to sand only the area that has been coated with joint cement, because sanding the paper layer will result in a roughness that will be visible, particularly when a painted semigloss or gloss finish is applied. In fact, the Gypsum Association suggests that a thin, skim coat of joint compound be applied over the entire surface to provide a uniform surface for these paints. The drywall installer should be informed of the final finish so that attention can be paid to special finishing.

The surface of the gypsum board may be left smooth, ready for painting or a wallcovering, or it may have some type of texture applied. The latter is done for several reasons. Aesthetically, a texture may eliminate glare and is likely to hide any surface discrepancies caused by warping studs and/or finishing of joints. The lightest texture available is called an orange peel (the surface has the texture of the skin of an orange). Another finish is a skip-troweled surface: After the texture has been sprayed on, a metal trowel is used to flatten some areas. The heaviest texture is a heavily stippled or troweled appearance, similar to rough-finished plaster. A texture is preferred whenever there is a **raking light** on the wall surface; the texture helps hide surface discrepancies.

When water may be present, such as in bathrooms and kitchens, most building codes require the use of a water-resistant gypsum board. Its facing paper is colored light green so as to make it readily distinguishable from regular gypsum wallboard.

> Moisture-prone areas like basements and bathrooms call for highly mold-resistant interior gypsum panels. DensArmor® Plus Interior Panels fill the bill. Coated glass mats resist mold both inside the wall cavity and in room interiors. The core is reinforced with glass fibers for added strength.[6]

When ceramic tile is used, special water-resistant tile backers are used. If a pliant wallcovering is used, all plaster board must be sealed or sized, because the paper of the gypsum board and the backing of the wallcovering would become bonded and the wallcovering would be impossible to remove.

Another type of gypsum board features fabric or vinyl wallcovering plastic in a variety of simulated finishes, including wood grains and other textures. This type of gypsum board can be applied directly by adhesive to the studs or as a finish layer over a preexisting wall. The edges may be square or beveled. Wood or metal trim must be applied at both floor and ceiling to create a finished edge. National Gypsum manufactures Durasan®, a vinyl-covered wall panel (also available in 30-yard rolls). Durasan yardage is for use on columns, curved surfaces, or where extensive cutouts would make Durasan panels difficult to use. Because field-applied vinyl is fabric backed, the Durasan panels and the complementary vinyl roll goods may vary slightly in color and texture.

> Micore® Mineral Fiber Board is designed to be used as a substrate for fabric and vinyl-covered wall panels, office dividers, tack boards and similar products. It also serves as an excellent core for chalkboards and stoveboards.[7]

FIGURE 5.9
A bamboo curved tambour
is used in this restaurant.
(Photo courtesy of Smith &
Fons)

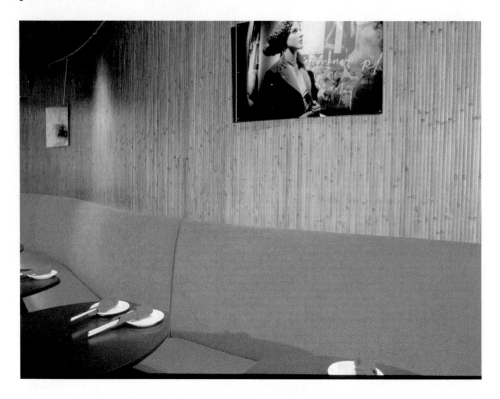

TAMBOURS

Tambours (Figure 5.9) are vertical slats of any material attached to a flexible backing, as in the front of a roll-top desk. The slats may be solid wood or hardboard. Other materials, such as wood veneer, bamboo, high-pressure laminate, metal, metallic mylar, melamine, and melamine/ mylar, real glass mirror, are laminated to a tempered hardboard core with a flexible brown fabric backing approximately 3/16 of an inch thick over-all. Slats are cut 1/2 to 1 inch o.c. with the angle of the groove varying between 30 and 90 degrees. Depending on the face material and use, dimensions vary from 18 inches wide by 15 inches long for roll-top desks, to 48 inches by 120 inches long. Because of their flexibility, tambours are used for curved walls as well as for roll-up doors in kitchen appliance garages (See Figure 9.13).

Installation

The method of installation depends on the surface to which the tambour is to be attached. A special adhesive is usually required, but the manufacturer's instructions should always be followed.

WOOD

When selecting a wood or veneer, designers should ascertain whether it comes from a renewable source. It is possible for some woods to be sustainable with proper management.

Wood is a good natural insulator because of the millions of tiny air cells within its cellular structure. At equal thickness, it is 4 times as effi-cient of an insulator as cinder block, 6 times as efficient as brick, 15 times as efficient as stone, 400 times as efficient as steel, and 1,770 times as efficient as aluminum. The production of the final wood product is also energy efficient: One ton of wood requires 1,510 kilowatt-hours to manufacture, whereas one ton of rolled steel requires 12,000 kilowatt-hours, and one ton of aluminum requires 67,200 kilowatt-hours.

Wood for walls comes in two different forms: solid wood strips (dimensional lumber) and plywood. Solid wood may be used on the walls of residences, but it is not usually used for commercial applications, unless treated, because of fire and building code restrictions. For residences, redwood, cedar, and knotty pine are the most commonly used woods, but walnut, pecan, and many others may also be used.

There are several grades of redwood from which to choose. The finest grade of redwood is Clear All Heart, with the graded face of each piece free of knots. Clear All Heart gives a solid red color, whereas Clear redwood is also top quality but does contain some cream-colored sapwood and may also contain small knots. The cream-colored sapwood may be attractive to some, but to others its random appearance is bothersome; therefore, the clients need to know the difference in appearance as well as cost between Clear All Heart and Clear. Clear B Heart is an economical, all-heartwood grade containing a limited number of tight knots and other characteristics not permitted in Clear or Clear All Heart. Clear B Grade is similar to B Heart except that it permits sapwood as well as heartwood.

Redwood is available in vertical grain, which has straight vertical lines, and flat grain, which is cut at a tangent to the annual growth rings, exposing a face surface that appears highly figured or marbled. Smooth-faced redwood is referred to as surfaced; saw-textured lumber has a rough, textured appearance.

There are two types of cedar: aromatic cedar, which is used for mothproof closets, and regular cedar, which is used for both interior and exterior walls. Another soft wood frequently used for residential interiors is knotty pine, in which knots are part of the desired effect (unlike the top-grade redwood).

Boards may be anywhere from 4 to 12 inches wide, with tongue and groove for an interlocking joint or **shiplap** for an overlapping joint. The tongue and groove may have the beveled edges for a V-joint or may be rounded or even elaborately moulded for a more decorative effect. Shiplap boards come with their top edges beveled to form a V-joint or with straight edges to form a narrow slot at the seams.

Square-edged boards are used in contemporary settings and may be board and batten, board on board, reverse board and batten, or contemporary vertical. Board and batten consists of wide boards spaced about 1 inch apart; a narrow 1″ × 2″ strip of batten is nailed on top to cover the 1-inch gap. Board on board is similar to board and batten except that both pieces of wood are the same width. Reverse board and batten has a narrow strip under the joint or gap. In contemporary vertical installations, the battens are sometimes placed on edge between the wider boards.

For acoustical control, boards are often placed on edge and spaced about 2 to 3 inches apart on an acoustical substrate (Figure 5.10).

The National Oak Flooring Manufacturer's Association (NOFMA) suggests using oak flooring on walls and ceilings. It is now possible to

FIGURE 5.10
Board and batten.

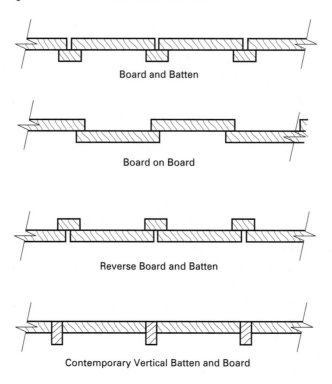

Board and Batten

Board on Board

Reverse Board and Batten

Contemporary Vertical Batten and Board

obtain a Class A 0 to 25 flame spread rating (often required in commercial structures) by job-site application of an intumescent coating. Beveled oak strip flooring gives a three-dimensional effect when installed on a wall.

Several companies manufacture paneling that comes prepackaged in boxes containing approximately 64 square feet. The longest pieces are 8 feet and the shortest 2 feet, with beveled edges and tongue-and-grooved sides and ends. This type of paneling, although more expensive than regular strips, eliminates waste in a conventional 8-foot-high room.

Installation

Wood may be installed horizontally, vertically, or diagonally. Each type of installation will give a completely different feeling to the room. Horizontal planking will appear to lengthen a room and draw the ceiling down, whereas vertical planking adds height to a room and is more formal. Diagonal installations appear a little more active and should be used with discretion or as a focal point of a room. Diagonal or herringbone patterns look best on walls with few doors or windows. Each application method requires its own type of substrate.

If installed horizontally or diagonally over bare studs or gypsum board, no further preparation of the surface is needed. The strips are attached to the wall in the tongue area, as with hardwood flooring, except that with wall applications the nails penetrate each stud.

Vertical installations require the addition of nailing surfaces. The two types of nailing surfaces are blocking and furring. Blocking involves filling in horizontally between the studs with 2- to 4-inch pieces of wood in order to make a nailing surface. Blocking also acts as a fire stop. Furring features thin strips of wood nailed across the studs (Figure 5.11).

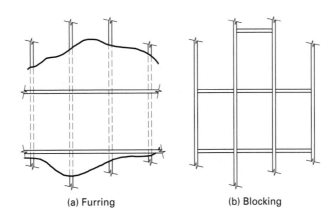

FIGURE 5.11
Furring and blocking.

(a) Furring   (b) Blocking

When wood is used on an outside wall, a vapor barrier such as a polyethylene film is required. In addition, wood should be stored for several days in the area in which it is to be installed so it may reach the correct moisture content. Some manufacturers suggest several applications of a water-repellent preservative to all sides, edges, and especially the porous ends (this is particularly important in high-humidity installations).

There are several suggested finishes for wood walls: wax, which adds soft luster to the wood, or a sealer and a matte varnish, for installations that will require cleaning. Paneling may also be stained, but it is important to remember that if solid wood is used, the natural beauty of the wood should be allowed to show through.

PLYWOOD PANELING

Plywood is produced from thin sheets of wood veneer, called plies, which are laminated together under heat and pressure with special adhesives. This process produces a bond between plies that is as strong as or stronger than the wood itself.

Plywood always has an odd number of layers that are assembled with their grains perpendicular to each other. Plywood may also have a lumber core, veneer core, medium-density fiberboard core, or particle-board core (see page 85 for information of particleboard); however, lumber-core plywood is virtually never used today in fine architectural woodworking (Figure 5.12). The face veneer is the best side, with the back veneer being a balancing veneer. One of the latest materials used for plywood paneling is bamboo, as seen in Figure 5.9.

The Architectural Woodwork Institute (AWI) is a not-for-profit organization that represents the architectural woodwork manufacturers located in the United States and Canada. The discussion in this section would not be possible without the assistance and cooperation of AWI.

The side of the plywood panel with the best-quality veneer is designated as the face, and the back may be of the same or of lesser quality depending on its projected uses.

AWI's *Architectural Woodwork Quality Standards* provide for three grades of plywood panel construction: Premium, Custom, and Economy:

Premium Grade—The grade specified when the highest degree of control over the quality of workmanship, materials, installation,

FIGURE 5.12
Types of plywood.

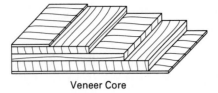

Veneer Core

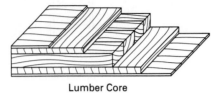

Lumber Core

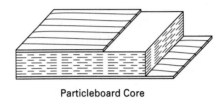

Particleboard Core

and execution of the design intent is required. Usually reserved for special projects, or feature areas within a project.

Custom Grade—The grade specified for most conventional architectural woodwork. This grade provides a well-defined degree of control over the quality of workmanship, materials, and installation of a project. The vast majority of all work produced is Custom Grade.

Economy Grade—The grade which defines the minimum expectation of quality, workmanship, materials, and installation within the scope of the standards.

Prevailing Grade—When the Quality Standards are referenced as part of the contract documents and no grade is specified, Custom Grade standards shall prevail.[8]

Types of Veneer Cuts

According to the AWI:

The manner by which a log segment is cut with relation to the annual rings will determine the appearance of the veneer. When sliced, the individual pieces of veneer, referred to as **leaves,** are kept in the order in which they are sliced, thus permitting a natural grain progression when assembled as veneer faces. The group of leaves from one slicing is called a **flitch** and is usually identified by a flitch number and the number of gross square feet of veneer it contains. The faces of the leaves with relation to their position in the log are identified as the *tight face* (toward the outside of the log) and the *loose face* (toward the inside or heart of the log).

During slicing the leaf is stressed on the loose face and compressed on the tight face. When this stress is combined with the natural variation in light refraction caused by the pores of the wood, the result is a difference in the human perception of color and tone between tight and loose faces.

Plain or (Flat Slicing) is the slicing method most often used to produce veneers for high-quality architectural woodworking. Slicing is done parallel to a line through the center of the log. A combination of cathedral and straight grain patterns result, with a natural progression of pattern from leaf to leaf. [emphasis added][9]

Walnut is usually cut by this method. Figure 5.13 shows different methods of slicing.

The AWI also details the following slicing methods:

Quarter Slicing or (Quarter Cut) simulates the quarter sawing process of solid lumber, roughly parallel to a radius line through the log segment. In many species the individual leaves are narrow as a result. A series of stripes is produced, varying in density and thickness from species to species. "Fleck" (sometimes called **flake**) is a characteristic of this slicing method in red and white oak.

Rift Slicing or (Rift Cut Veneers) are produced most often in red and white oak, rarely in other species. Note that rift veneers and rift sawn solid lumber are produced so differently that a "match" between rift veneers and rift sawn solid lumber is highly unlikely. In both cases the cutting is done slightly off the radius lines, minimizing the "fleck" (sometimes called flake) associated with quarter slicing.

Comb Grain is limited in availability, and is a select product of the rift process distinguished by tight, straight grain along the entire length of the veneer. Slight angle in the grain is allowed. Comb grain is restricted to red and white oak veneers.

Rotary. The log is center mounted on a lathe and "peeled" along the general path of the growth rings like unwinding a roll of paper, providing a generally bold, random appearance. Rotary cut veneers may vary in width, and matching at veneer joints is extremely difficult. Almost all softwood veneers are cut this way. Except for a specific design effect, rotary veneers are the least useful in fine architectural woodwork.[10]

Other decorative veneer patterns may be obtained by using the crotch, burl, or stump of the tree. The crotch pattern is always reversed so that the pointed part, or V, is up. Burl comes from a damaged area of the tree, where the tree has healed itself and grown over the injury; it is a very swirly pattern. Olive burl is frequently used in contemporary furniture.

Matching Between Adjacent Veneer Leaves

It is possible to achieve certain visual effects by the manner in which the leaves are arranged. As noted, rotary cut veneers are difficult to match; therefore, most matching is done with sliced veneers. The matching of adjacent veneer leaves must be specified. Special arrangements of leaves such as "diamond" and "box" matching are available. Consult

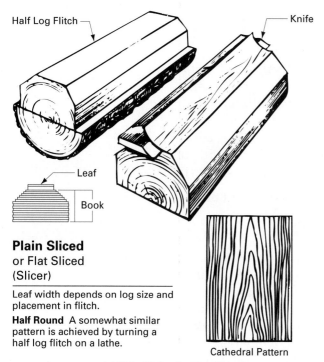

Plain Sliced
or Flat Sliced
(Slicer)

Leaf width depends on log size and placement in flitch.

Half Round A somewhat similar pattern is achieved by turning a half log flitch on a lathe.

Cathedral Pattern

(a) Plain Slicing (or Flat Slicing)

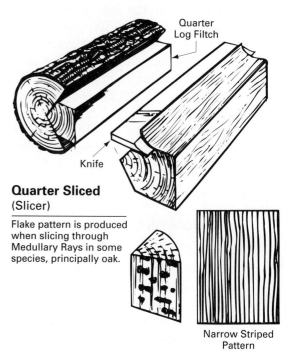

Quarter Sliced
(Slicer)

Flake pattern is produced when slicing through Medullary Rays in some species, principally oak.

Narrow Striped Pattern

(b) Quarter Slicing (or Quarter Cut)

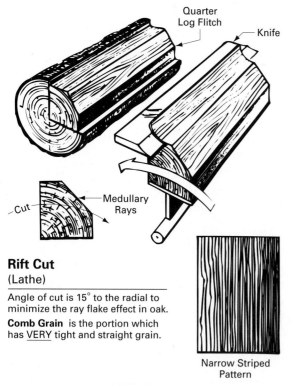

Rift Cut
(Lathe)

Angle of cut is 15° to the radial to minimize the ray flake effect in oak.

Comb Grain is the portion which has <u>VERY</u> tight and straight grain.

Narrow Striped Pattern

(c) Rift Slicing (or Rift Cut)

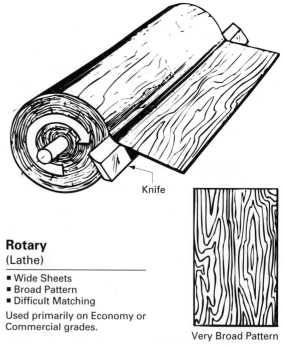

Rotary
(Lathe)

- Wide Sheets
- Broad Pattern
- Difficult Matching

Used primarily on Economy or Commercial grades.

Very Broad Pattern

(d) Rotary

FIGURE 5.13
Veneer cuts. (Courtesy of Architectural Woodwork Institute)

176

your woodworker for choices. The more common types are book matching, random matching, and end matching.

Book matching is the most commonly used match in the industry. Every other piece of veneer is turned over so adjacent pieces (leaves) are opened like the pages of a book (Figure 5.14).

Visual effect: Veneer joints match, creating a symmetrical pattern. Yields maximum continuity of grain. When sequenced panels are specified, prominent characteristics will ascend or descend across the match as the leaves progress from panel to panel (Figure 5.14a–f).

Barber Pole effect Book Match. Because the *tight* and *loose* faces alternate in adjacent pieces of veneer, they may accept stain differently, and this may result in a noticeable color variation in some species or flitches.

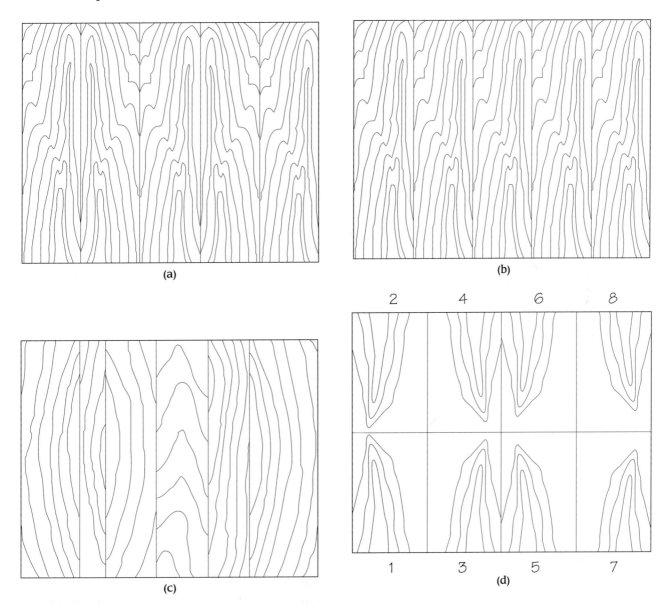

FIGURE 5.14
Matching of veneers. (Drawings courtesy of the Architectural Wood Institute) *Continued*

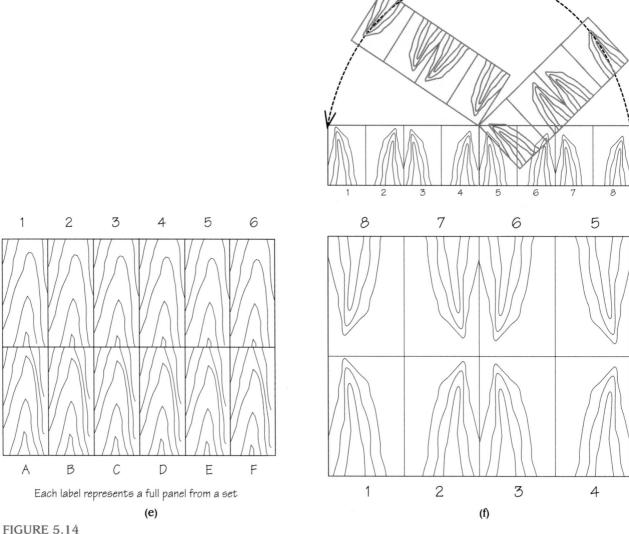

Each label represents a full panel from a set

(e)

(f)

FIGURE 5.14
Continued

Slip matching is often used with quarter-sliced and rift-sliced veneers. Adjoining leaves are placed (slipped out) in sequence, without turning, resulting in all the same face sides being exposed (Figure 5.14b).

Visual effect: Grain figure repeats but joints do not show grain match. NOTE: The lack of grain match at the joints can be desirable. The relatively straight grain patterns of quartered and rift veneers generally produce pleasing results and a uniformity of color because all faces have the same light refraction.

In *random matching*, veneer leaves are placed next to each other in a random order and orientation, producing a "board-by-board" effect in many species.

Visual effect: Casual or rustic appearance, as though individual boards from a random pile were applied to the product. Conscious effort is made to mismatch grain at joints (Figure 5.14c).

End matching is often used to extend the apparent length of available veneers for high wall panels and long conference tables. End matching occurs in two types: architectural end match in which leaves are individually book (or slip) matched, first end-to-end and then side-to-side, alternating end and side. Visual effect is the best for continuous-grain patterns for length as well as width (Figure 5.14d).

Continuous end match leaves are individually book (or slip) matched, and separate panels are stacked in sequenced order, either horizontally or vertically in the elevation. (Horizontal sequence is illustrated.)

Visual effect: Yields sequenced grain patterns for elevations, with a pleasing blend of figure horizontally or vertically (Figure 5.14e).

Panel end match leaves are book (or slip) matched on panel subassemblies, with sequenced subassemblies end matched, resulting in some modest cost savings on projects where applicable. The visual effect for most species is a pleasing, blended appearance and grain continuity (Figure 5.14f).

Matching within Individual Panel Faces

The individual leaves of veneer in a sliced flitch increase or decrease in width as the slicing progresses. Thus, if a number of panels are manufactured from a particular flitch, the number of veneer leaves per panel face will change as the flitch is utilized. The manner in which these leaves are "laid-up" within the panel requires specification, and is classified as follows:

Running Match. Each panel face is assembled from as many veneer leaves as necessary. This often results in a nonsymmetrical appearance, with some veneer leaves of unequal width. Often, the most economical method at the expense of aesthetics is the standard for Custom Grade and must be specified for other grades. Running matches are seldom "sequenced and numbered" for use as adjacent panels. Horizontal grain "match" or sequence cannot be expected. (See Figure 5.15a.)

Balance Match. Each panel face is assembled from veneer leaves of uniform width before edge trimming. Panels may contain an even or odd number of leaves, and distribution may change from panel to panel within a sequenced set. Although this method is the standard for Premium Grade it must be specified for other Grades, and it is the most common assembly method at moderate cost. (See Figure 5.15b.)

Balance and Center Match. Each panel face is assembled of an even number of veneer leaves of uniform width before edge trimming. Thus, there is a veneer joint in the center of the panel, producing horizontal symmetry. A small amount of figure is lost in the process. This match is considered by some to be the most pleasing assembly at a modest increase of cost over balance match.[11]

Figure 5.15c shows different types of matching within panel faces.

Methods of Matching Panels

Veneered panels used in casework or paneling in the same area may be matched to each other. This important component of the project must be carefully detailed and specified. The natural growth patterns of the

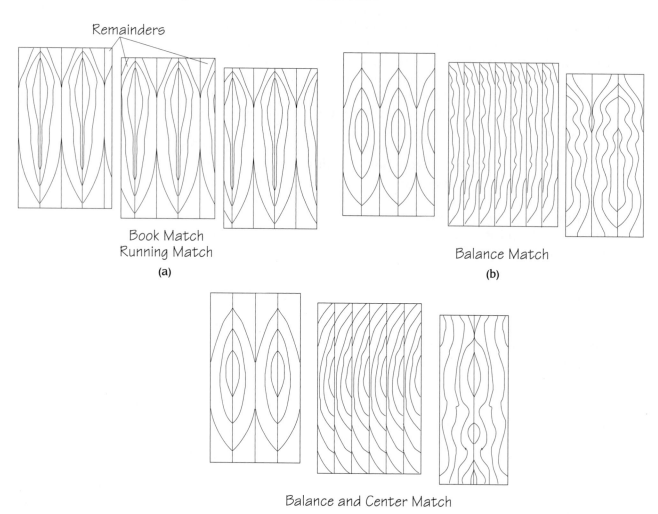

Remainders

Book Match
Running Match
(a)

Balance Match
(b)

Balance and Center Match
(c)

FIGURE 5.15
Matching within individual panel faces.
(Drawings courtesy of the Architectural Wood Institute)

tree will cause the figure on the sequential panels to ascend, descend, or show a "grain progression" as the eye moves from panel to panel. (These illustrations were developed in Imperial measure and have not been converted for this edition.) The four common methods are:

1. *Premanufactured sets—full width.* These are one step above stock plywood panels, usually made and warehoused in 4′ × 8′ or 4′ × 10′ sheets in sequenced sets. They may be produced from a single flitch or a part of a flitch, usually varying in number from 6 to 12 panels. If more than one set is required, matching between sets cannot be expected. Similarly, doors or components often cannot be fabricated from the same flitch materials, resulting in noticeable mismatch. This is often the most economical type of special panel product. (See Figure 5.16a.)

2. *Premanufactured sets—selectively reduced in width.* These are panels just like premanufactured sets—full width, usually made and warehoused in 4′ × 8′ and 4′ × 10′ sheets in sequenced sets. They are often selected for continuity, recut into modular widths, and numbered to achieve the appearance of greater symmetry. If more than one set is required, matching between the sets cannot be expected.

a - Pre-manufactured Sets - Full Width

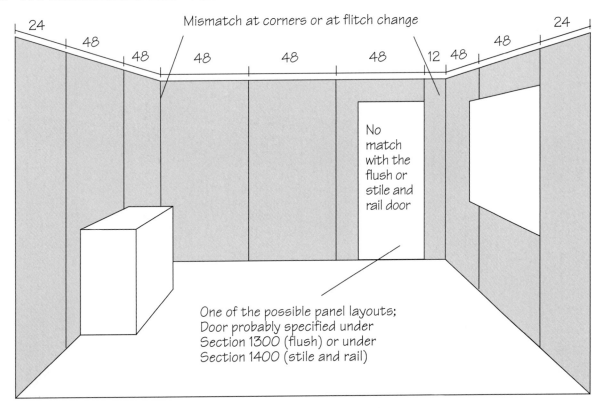

Mismatch at corners or at flitch change

24   48   48   48   48   48   12   48   48   24

No match with the flush or stile and rail door

One of the possible panel layouts;
Door probably specified under
Section 1300 (flush) or under
Section 1400 (stile and rail)

b - Pre-manufactured Sets - Selectively Reduced in Width

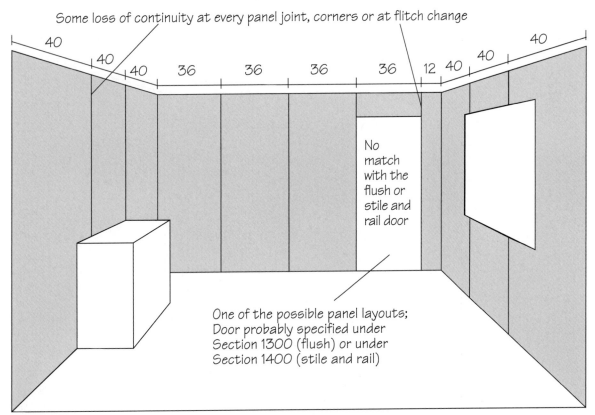

Some loss of continuity at every panel joint, corners or at flitch change

40   40   40   36   36   36   36   12   40   40   40

No match with the flush or stile and rail door

One of the possible panel layouts;
Door probably specified under
Section 1300 (flush) or under
Section 1400 (stile and rail)

FIGURE 5.16
Matching of panels within an area. (Drawings courtesy of the Architectural Wood Institute) *Continued*

181

c - Sequence-Matched Uniform Size Set

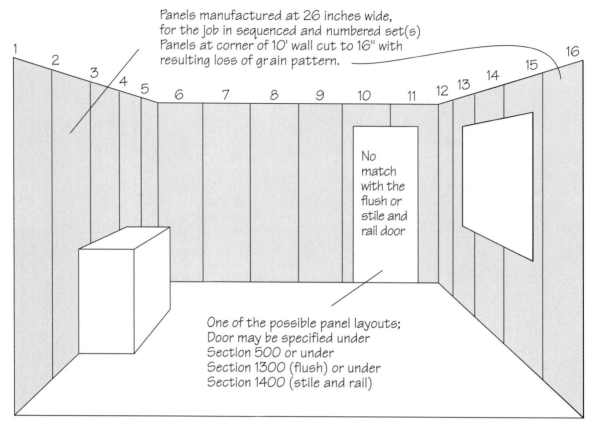

Panels manufactured at 26 inches wide,
for the job in sequenced and numbered set(s)
Panels at corner of 10' wall cut to 16" with
resulting loss of grain pattern.

1 2 3 4 5 6 7 8 9 10 11 12 13 14 15 16

No match with the flush or stile and rail door

One of the possible panel layouts;
Door may be specified under
Section 500 or under
Section 1300 (flush) or under
Section 1400 (stile and rail)

d - Blueprint-Matched Panels and Components

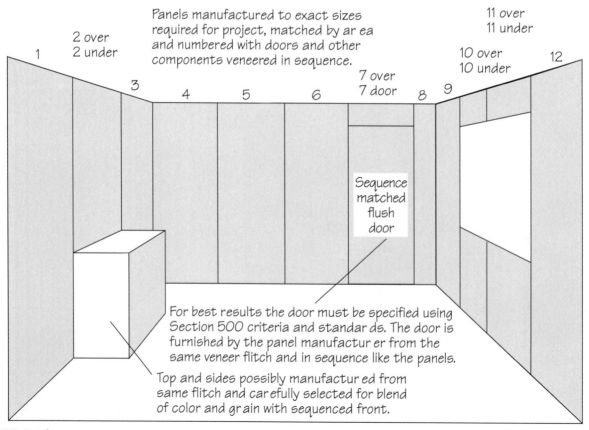

Panels manufactured to exact sizes
required for project, matched by area
and numbered with doors and other
components veneered in sequence.

2 over 2 under

1 3 4 5 6

7 over 7 door

8 9

10 over 10 under

11 over 11 under

12

Sequence matched flush door

For best results the door must be specified using
Section 500 criteria and standards. The door is
furnished by the panel manufacturer from the
same veneer flitch and in sequence like the panels.

Top and sides possibly manufactured from
same flitch and carefully selected for blend
of color and grain with sequenced front.

FIGURE 5.16
Continued

182

Similarly, doors or components often cannot be fabricated from the same flitch materials, resulting in noticeable mismatch. (See Figure 5.16b.)

3. *Sequence matched uniform size set.* These sets are manufactured for a specific installation to a uniform panel width and height. If more than one flitch is necessary to produce the required number of panels, similar flitches will be used. This type of panel matching is best used when panel layout is uninterrupted and when the design permits the use of equal-width panels. Some sequence will be lost if trimming is required to meet field conditions. Doors and components within the wall cannot usually be matched to the panels. Moderate in cost, sequenced uniform panels offer a good compromise between price and aesthetics. (See Figure 5.16c.)

4. *Blueprint-matched panel and components.* This method of panel matching achieves maximum grain continuity, since all panels, doors, and other veneered components are made to the exact sizes required and in exact veneer sequence. If possible, flitches should be selected that will yield sufficient veneer to complete a prescribed area or room, if more than one flitch is needed, flitch transition should be accomplished at the least noticeable predetermined location. This method requires careful site coordination and relatively long lead times. Panels cannot be manufactured until site conditions can be accurately measured and detailed. This panel matching method is more expensive and expresses veneering in its most impressive manner.[12] (See Figure 5.16d.)

Rooms treated with paneling always produce a feeling of permanency. Architectural paneling is as different from ready-made paneling as a custom-made Rolls Royce is from an inexpensive production car. Ready-made paneling is discussed later in this chapter.

Fire-Retardant Panel Flame Spread Classification

The various codes utilize flame spread classifications for wood and other materials. It is the responsibility of the specifier to determine which elements, if any, of the woodworking require special treatment to meet local codes. Generally fire codes limit untreated wood trim to 10 percent of the wall area. If over 10 percent, wood trim must be treated. In most codes, the panel products used to fabricate casework and furniture are not regulated. For more detailed information, please refer to the AWI publication *Fire Code Summary* and your local code book. Flame spread ratings are as follows:

Class I or A   0–25
Class II or B   26–75
Class III or C   76–200

Flame Spread Factors

A. **Core**—The fire rating of the core material determines the rating of the assembled panel. Fire-retardant veneered panels must have a fire-retardant core. Particleboard core is available with a Class I

(Class A) rating and can be used successfully with veneer or rated high-pressure decorative laminate faces. Medium density fiberboard (MDF) is currently available with a fire rating in some markets.

B. Face—Some existing building codes, except where locally amended, provide that facing materials 1/28″ or thinner are not considered in determining the flame spread rating of the panel. If state and local codes move toward adoption of the International Building Code provisions, it is possible that the 1/28″ exemption may not be available.

Note: In localities where basic panel building codes have been amended, it is the responsibility of the specifier to determine whether the application of the facing material specified will meet the code.

Traditionally, face veneers are not required to be fire-retardant treated, and such treatment will adversely affect the finishing process.[13]

There are several methods of installing panels for acoustical control. The panels may be floated or raised, or batten mouldings of wood, metal, or plastic may also be used.

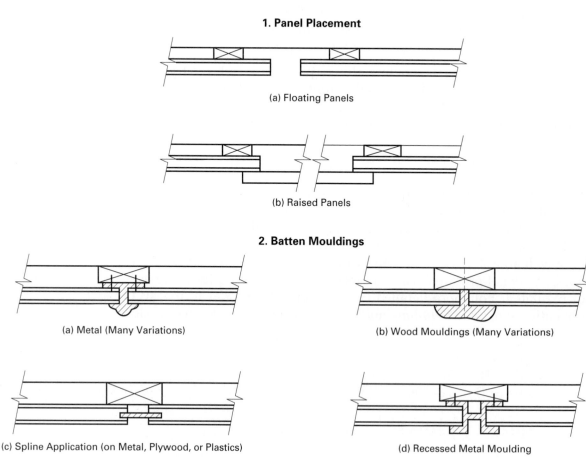

1. Panel Placement

(a) Floating Panels

(b) Raised Panels

2. Batten Mouldings

(a) Metal (Many Variations)

(b) Wood Mouldings (Many Variations)

(c) Spline Application (on Metal, Plywood, or Plastics)

(d) Recessed Metal Moulding

FIGURE 5.17
Panel installation for acoustic control.

Finishing

The Architectural Woodwork Institute has specific standards for factory finishing of woodwork, and its publication entitled *Architectural Woodwork Quality Standards* should be consulted.

PREFINISHED PLYWOOD

Prefinished plywood paneling varies from 1/4 to 1/2 inch thick. Standard panel size is 4 × 8 feet but panels are also available in 7- and 10-foot heights. The face of the plywood is grooved in random widths to simulate wood strips. This feature also hides the joining, where each panel is **butted** up to the next, because outside edges are beveled at the same angle as the grooves. The finish on prefinished plywood paneling is clear acrylic over a stained surface.

Some plywood paneling features a wood grain reproduction on the plywood or a paper overlay applied to **lauan mahogany** plywood and then protected with an oven-baked topcoat.

Installation

As with all wood products, paneling should be stored in the room it will be installed in for 24 hours to condition for humidity and temperature. Paneling may be applied directly to the stud framing, but it is safer, from a fire hazard point of view, to install it over gypsum board. A 1/4-inch sound-deadening board used as a backing decreases sound transmission. Nails or adhesive may be used to install the panels. If nails are used, they may be color coated when exposed fasteners are acceptable, or countersunk and filled with colored putty.

Maintenance

Prefinished plywood panels require frequent dusting in order to prevent a buildup of soil, which dulls the finish. Each manufacturer supplies instructions for maintenance of its particular product, and these should be followed.

PARTICLEBOARD

Industrial Grade Particleboard Core has wood particles of various sizes that are bonded together with a synthetic resin or binder under heat and pressure.

Medium-density Industrial Particleboard is used in the broadest applications of architectural woodwork. It is especially well suited as a substrate for high-quality veneers and decorative laminates.

When used as panels without any surface plies, the product is referred to as particleboard. *When used as an inner core with outer wood veneers, the panel is referred to as particle core plywood.*

Industrial particleboard is commercially classified by "density," which is measured by the weight per cubic foot of the panel product.

- Low Density (LD series) = generally less than 640 kg per m^3 (40 pounds per ft^3)
- Medium Density (M series) = generally between 640–800 kg per m^3 (40–50 pounds per ft^3)
- High Density (H series) = generally above 800 kg per m^3 (50 pounds per ft^3)

Some medium-density industrial particleboard is bonded with resins more resistant to swelling when exposed to moisture. . .

Medium-density Fiberboard (MDF) core has wood particles reduced to fibers in a moderate-pressure steam vessel, combined with a resin, and bonded together under heat and pressure. Due to the finer texture of the fibers used in manufacturing medium-density fiberboard (MDF), it is smoother than medium-density particleboard. The uniform texture and density of the fibers create a homogenous panel that is very useful as a substrate for paint, thin overlay materials, veneers, and decorative laminates. MDF is among the most stable of the mat-formed panel products. *When used as an inner core with outer wood veneers, the panel is referred to as MDF core plywood.*[13]

Marlite Displawall is a slotted panel merchandising system that can be used to cost effectively and quickly establish a retail environment. The panels are available in a wide range of sizes and groove configurations and may be horizontally or vertically oriented. Custom panel sizes and configurations may be specified as well. Groove insert, trim, and accessory options are abundant and help create a professional, finished appearance. Marlite has the largest manufacturing commitment in the slotted merchandising wall panel industry.

Installation

Displawall panels may be applied directly to open studs or over drywall. Care must be taken to prevent moisture penetration through the walls.[14]

HARDBOARD

Hardboard is a high-quality panel manufactured from specially engineered fibers that are compressed under heat and pressure. These panels are produced by a "wet" or "dry" process.

Hardboard sheets or planks consist of a hardboard base that is textured during the pressing process, usually in a wood grain pattern. A dark base coat is then placed on top of the base. This layer gives the dark color to the V-joints. A light precision coat is applied next; it does not cover the V-joints. This precision coat is grained and coated with a melamine topcoat that is baked on and is resistant to most household chemicals and staining agents such as cosmetics and crayons. Tape should not be applied to the panel surface because it may damage the surface.

Hardboard paneling is also available in 4′ × 8′ sheets and may utilize harmonizing mouldings between panels or may be butted. Pigmented vertical grooves simulate joints of lumber planks, and edges are also pigmented to match face grooves and to conceal butt joints. Hardboard panels are not used below grade, over masonry walls, in bathrooms, or in any area of high humidity.

When hardboard is covered with a photo reproduction of wood, it does not have the depth or richness of real wood and is probably best used for inexpensive installations where price and durability are more important than the appearance of real wood. Because this paneling is not wood veneered but rather a reproduction, the same manufacturing methods may be used for solid colors or patterns. Fast-food restaurants and many businesses requiring the feature of durability and easy cleaning use Marlite plank. The plank may be used vertically, horizontally, or diagonally, provided that furring strips have been installed over any sound, solid substrate.

Some hardboard is available in a stamped grille-type pattern or with holes. The grille types are framed with wood and used for dividers. The perforated board is useful for hanging or storing items. Special hooks and supports are available for this purpose and are easily installed and removed for adjustment.

Installation

Thicknesses of hardboard vary from 1/8 and 3/16 of an inch to 1/4 of an inch. The 1/8-inch and 3/16-inch thicknesses must be installed over a solid backing, such as gypsum board. Panels are glued or nailed to the substrate.

Maintenance

To remove surface accumulation such as dust and grease, a lint-free soft cloth dampened with furniture polish containing no waxes or silicones may be used. More stubborn accumulations may require wiping with a soft cloth dampened in a solution of lukewarm water and a mild detergent. The hardboard must be wiped dry with a clean, dry cloth immediately following this procedure. (An inconspicuous area or scrap paneling should be used for experimental cleaning.)

DECORATIVE LAMINATE

Decorative laminate is often mistakenly referred to as Formica®, but that is the brand name of a manufacturer of decorative laminate. Decorative laminates for walls are the same as for floors (see page 108). Laminates will not promote the growth of bacteria.

The vertical surface of decorative laminate may be 0.050 inch (general purpose) or 0.030 inch (vertical surface). The 0.030 inch, vertical-surface type is not recommended on surfaces exceeding 24 inches in width. Decorative laminate for walls is often installed at the job site.

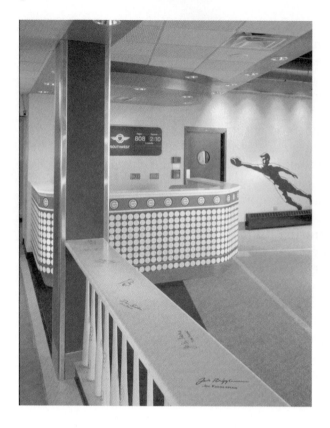

Balancing or backing laminates are used to give structural balance and **dimensional stability.** They are placed on the reverse side of the substrate to inhibit moisture absorption through the back surface.

Wilsonart Metalaminates™ consist of 13 dazzling surfaces in colors that duplicate all types of reflective metals. (See Figure 5.18.)

There are other specialty types of decorative laminate. Where anti-static properties are required, a standard-grade laminate is available. Most manufacturers of high-pressure decorative laminate (**HPDL**) produce a fire-resistant type that, when applied with approved adhesives to a fire-resistant core, results in wall paneling with Class I or A flame spread rating.

Installation

When decorative laminates are to be used on a wall, 3/4-inch hardwood-faced plywood or particleboard should be used as a core. The use of an expansion-type joint is suggested. To permit free panel movement and to avoid visible fastenings, the AWI recommends that panels be hung on the walls, utilizing metal panel clips or interlocking wood wall cleats.

Maintenance

To clean the surface, use a damp cloth or sponge and a mild soap or detergent. Difficult stains such as coffee or tea can be removed using a mild household cleaner and baking soda, mixing to achieve a paste consistency. Use a stiff nylon-bristle brush, scrubbing (approx. 15–20 strokes) the affected area. Do not scrub so as to mar (damage, scratch) the surface finish. If spots remain, an all-purpose cleaner or bathroom cleaner, such as Formula 409®, Glass Plus®, or Mr. Clean®, should be used.

For stubborn stains, a paste of baking soda and water should be applied to the stain with a soft bristle brush. The last resort is undiluted household bleach such as Clorox®, followed by a clean-water rinse. Use of abrasive cleansers or special cleansers should be avoided because they may contain abrasives, acids, or alkalines.

Metallic laminates other than solid polished brass may be cleaned as described previously. The surface of metallic laminates, however, should always be wiped completely dry with a clean soft cloth after washing. Stubborn smudges may be removed with a dry cloth and a thin, clean oil. For solid polished brass surfaces, only glass cleaners free of petroleum products should be used. The surface may be touched up with Fill 'n Glaze™ and a good grade of automobile wax. The manufacturer's instructions must be followed carefully during application.

PORCELAIN ENAMEL

Porcelain enamel is baked-on 28-gauge steel, laminated to 3/16 to 21/32 of an inch gypsum board or hardboard. It comes in many colors and finishes for use in high-abuse public areas such as hospitals and food processing and preparation areas. It is also available with writing board surfaces that double as projection screens. Widths are from 2 to 4 feet, and lengths are from 6 to 12 feet. Weight varies from 1.60 to 2.7 pounds per square foot. Porcelain enamel is also used for toilet partitions in public restrooms.

Maintenance

Maintenance is the same as that for ceramic tile.

GLASS

Glass, one of our most useful products, is also one of the oldest (it was first used about 4000 B.C). In ancient times, formed pieces of colored glass were considered as valuable as precious stones. In the past, glass was used mainly for windows, permitting light and sun to enter a home or building.

Glass can open up a space and enclose it at the same time. Glass is transformational in its ability to change the atmosphere of a space by letting in light, by extending interior visual horizons. . . . Today, as glass design evolves, innovative textured glass products are presenting new possibilities for reflecting the focus of architecture in the 21st century.[15]

Skyline Design has protective coating, Etch Sealer™, on all its etched glass products that makes them virtually maintenance free.

In response to architects' requests, Skyline created Fosil-Glas™, a collection of 10 organic textured designs available in clear, frosted or color finishes. . . . The translucent texture glass collection is created using a cold process that produces the beauty and texture of kiln glass much more cost effectively. . . .

Textured glass is being used for feature walls, frameless doors, door lites, side lites, conference rooms, privacy panels, partitions,

FIGURE 5.19
An interesting wall of
etched glass from Skyline
Design. Client eGM, San
Francisco. Design by
Ottolini Booth & Associates
Architects. Photo: John
Sutton. (Photo courtesy of
Skyline Design)

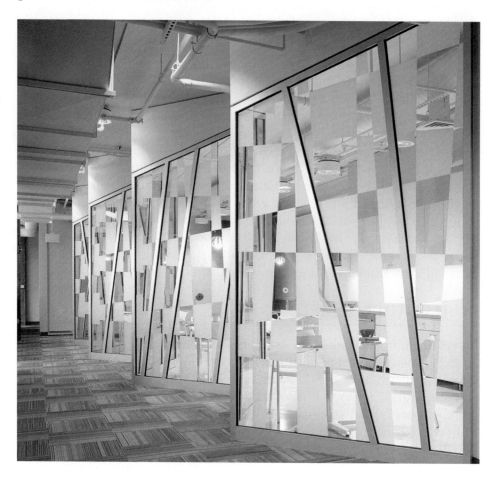

transom panels, partition walls, shelving, stair rails and as art with great design impact.[16] (See Figure 5.19.)

UltraGlas® textures create natural diffusion, which provides privacy without restricting light transmission. UltraGlas is kiln-formed embossed glass that is decorative and functional. It is available in many standard textures, designs, patterns, and colors; it can also be custom created to incorporate theme elements and color palettes. UltraGlas may be used for interior or exterior applications, and requires very little maintenance.[17] Of course, one disadvantage of glass is that it is breakable, but there are products specially made to reduce this problem.

There are three methods of manufacturing glass. The first is sheet or window glass, in which the molten glass is drawn out and both sides are subjected to open flame. This type of glass, which is not treated after manufacture, can show distortions and waviness. The second, plate glass, has both surfaces ground and polished, which renders its surfaces virtually plane and parallel. The third, float glass, is a more recently developed and less expensive process of manufacturing; molten glass is floated over molten metal and is used interchangeably with plate glass.

Insulating glass consists of two or three sheets of glass separated by either a dehydrated air space or an inert gas-filled space, together with a **desiccant.** Insulating glass limits heat transference and, in some areas of the country, may be required by the building codes in all new construction for energy conservation purposes. It also helps eliminate the problem of condensation caused by a wide difference in outside and inside temperatures.

There are various types of safety glass. The one with which we are most familiar is **tempered glass,** the kind used for windshields, in entry doors, or shower doors. In tempered glass, a heavy blow breaks the glass into small grains rather than sharp, jagged slivers. Another type of tempered glass, which has a wire mesh incorporated into its construction, can break under a blow but does not shatter.

Laminated glass can control sound, glare, heat . . . , and light transmission. It offers security and safety through high resistance to breakage and penetration. In interior areas where transparency is desired, laminated acoustical glass is effective in reducing sound transmission. When exterior sounds (traffic, airplanes, etc.) are present and distracting, laminated acoustical glass may be used. Acoustical glass may be clear or colored.

Another form of glass used for energy conservation is a laminated glass with a vinyl interlayer that, depending on the color of the interlayer, may absorb or transmit light in varying degrees. The tinted glass may have a bronze, gray, green, blue, silver, or gold appearance, and these tints cut down on glare in a manner similar to sunglasses or the tinted glass in an automobile. Where 24-hour protection is required, such as in jewelry stores, banks, and detention areas, a security glass with a high-tensile polyvinyl butryal inner layer is effective. There are even bullet-resistant glasses on the market.

For those involved in historical restorations, Bendheim Corporation offers Restoration Glass®. This glass is handmade using the original cylinder method, yet the glass easily meets today's tougher building codes. It is available in two levels of distortion: full, for thicker and more distorting effects; and light, for thinner and less distorting effects. Restoration Glass is available in laminated form if safety glass is required.

The Nippon Electric GlassCo. Ltd. has NeoClad, a product manufactured by the crystallization of specially formulated sheet glass. In the manufacturing process, the glass gains remarkable strength, a soft color, and a smooth high-gloss surface. The edges can be shaped with various types of bevels on the front or back. NeoClad is for both interior and exterior use and is extremely resistant to environmental pollution and graffiti.

Office configurations are always changing. Transwall is the manufacturer of ZWall, movable floor-to-ceiling and architectural (relocatable) wall systems. This is a revolutionary movable wall concept that will open new doors for business with its flexibility, durability, and individuality. ZWall has solid design, nearly endless panel options, and the ability to change and grow with needs (Figure 5.20).

GLASS TILE

ArchiTextures may be used alone, for a sophisticated, neutral architectural effect, or as backgrounds for more dimensional textures and/or designs. These textures occur on one side of the glass, leaving the other side almost smooth. Most of the time, due to lighting conditions, both sides of the glass will appear the same—there is no "wrong" side of the glass.[18]

The thickness is from 1/8″ to 3/4″.

FIGURE 5.20
Easily demountable walls
such as these office dividers
from Transwall, can be
changed into another
configuration. (Photo
courtesy of Transwall)

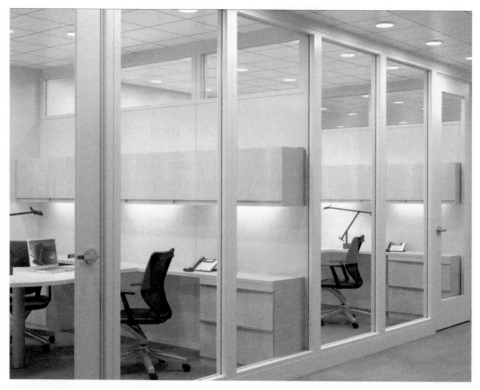

Installation

Glass tiles should not be used in areas where extreme rapid temperature changes may occur. Glass and the coatings can withstand extreme temperatures but only when they are achieved by uniform and gradual heating or cooling. As an example, cold glass tile should not be exposed to a hot shower. UltraGlas has specific recommendations as to the recommended setting materials which provide the best and most flexible bond between the substrate and UltraGlas in both wet and dry areas. Unlike some other materials, complete coverage of the UltraGlas tiles and the substrate is mandatory. The entire tile back surface should be completely back-buttered with a non-toothed plastic trowel or spreader. Much care should be taken not to scrape or mar the tile/s finish in any way.[19]

MIRROR

The mirrors used 2000 years ago by the Egyptians, Romans, and Greeks were highly polished thin sheets of bronze. Today, many of these metal mirrors may be seen in museums. The method of backing glass with a metallic film was known to the Romans, but it was not until 1507 that the first glass mirrors were made in Venice. Plate glass was invented in France in 1691, enabling larger pieces of glass to be manufactured. The shapes of mirrors used in various periods of design should be studied by interior designers, such as those of Robert and James Adam. Mirrors are no longer just accessories hung on the wall for utilitarian or decorative purposes. Walls are often completely covered with these highly reflective surfaces.

Quality mirrors are made of float glass and are silvered on the back to obtain a highly reflective quality. Also used in certain circumstances are two-way mirrors, which permit viewing from one side but not from the other (they appear to be an ordinary mirror). These two-way mirrors have many uses, such as in apartment doors, child observation areas, department stores, banks, and prison security areas.

Mirrors used on wall installations may be clear and brightly reflective or grayed or bronze hued. The latter are not as bright, but do not noticeably distort color values. The surface may also be antiqued, which produces a smoky, shadowy effect. Mirrored walls always enlarge a room and may be used to correct a size deficiency or to duplicate a prized possession, such as a candelabra or chandelier. Mirrored walls may also display all sides of a piece of sculpture or double the light available in a room.

Mirrors are available for wall installations in many sizes, ranging from large sheets to small mosaic mirrors on sheets similar to mosaic tile. Sometimes a perfect reflection is not necessary and the mirrors may be in squares, **convex** or **concave**, acid etched, engraved, or beveled.

Mirror Terminology

The following terminology was provided by the North American Association of Mirror Manufacturers.

Acid etch— A process of producing a specific design or lettering on glass, prior to silvering but cutting into the glass with a combination of acids. This process may involve either a frosted surface treatment or a deep etch. This process can also be done on regular glass.

Antique mirror—A decorative mirror in which the silver has been treated to create a smoky or shadowy effect. The antique look is often heightened by applying a veining on the silvered side in any one of more of a variety of colors and designs.

Backing paint—The final protective coating applied on the back of the mirror, over copper, to protect the silver from deterioration.

Concave mirror—Surface is slightly curved inward and tends to magnify reflected items or images.

Convex mirror—Surface is slightly curved outward to increase the area that is reflected. Generally used for safety or security surveillance purposes.

Edge work—Among numerous terms and expressions defining types of edge finishing, the five in most common usage are as follows:

Clean-cut edge—Natural edge produced when glass is cut. It should not be left exposed in installation.

Ground edge—Grinding removes the raw cut of glass, leaving a smooth satin finish.

Seamed edge—Sharp edges are removed by an abrasive belt.

Polished edge—Polishing removes the raw cut of glass to give a smooth-surfaced edge. A polished edge is available in two basic contours.

Beveled edge—A tapered polished edge, varying from 1/4 of an inch to a maximum of 1 1/4 inches thick, produced by machine in a rectangular or circular shape. Other shapes or ovals may be beveled by hand, but the result is inferior to machine bevel. Standard width of bevel is generally half an inch (Figure 5.21).

FIGURE 5.21
Glass bevels.

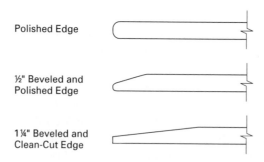

Polished Edge

½" Beveled and
Polished Edge

1¼" Beveled and
Clean-Cut Edge

Electro-copper-plating—Process of copper-plating by electrolytic deposition of copper on the back of the silver film, to protect the silver and to assure good adherence of the backing paint.

Engraving—The cutting of a design on the back or face of a mirror, usually accomplished by hand on an engraving lathe.

Finger pull—An elongated slot cut into the glass by a wheel, so that a mirrored door or panel, for instance, may be moved to one side.

First-surface mirror—A mirror produced by deposition of reflective metal on the front surface of glass, usually under vacuum. Its principal use is as an automobile rear-view mirror or transparent mirror.

Framed mirror—Mirror placed in a frame that is generally made of wood, metal, or composition material and equipped for hanging.

Hole—Piercing of a mirror, usually ½ inch in diameter and generally accomplished by a drill. Often employed in connection with installations involving rosettes.

Mitre cutting—The cutting of straight lines by use of a wheel on the back or face of a mirror for design purposes. Available in both satin and polished finishes.

Rosette—Hardware used for affixing a mirror to a wall. A decorative rose-shaped button used in several places on the face of a mirror.

Sandblasting—Engraving or cutting designs on glass by a stream of sand, usually projected by air.

Shadowbox mirror—Mirror bordered or framed at an angle on some or all sides by other mirrors, creating multiple reflections of an image.

Stock-sheet mirrors—Mirrors of varying sizes over 10 square feet, and up to 7 square feet, from which all types of custom mirrors are cut. Normally packed 800 to 1,000 square feet to a case.

Transparent mirror—A first surface mirror with a thin film of reflective coating. To ensure most efficient use, the light intensity on the viewer's side of the mirror must be significantly less than on the subject side. Under such a condition, the viewer can see through the mirror as through a transparent glass, while the subject looks into a mirror.

Installation

Both mastic and mechanical devices, such as clips or rosettes, should be used to install a mirror properly. Clips are usually of polished chrome and are placed around the outside edges. Rosettes are clear plastic fasteners and require a hole to be drilled several inches in from the edge so the mirror will accept the fastening screws and rosettes. Because of the fragile quality of mirrors, their use should be limited to areas where the likelihood of breakage is minimal.

CERAMIC TILE

Ceramic tile is frequently used on walls when an easily cleaned, waterproof, and durable surface is desired. One use of ceramic tile is as a **backsplash** in the kitchen or as a countertop. When ceramic tile is used for these purposes, the grout may be sealed by use of a commercial sealer or by using a lemon oil furniture polish. Ceramic tile is also used for the surrounds of showers and bathtubs and for bathroom walls in general (see Chapter 10). These three uses are probably the most common ones, but ceramic tile may also be used on the walls in foyers and hallways—plain, patterned, or displaying a logo—and as a heat-resistant material around fireplaces and stoves. Ceramic tile for countertops is discussed in Chapter 9.

If walls are completely covered with ceramic tile, there will be no need for trim pieces. In bathrooms or kitchens, however, or anyplace where tiling will not be continued from wall to wall or from ceiling to floor, trim pieces must be added. The type of tile trim used will vary with the method of installation. A thin-set installation will require a surface bullnose. With the thick-set method, a separate piece of trim is used to finish off the edge and corners (Figure 5.22).

A bullnose for thick-set installations has an overhanging curved piece, whereas a bullnose for thin-set installations is the same thickness as the surrounding tiles but has a curved finished edge. For bath and shower installations, angle trims for the top and inside edges are used, and for walls meeting the floor, a cove is used (Figure 5.22).

One of the more recent decorative treatments with ceramic tile installations is adding borders, accent tiles, and **listellos**, which are narrow mouldings or bands. These can be used anywhere but are mainly used in bathrooms or in kitchens as backsplashes.

The TCNA offers the following installation advice:

> Use of wall-washer and cove type lighting, where the lights are located either at the wall/ceiling interface, or mounted directly on the wall, are popular techniques of producing dramatic room lighting effects. When proper backing surfaces, installation materials and methods, and location of light fixtures are not carefully coordinated, these lighting techniques may produce shadows and undesirable effects with ceramic tiles. Similar shadows are created from side lighting interior walls and floors when light shines at that angle through windows and doors.[20]

Installation of Ceramic, Metal, and Mirror Tile

Because of the force of gravity, mortar cement cannot be troweled directly onto the wall without sagging. To prevent this sagging, a metal lath, similar to the one used for a plaster wall, is attached to the solid backing and then troweled with mortar. The metal lath acts as a stabilizing force.

FIGURE 5.22
Wall trim from Crossville.
(Reproduced courtesy of
Crossville Ceramics)

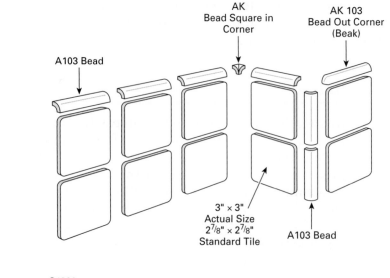

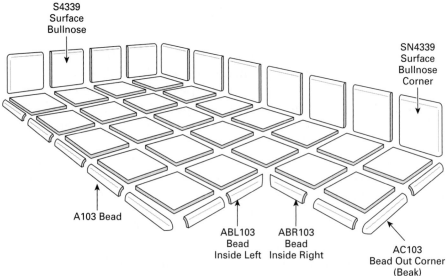

The backing may be wood, plaster, masonry, or gypsum board. This procedure is equivalent to the thick-set method of floor installation. For wall use over gypsum board, plaster, or other smooth surfaces, an organic adhesive may be used. This adhesive should be water resistant for bath and shower areas (see Table 5.2).

The Handbook of Ceramic Tile Installation, available from the TCNA, contains the nationally accepted guidelines for tile installation, even for materials other than ceramic tile.

METAL

In the latter part of the 19th century, during the Victorian era, stamped tin panels were used on ceilings and **dadoes.** The dadoes even had a molded chair rail incorporated into them. (See Chapter 6 for more details on stamped metal.) Though stamped metal is used primarily for ceilings, it can be used on walls.

Crossville's Questech® metal floor borders are suitable for kitchens, entrance halls, showers, and other wet areas of the house.

Simplest methods are indicated; those for heavier services are acceptable. Very large or heavy tiles may require special setting methods. Consult ceramic tile manufacturer.

Service Requirements	Wall Type (numbers refer to Handbook method numbers)					
	Masonry or Concrete	Page	Wood Studs	Page	Metal Studs	Page
Commercial Construction—Dry or limited water exposure: dairies, breweries, kitchens	W202	41	W223	42	W223	42
	W221*	42	W231	44	W241	44
	W223	42	W243	45	W242, W243	45
			W244	46	W244	46
			W246	47	W246	47
Commercial Construction—Wet: gang showers, tubs, showers, laundries	W202	41	W231	44	W241	44
	W211	43	W244	46	W244	46
	W221*	42	W246	47	W246	47
			B411	50	B411	50
			B414	52	B414, B415	52
					B425	51
					B426	53
Residential & Light Construction—Dry or limited water exposure: kitchens and toilet rooms, commercial dry area interiors and decoration			W222*, W223	42	W222*	42
	W221*	42	W243	45	W242, W243	45
	W223	42	W244, W245	46	W244, W245	46
			W246, W247	47	W246, W247	47
			B430	49	B430	49
Residential & Light Construction—Wet: tub enclosures and showers	W202	41	W222*, W223	42	W222*	42
	W211	43	W244, W245	46	W241	44
	W223	42	W246	47	W244, W245	46
			B412	50	W246	47
			B413	49	B412	50
			B415	52	B413	49
			B419	51	B415	52
			B420	53	B419	51
			B421, B422	54	B420	53
			B425	51	B421, B422	54
			B426	53	B425	51
					B426	53
Exterior (See notes on page 41.)	W201, W202	41	W231	44	W241 (Refer to page 9.)	44

*Use these details where there may be dimensional instability and possible cracks developing in, or foreign coating (paint, etc.) on, the structural wall since these details include a cleavage membrane (15 lb. felt or polyethylene) between the wall surface and tile installation.

Source: Reproduced with permission of the Tile Council of North America.

TABLE 5.2
Wall Tiling Installation Guide

Perforated metal was developed for use in ventilation grilles, drainage grates, and similar applications. Today it has many interior uses. It can be used instead of a solid wall, providing a feeling of privacy yet with a slight see-through quality. A partition made from perforated metal gives a sense of separation without the thickness of a solid wall. Another use is metal for the doors of wood-framed kitchen cabinets. Perforated metal is made by stamping out holes of various sizes and shapes. The perforations can form almost any small geometrical pattern.

FIGURE 5.23
The AlphaSorb™ Fabric
Wrapped Wall Panel is class
1 fire-rated, offers a variety
of colors, edge details, as
well as installation options.
(Photo courtesy of
Acoustical Solutions, Inc.)

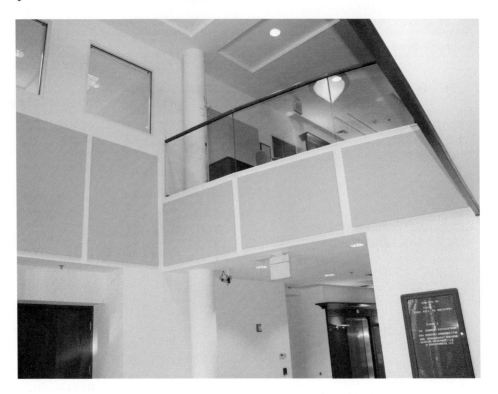

A similar material is expanded metal, which, because of the manufacturing process, is always diamond shaped.

ACOUSTICAL PANELS

Several manufacturers produce a mineral fiberboard or fiberglass panel that, when covered with fabric, absorbs sound and provides an attractive and individually designed environment. Because of the textured, porous surface of acoustical panels and the absorbent substrate, sound is absorbed rather than bounced back into the room. These panels may also be used as tack boards for lightweight pictures and graphics. In open-plan office areas, different colors of acoustical panels can be used to direct the flow of traffic through an open office and to differentiate between work areas. In addition to the acoustical qualities of these panels, there are two other beneficial features: (1) The panels are fire retardant, and (2) when installed on perimeter walls, there is a sound-insulating factor that varies with the thickness of board used.

The acoustical panels may take the form of appliques in sizes of 2 × 4 feet or 2 × 6 feet, or they may cover the wall completely, in panel sizes of 24 or 30 inches × 9 feet.

Vinyl- or fabric-faced acoustical panels may be designed for various types of installation, so for use on an existing wall, only one side needs to be covered. For open-plan landscapes, both surfaces are covered to absorb sound from both sides. Some panels are covered on the two side edges for butted installation, whereas another portable type is wrapped on all surfaces and edges.

Fabri-*Trak*® Wall System utilizes fabric as an architectural finish. It is a cost effective tool for creating and enhancing interior environments with function, form, color and texture. Panels are created per specification—shape, width and height. The subsurfaces (acoustical, rigid, tackable, nailable or combinations) are installed within the perimeter of the 3/8″ deep framework and secured between the fabric and the substrate. Fabric is then stretched over the framework. A patented tool inserts the fabric border through the inlet jaws and locks it into the framework's hidden storage channel, leaving a perfectly crisp, smooth, finished edge.[21]

Puff Panels: Pillow-like panels are created with one layer of 3/8″ rigid subsurface for an effective sound barrier and an extra layer of acoustical FABRI-FILL™ to provide dimension, softness and additional quietude. Columns: The Fabri-*Trak* System may be **kerfed** for radiused surface designs such as columns, arches, circles, etc. Obtrusive columns may be fabric covered and blended into the total design concept. [emphasis added][22]

See Figure 5.23 for an example of Fabri-*Trak*.

Another product from the same company is Acousticotton, an acoustic core material that is direct-applied or in stand-alone panels. These panels have sound-control, noise-control, and acoustic qualities. Composed of reclaimed and recycled cotton fibers, this "green" product offers excellent sound absorption and a superior NRC in bonded, recyclable sheets. It meets all fire and safety tests and gives a building L.E.E.D points. Installation is done by factory-trained installers and any adjustments needed can be made at the site. (See Figure 5.24.)

Installation

Because there are numerous types of acoustical panels, no single installation method covers all panels. Depending on the type of panel, panels may be attached to the wall by means of an adhesive and/or may

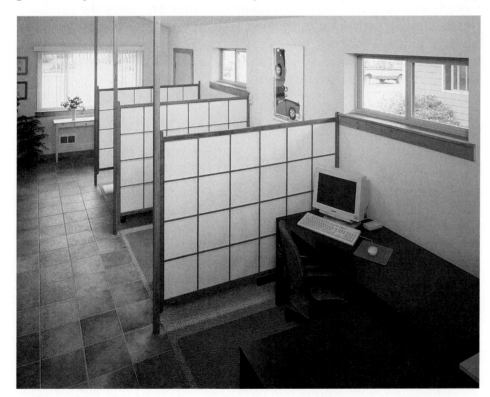

FIGURE 5.24
These office dividers are made with Shoji screens. Design © Cherry Tree Design. (Photo courtesy Cherry Tree Design)

have moulding concealing the seams. Manufacturers' recommended installation methods should be followed.

Maintenance

Surface dirt is removed by vacuuming or light brushing. Spots can be treated with dry-cleaning fluid or with carpet shampoo. Damaged fabric panels can easily be replaced by recovering just the damaged panel. Be sure to order extra fabric so that repairs can be easily made.

CORK

Cork tiles or panels are available in a 12″ × 36″ size and in thicknesses of 1/2, 3/4, 1, and 1 1/2 inches. They may be used in residential, commercial, educational, and institutional buildings. Because of its porous nature, cork can breathe, and therefore can be used on basement walls or on the inside surface of exterior support walls without the risk of moisture accumulation. Because of the millions of dead-air spaces in the cork particles, cork also has good insulating properties.

Installation

Cork panels are applied by using a 1/8″ × 1/8″ notched trowel and the manufacturer-recommended adhesive.

Maintenance

Vacuuming periodically with the brush attachment is recommended. A light, dust-free sealing coat of silicone aerosol spray will give dust protection; a heavier spray protects against dust and gives the surface a glossier finish, providing more light reflection. A heavy spray tends to close the pores of the cork, however, thus decreasing its sound-deadening and insulating qualities. An alternative to the silicone spray is a 50–50 blend of clear shellac and alcohol.

OTHER MATERIALS

Fixed Shoji panels can be used for walls. Bamboo Hardwoods offers Shoji screens made with bamboo dividers (Figure 5.24).

> QuarryCast® is a molded "Faux Stone" with a sandstone look available in a range of standard earthtone colours. It may be customised to meet designers criteria for colour or texture, but for small quantities this may be expensive. *QuarryCast*® is *FOR INTERIOR APPLICATIONS ONLY.* Using real metal powders in the surface, with a gypsum back up, MetalCast® provides the design community an opportunity to use cast metal features without the associated cost of metal castings.[23]

Installation

QuarryCast and MetalCast should be installed by a finish carpenter.

BIBLIOGRAPHY

Ackerman, Phyllis. *Wallpaper, Its History, Design and Use*. New York: Frederick A. Stokes Company, 1923.

Architectural Woodwork Institute. *Architectural Woodwork Quality Standards Illustrated*, 7th ed., Version 1.0, Reston, VA: Architectural Woodwork Institute, 2003.

Byrne, Michael. *Setting Tile*. Newton, CT: Taunton Press, 1996.

Pittsburgh Corning Corporation. *PC Glass Block® Products Specification Guidelines*. Pittsburgh, PA: Pittsburgh Corning, 2005.

Plumridge, Andrew, and Meulenkamp, Wlm. *Brickwork, Architecture and Design*, New York: Harry N. Abrams, 1993.

GLOSSARY

ashlar. Rectangular cut stone.

backsplash. The vertical wall area between the kitchen counter and the upper cabinets.

bond. Patterns formed by exposed surface of the brick.

book matching. Every other leaf is turned over, so the right side of a leaf abuts a right side and a left side abuts a left side.

butt. Two pieces of material placed side by side so there is no space between the pieces.

casing bead. A carved protective reinforcement strip to protect the edge from damage.

cobble. Similar in appearance to fieldstone.

compound curve. Curving in two different directions at the same time.

compressive strength. Amount of stress and pressure a material can withstand.

concave. Hollow or inward-curving shape.

convex. Arched or outward-curving shape.

course. One of the continuous horizontal layers of bricks, bonded with mortar.

cramps. U-shaped metal fastenings.

dado. The lower part of the wall below the chair rail.

desiccant. Substance capable of removing moisture from the air.

dimensional stability. Ability to retain shape regardless of temperature and humidity.

drywall. Any interior covering that does not require the use of plaster or mortar.

efflorescence. A powder or stain sometimes found on the surface of masonry, resulting from deposition of water-soluble salts.

evacuated. Air is removed.

feathering. Tapering off to almost nothing.

fieldstone. Rounded stone.

flake. A pattern produced when slicing through the medullary rays in some species, principally oak.

flitch. Portion of a log from which veneer is cut.

head. Horizontal cross-member supported by the jambs.

header. End of an exposed brick.

header course. Headers used every sixth course.

HPDL. High-pressure decorative laminate.

jamb. Vertical member at the sides of a door.

kerf. Slots cut into a material so that it will bend toward the kerfed edge.

laminated glass. Breaks without shattering. Glass remains in place.

lauan mahogany. A wood from the Philippines that, although not a true mahogany, resembles mahogany in grain.

leaves. Individual pieces of veneer.

listello. Narrow, horizontal, decorative tile.

load bearing. A wall that supports any vertical load in addition to its own weight.

mortar. A plastic mixture of cementitious materials, fine aggregate, and water.

mortar stain. Stain caused by excess mortar on the face of brick or stone.

raking light. Light shining obliquely down the length of a wall.

reveal. A recessed space left between two adjoining panels for design purposes.

rowlock. The end of a brick installed vertically.

rubble. Uncut stone.

scratch coat. In three-coat plastering, the first coat.

shiplap.   An overlapping wood joint.

stretcher.   Brick with the largest dimension horizontal and parallel to the wall face.

struck.   Mortar joint where excess mortar is removed by a trowel.

suction.   Absorption of water by the gypsum board from the wet plaster.

tambours.   Thin strips of wood or other materials attached to a flexible backing for use on curved surfaces. Similar in appearance to a roll-top desk.

tempered glass.   Glass having two to four times the strength of ordinary glass as the result of being heated and then suddenly cooled.

NOTES

[1]Website, www.stone-panels.com.

[2]Dr. Oliver Graydon, "Concrete Casts New Light in Dull Rooms," editor of Optics.org and *Opto & Laser Europe* magazine, March 2002.

[3]Website, www.pittsburghcorning.com.

[4]Website, www.ecobydesign.com.

[5]Website, www.nationalgypsum.com.

[6]Website, www.georgiapacific.com.

[7]Website, www.usgypsum.com.

[8]Architectural Woodwork Institute Quality Standards.

[9]Ibid, p. 36.

[10]Ibid, pp. 47–49.

[11]Ibid, pp. 50–53.

[12]Ibid, p. 47.

[13]Website, www.marlite.com.

[14]Melissa Wadsworth, "Looking at Glass," *Interior & Sources*, March 2001, p. 22.

[15]Website, www.skydesign.com.

[16]Skyline Design UltraGlas Inc., "The Artful Dimension in Architectural Glass," Chatsworth, CA, 2001.

[17]UltraGlas, Inc., "UltraGlas Embossed Glass Tile," Chatsworth, CA, 2001.

[18]UltraGlas, Inc., "UltraGlas Installation Procedures," Chatsworth, CA, 2001.

[19]Tile Council of America Inc., *2005 Handbook for Ceramic Tile Installation,* Clemson, SC: Author, 2005, p. 11.

[20]FabriTrak "Fabric as an Architectural Finish. The Solution . . . FABRI*TRAK*®". South River, NJ: Fabri*Trak*, Systems, Inc., 2000, p. 1.

[21]Ibid, p. 6.

[22]Website, www.formglas.com.

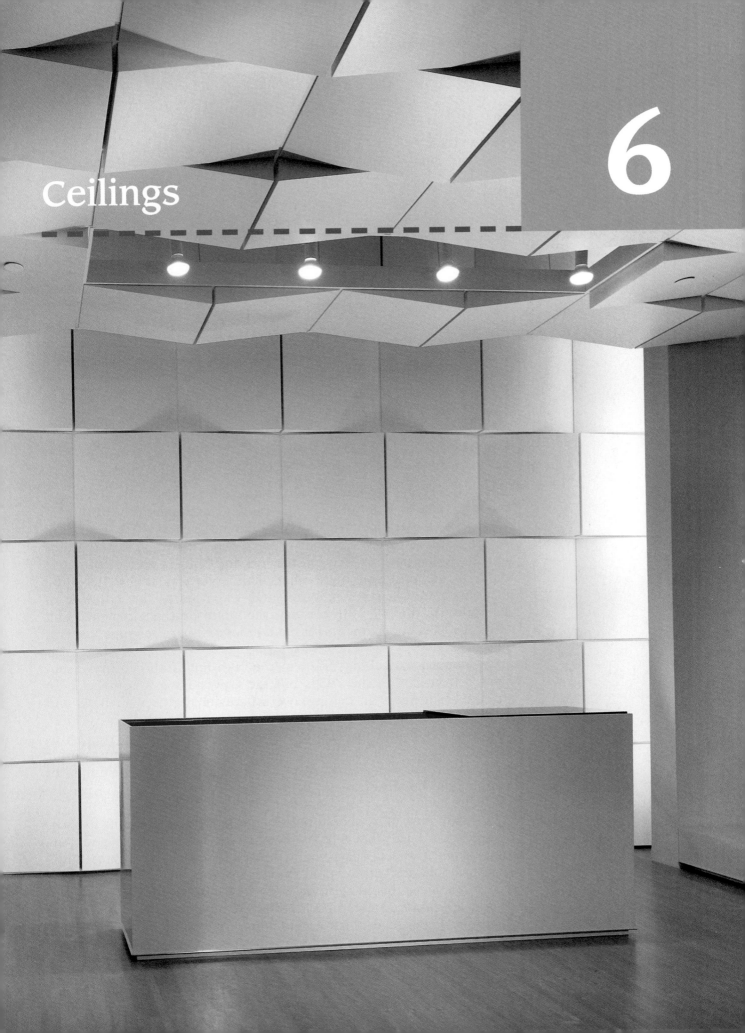

Ceilings

6

FIGURE 6.1
Pressed-tin sheets for
walls and ceilings give a
nostalgic ambience to a
room. (Photo courtesy of
AA Abbingdon, Inc.)

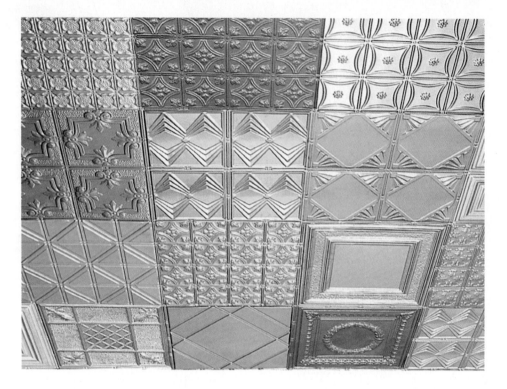

Early Greeks and Romans used lime stucco for ceilings, on which low, medium, and high **reliefs** were carried out. Italians in the 15th century worked with plaster, and in England Henry VIII's Hampton Court featured highly decorative plasterwork ceilings. In the Tudor and Jacobean periods, the plasterwork for ceilings had a geometric basis in medium and high relief. This style was followed by the classicism of Christopher Wren and Inigo Jones (an admirer of Palladio). In the late 18th century, the Adam brothers designed and used cast plaster ornaments for medallions, with **arabesques, patera,** and urns.

Stamped tin ceilings used in the 19th and 20th century disappeared from use in the 1930s but are now staging a comeback. In private residences, tin ceilings were occasionally used in halls and bathrooms. Stamped metal ceilings now come in 1 foot square, 1′ × 2′, 2′ × 4′, or 2′ × 8′ and are installed by tacking the units to furring strips nailed 12″ apart. These stamped metal ceilings are very suitable for Victorian restoration work. Also available are cornice moldings. In commercial buildings, metal ceilings were used to comply with the early fire codes.

Today, the ceiling should not be considered as merely the flat surface over our heads that is painted white. The ceiling is an integral part of a room; it affects space, light, heat, and sound, and the ceiling's design should reflect the overall ambience of the room. There are many ways to achieve this integration, such as beams for a country or Old World appearance, a stamped ceiling for a Victorian ambience (see Figure 6.1), a wood ceiling for contemporary warmth, or an acoustical ceiling for today's noisier environments. Ceiling treatments are limited only by the designer's imagination.

PLASTER

There are times when the ceiling should be an unobtrusive surface in a room. If this is the case, plastering is the answer. The plaster surface may be smooth or highly textured or somewhere in between. A smooth surface will reflect more light than a heavily textured one of the same color.

The plaster for a ceiling is applied in the same manner as for walls, although scaffolding must be used in the application process so the surface will be within working reach. It will take longer to plaster a ceiling than it will to plaster a wall area of similar size, because of the overhead reach.

The ornately carved ceilings of the past are obtained today using one of three means:

1. Precast plaster, either in pieces or **tiles**
2. Molded polyurethane foam
3. Wood mouldings, mainly used as **crown mouldings**

Urethane foam mouldings are discussed in detail in Chapter 7, in the section titled "Mouldings." Monarch™ ceiling panels from Chicago Metallic are glass-reinforced gypsum panels with ornately intricate patterns, detailed after turn-of-the-century styling, to provide today's modern interior with a distinguishing sense of elegance and refinement.

GYPSUM BOARD

The main difficulty with installing gypsum board for ceilings is the weight of the board. Ceiling **panels** are 1/2-inch thick and are specially designed to resist sagging and are equal to a 5/8-inch wallboard, installed perpendicular to framing. Gypsum board does require more labor and, again, scaffolding. It may be applied to a flat or curved surface. Spacing, whether using nails or screws, is 6 to 8 inches apart. The seams and screw holes are filled in the same manner as for gypsum board walls. The surface may be perfectly smooth, lightly textured, or heavily textured. A smooth surface not only reflects the most light but also shows any unevenness of ceiling joists. Wallpaper may also be used on the ceiling.

BEAMS

Although technically not a ceiling treatment, beams are probably the oldest form of ceiling construction, with the ceiling beams of the lower floor being the floor joists of the room above. The Colonial New England houses had hand-hewn timbers that ran the length of the room; a larger **summer beam** ran across the width. The area between the beams was covered by the floor boards of the room above or in the case of a sloping ceiling, the wood covering the outside of the roof timbers. Later these floorboards were covered with plaster and the timbers were left to darken naturally. The plaster in between the timbers had a rough or troweled surface. Today, instead of plaster, a plank ceiling is sometimes used in combination with beams.

The beams in early American homes were made of one piece of wood 12" or more square, but today, beams of this size are difficult to

FIGURE 6.2
The exposed beams give a southwestern adobe feeling to the room. The floor from Aged Woods is in keeping with the rustic character of the home. (Photo courtesy of Aged Woods)

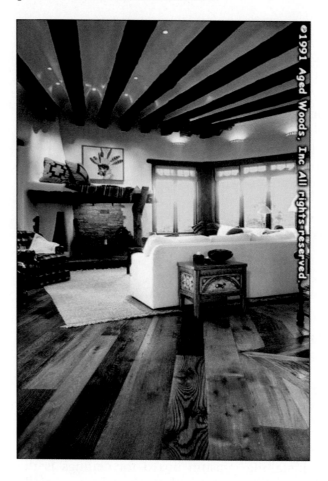

obtain. Trus Joist MacMillan, however, produces Parallam® PSL, which is available in dimensions up to 11 inches by 19 inches and lengths up to 60 feet. These beams are made from 3-foot-long to 8-foot-long veneer strands that are dried and then bonded using adhesives via a patented, microwave pressing process. Today, beamed ceilings are often used for a country setting with an Old World or contemporary feeling. (See Figure 6.2.) In southwestern style homes, rounded wood is used to imitate the **vigas** of the original adobe homes. These beams are sometimes filled in with smaller round pieces of wood called latillos.

There are several methods of imitating the solid, heavy look of hand-hewn beams. For example, box beams may be built as part of the floor joists or as a surface addition. To make a box beam appear similar to a hand-hewn beam, the surface must be treated to avoid the perfectly smooth surface of modern lumber.

In contemporary homes, **laminated beams** are used. These consist of several pieces of lumber (depending on the width required) glued together (on the wider surfaces). Because of this type of construction, laminated beams are very strong. Laminated beams are commonly referred to as "lam" beams.

WOOD

A natural outgrowth of a beamed ceiling is to use wood planks or strips to cover ceiling joists. With the many types of wood available on the market today, wood ceilings are used in many homes, particularly contemporary ones.

Almost all types of strip flooring or solid wood for walls may be used on a ceiling. Because of the darkness of wood, it is more suitable for a cathedral or shed ceiling (the dark color appears to lower the ceiling).

ACOUSTICAL CEILINGS

Residential

Because the ceiling is the largest unobstructed area in a room, sound is bounced off its surface without much absorption. Just as light is reflected from a smooth, high-gloss surface, so sound is reflected or bounced off the ceiling. Uncontrolled reverberations transform sound into noise, muffling music and disrupting effective communication. Textured ceiling tiles help reduce this reverberation and are often used in both residential and commercial interiors.

Acoustical ceilings, however, do not prevent the transmission of sound from one floor to another. The only answer to sound transmission is mass—the actual resistance of the material to vibrations caused by sound waves.

Sound absorption qualities may be obtained by using different materials and different methods. The most well-known is the acoustical tile (a 12-inch square) or panel (larger than 1 square foot) composed of mineral fiberboard. Other materials, such as fiberglass, metal, plastic-clad fiber, and fabric, may also be used. Sound absorption properties are produced by mechanical dies that perforate the mineral fiberboard after curing. Metal may also be perforated to improve its acoustical qualities if backed with an absorptive medium. An acoustical ceiling installation would be suitable in a basement playroom.

Installation

In private residences, any of three installation methods may be used: (1) If the tiles are to be used over an existing ceiling, they may be cemented to that ceiling provided the surface is solid and level. (2) Tiles have interlocking edges that provide a solid joining method as well as an almost seamless installation. If the existing ceiling is not solid or level, furring strips are nailed up so that the edges of the tile may be glued and stapled to a solid surface. (3) A suspended ceiling, may be used, which consists of a metal spline suspended by wires from the ceiling or joists. (This is the method used in commercial applications.) (See Figure 6.3.) The tiles are laid in the spline so that the edges of the panels are supported by the edge of the T-shaped spline. The splines may be left exposed or they may be covered by the tile. There are two advantages to using a suspended ceiling:

1. Damaged panels are easily replaced.
2. The height of the ceiling may be varied according to the size of the room or other requirements. With an exposed spline, it is easy to replace a single panel; the damaged panel is merely lifted out. However, if the spline is covered, the damaged panel or panels are removed and when replacing the last panel, the tongue is removed.

FIGURE 6.3
Suspension systems. Each type gives a different look to the ceiling. (Photos courtesy of Armstrong Ceilings)

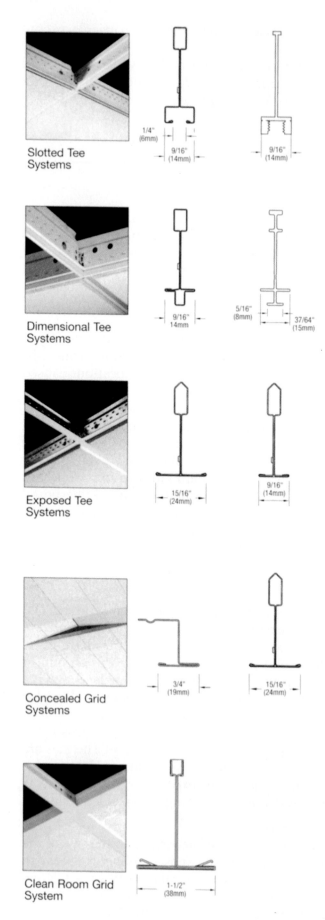

Slotted Tee Systems

1/4" (6mm)
9/16" (14mm)
9/16" (14mm)

Dimensional Tee Systems

9/16" 14mm
5/16" (8mm)
37/64" (15mm)

Exposed Tee Systems

15/16" (24mm)
9/16" (14mm)

Concealed Grid Systems

3/4" (19mm)
15/16" (24mm)

Clean Room Grid System

1-1/2" (38mm)

Maintenance

A soft gum eraser should be used to remove small spots, dirt marks, and streaks from acoustical tiles. For larger areas, or larger smudges, a chemically treated sponge rubber pad or wallpaper cleaner is used. The sponge rubber pad or wallpaper cleaner must be in fresh condition. Nicks and scratches may be touched up with colored chalks. Dust is removed by brushing lightly with a soft brush or clean rag or by vacuuming with a soft brush attachment.

Acoustical tiles must not be soaked with water. They should be washed by light application of a sponge dampened with a mild liquid detergent solution: 1/2 cup detergent in 1 gallon of water. After the sponge is saturated, it should be squeezed nearly dry and then lightly rubbed on the surface to be cleaned using long, sweeping, gentle strokes. The strokes should be in the same direction as the texture if the tile is ribbed or embossed.

Surface openings must not be clogged or **bridged** when acoustical tiles are painted. A paint of high hiding power should be used because it is desirable to keep the number of coats to a minimum (paint greatly affects the noise reduction coefficient of the acoustical material). Some paint manufacturers provide specific formulations that have high hiding power and low combustibility and are not likely to bridge openings in the tile. The paint must be applied as thinly as possible.

Commercial

Acoustical ceiling products have become a mainstay of commercial installations. Movable office partitions are prevalent today, so sound privacy is necessary. In this day of electronic word processors and data processing equipment, office din is somewhat less than in the days of noisy typewriters, but telephones and voices still cause distracting sounds. Productivity is increased in a quieter environment, but a noiseless environment is easily disrupted.

The advantages of a residential suspended acoustical ceiling also apply to commercial installations, but the major reason for using a suspended ceiling in commercial work is the easy access to wiring, telephone lines, plumbing, and heating ducts.

When looking through the technical information on acoustical ceilings, the designer will find several of the following abbreviations.

The noise reduction coefficient (**NRC**) is a measure of sound absorbed by a material. The NRC of different types of panels may be compared. The higher the number, the more sound reduction is indicated. For purposes of comparison, tests must be made at the same **Hertz** (Hz) range.

The sound transmission class (**STC**) is a single number rating that is used to characterize the sound-insulating value of a partition (wall or ceiling). A partition prevents sound from being transmitted from one area to another; the STC rating denotes approximately how much the sound will be reduced when traveling through the partition. The higher the rating, the less sound will be transmitted through the wall or floor/ceiling.

The ceiling attenuation class (**CAC**) refers to the sound attenuation ability of ceiling systems. The CAC rates how much sound will be reduced when it is transmitted through the ceiling of one room into an adjacent room through a shared **plenum.** A higher rating indicates that the material will allow less sound transmission.

Another characteristic often included in acoustical mineral fiberboard charts is light reflectance (**LR**), which indicates the percentage of light reflected from a ceiling product's surface. This LR varies according to the amount of texture on the ceiling's surface and the value of the color. Some ceiling panels have a mineral fiber substrate with a needle-punched fabric surface.

i-ceilings®, a new generation of ceilings systems from Armstrong, allow architects and others to integrate sound and wireless systems into the ceiling plane without the systems being visible from below. The new "interactive" products thus create more effective commercial interiors by increasing speech privacy and providing easier access to information and people.

Armstrong's new i-ceilings Wireless Systems feature Antenna Panels, which have a suite of antennas embedded in the ceiling panel to enable the in-building of wireless connectivity for voice and data. The system helps increase employee and workplace effectiveness by providing occupants clearer, more reliable wireless telephone use and also access to the Internet and data networks, regardless of where they are in a building. Armstrong's new i-ceilings Sound Systems feature a unique Sound Panel that delivers sound masking, paging, and music simultaneously from one speaker. This system helps increase workplace effectiveness by enhancing speech privacy, which is a vital concern in both open- and closed-plan offices.

The Antenna and Sound Panels both look just like ordinary ceiling panels so that they blend in with the overall ceiling. This makes the interior space more aesthetically pleasing by eliminating unsightly speakers and surface-mounted antennas. (See Figure 6.4.)

Installation

The traditional approach to lighting is **luminaries** recessed at specific intervals in the acoustical ceiling. The fixtures are often covered by lenses or louvers to diffuse the light. Today, not only lighting but also heating and cooling are often incorporated into acoustical installations. This is done in several ways. The heating and cooling duct may be spaced between the modules in one long continuous line or individual vents may be used. In one interesting innovation, the entire area between the suspended ceiling and the joists is used as a plenum area, with the conditioned air entering the room through orifices in the individual tiles.

One word of warning: If you are replacing a ceiling that may contain asbestos, OSHA has some very stringent regulations and safety precautions that must be strictly adhered to.

EuroStone™ panels from Chicago Metallic® are the ideal acoustical ceiling choice for healthy buildings in education, health care, hospitality, corporate, and retail environments. Its unique, sculptured stone look is intrinsic to the material from which it comes, primarily volcanic perlite. This volcanic stone is fired in specially designed kilns to bond the stone particles together. The panels are totally inorganic in nature, which allows them to withstand fire, moisture, the invasion of microorganisms,

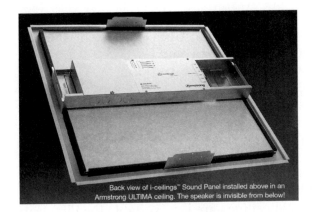

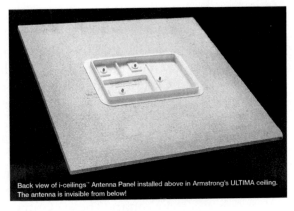

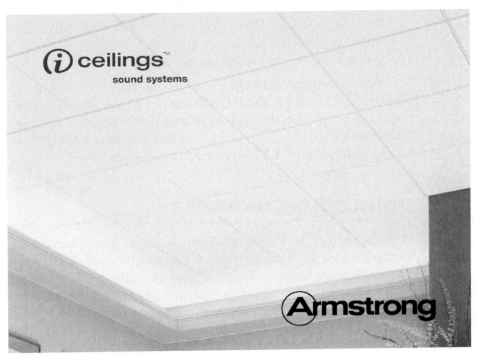

FIGURE 6.4

The components of the i-ceilings™ from Armstrong World industries, Inc. are shown above. Top photo (left) is the back view of i-ceilings Sound Panel installed above in an Armstrong ULTIMA ceiling. The speaker is invisible from below. Top right is a back view of the Antenna Panel installed above the same ceiling. The antenna is invisible from below. The large photo shows the completed ceiling. (© Copyright 2001 Armstrong World Industries, Inc. Photos courtesy of Armstrong World Industries, Inc.)

and to deliver good acoustical and insulating properties. The panels are also an ideal product for "building green" and are environmentally friendly and 100 percent recyclable with no man-made fibers. The paint-free surface has a permanent natural color. Dry-brushing, brush vacuuming, or washing with water (and a mild detergent) are distinct to EuroStone's moisture-resistant properties and integral coloring. Euro-Stone can even be washed with a hose! (See EuroStone in Figure 1.6.)

METAL

Metal ceilings were originally introduced in the 1860s as a replacement for the ornamental plasterwork that decorated the walls and ceilings of the most fashionable rooms of the day. Once in place, it was discovered that metal ceilings offered two important benefits: (1) Unlike plaster, the metal could withstand rough use, and (2) it could be more easily maintained than plaster, which would flake, crack, and peel. W. F. Norman Corporation uses 88-year-old dies to produce metal plates for ceiling and wall coverings. Available styles include Greek, Colonial, Victorian, Empire, Gothic, Oriental, and Art Deco. Many of today's metal ceilings are actually steel, which can be prepainted, or made of copper, brass, or chrome.

Stamped metal ceilings now come in 1-foot squares, $1' \times 2'$, $2' \times 4'$, or $2' \times 8'$, and are installed by tacking the units to furring strips nailed 12″ apart. These stamped metal ceilings are very suitable for Victorian restoration work. (See Figure 6.1.) Also available are cornice mouldings.

METALWORKS™ Open Cell systems offer decorative, durable, and 100% accessible solutions for open ceilings to help mask the plenum and create a unique design statement.[1]

Not all metal ceilings have to be flat. Another product from Armstrong Ceilings is the RH200 Curved Plank System, which offers a range of curved metal panel sizes and finish options. Chicago Metallic Corporation also has CurvGrid™, which provides a curve/wave look using standard 15/16″ T-bars painted on all sides.

OTHER CEILING MATERIALS

Mirrors are not recommended for ceilings. A vinyl-coated, embossed aluminum, bonded to a mineral fiber substrate, results in an easily maintained, corrosion-resistant, and durable ceiling product. Grease vapor concentrations may be wiped clean with a sponge or a mild detergent solution; these types of ceilings are suitable for commercial kitchens, laboratories, and hospitals.

Baffles are fabric-covered fiberglass panels hung from a ceiling by means of wire attached to eyelets installed in the top edge of the panel. Baffles are not only functional, but decorative too, with a sound rating

FIGURE 6.5
Sound Scapes Acoustical Canopies aesthetically define spaces, have high light reflectance and are adjustable to special heights and angles. (Photo courtesy of Armstrong Ceilings)

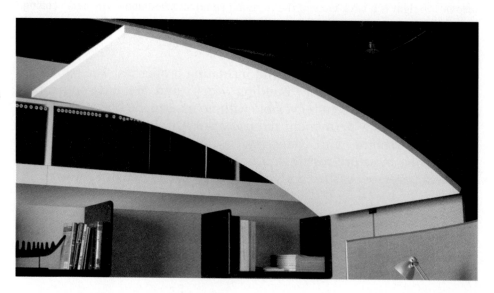

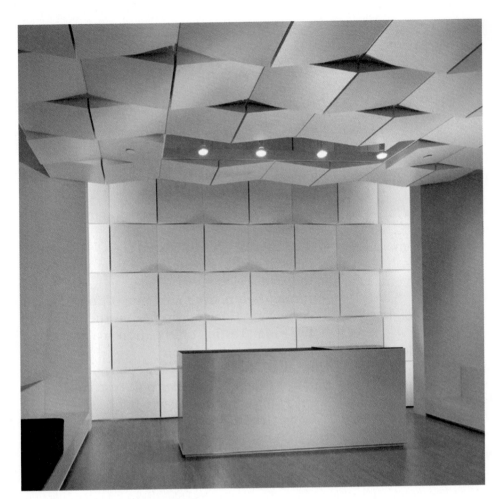

FIGURE 6.6
The Geometrix ceiling is
also used on the back wall,
creating a three-
dimensional effect.
(Photo courtesy of USG)

of NRC 0.80. Baffles hung perpendicular to a ceiling are an established and highly effective way to create additional sound-absorbing surfaces, especially in interiors lacking sufficient surfaces for wall-mounted panels. Baffles can be used for signage, and different colors can denote areas or departments within a larger space.

Not all acoustical ceilings are flat. Many are **coffered** in 2 - to 4-foot square modules. These panels may or may not include luminaries. (See Figure 6.6.)

CERAMIC TILE

For a ceiling that is easy to wipe clean, or in very moist areas such as bathrooms and showers, a ceramic tile may be installed. Ceramic tile is also used in restaurant kitchens.

BIBLIOGRAPHY

Rather, Guy Cadogan. *Ceilings and Their Deco-ration*. London, England: T. Werner Laurie, 1978.

Time-Life Books. *Walls and Ceilings*. Alexandria, VA: Author, 1980.

GLOSSARY

arabesque. Elaborate scroll designs either carved or in low relief.

bridged. Open pores covered by paint.

CAC. Ceiling attenuation class. The CAC rates how much sound will be reduced when it is transmitted through the ceiling of one room into an adjacent room through a shared plenum.

coffered. Recessed panels in the ceiling. May or may not be decorated.

crown moulding. The uppermost moulding next to the ceiling.

Hertz. Unit of frequency measurement. One unit per second. Abbreviation: Hz.

laminated beam. Several pieces of lumber glued to form a structural timber.

LR. Light reflectance. The amount of light reflected from the surface.

luminaries. A complete lighting fixture, with all components needed to be connected to the electric power supply.

NRC. Noise reduction coefficient. The average percentage of sound reduction at various Hertz levels.

panel. A ceiling unit larger than one square foot.

patera. A round or oval raised surface design.

plenum. The space between a suspended ceiling and the floor above.

relief. A design that is raised above the surrounding area.

STC. Sound transmission class. A number denoting the sound insulation value of a material.

summer beam. A main supporting beam in early New England homes, in the middle of the room, resting on the fireplace at one end and a post at the other.

tile. Ceiling tile (12 inches square).

vigas. The round wooden poles used in exposed in ceilings of southwestern adobe style homes and extending outside.

NOTE

[1]Website, www.armstrong.com.

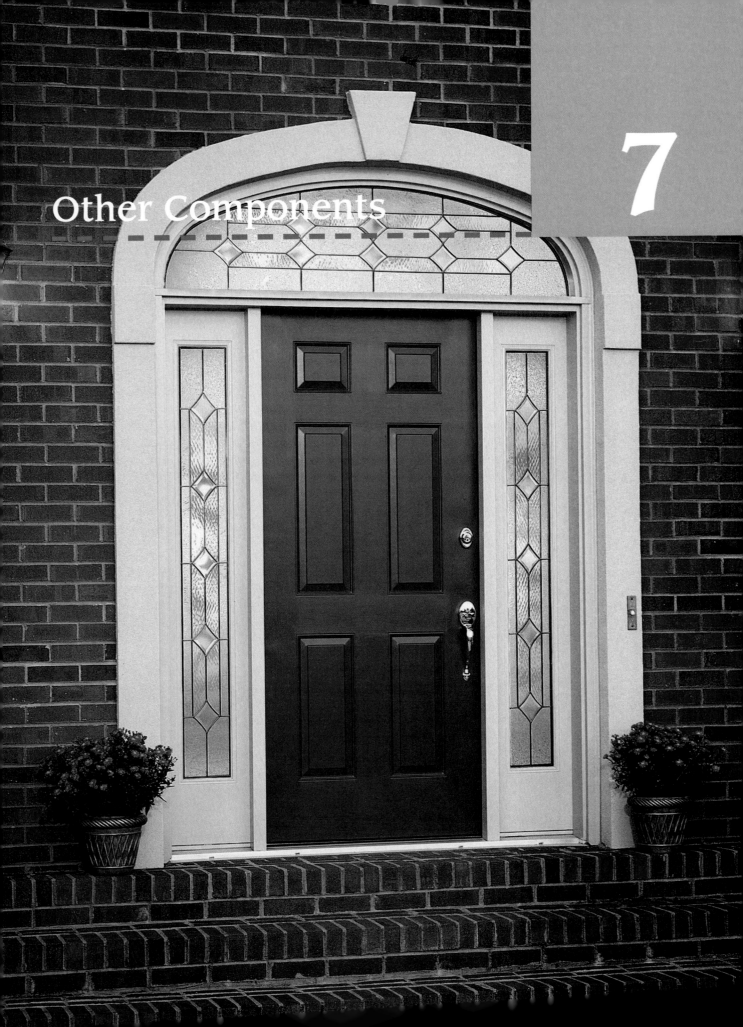

Other Components

7

MOULDINGS

To an interior designer, trim and mouldings are what icing is to a cake: They cover, enhance, and decorate a plain surface. Basically, heavily carved or ornate trim is used in a traditional setting, whereas simpler trim is used where a contemporary ambience is desired.

AWI lists four types of trim, all custom manufactured:

1. *Standing trim*—Custom-manufactured items of fixed length such as door and window **casings,** stops, **stools** or sills, **aprons,** and so on. These can usually be accomplished with single lengths of wood (depending on species).
2. *Running trim*—Custom-manufactured items of continuing length (depending on species) such as **cornices, fascias, soffits,** chair rails, baseboards, **shoe mouldings,** and so on.
3. *Rails*—Custom-manufactured rails used on corridor walls of hospitals, nursing homes, and other facilities, and guard rails at glass openings.
4. *Board paneling*—Custom-manufactured paneling applied in the form of multiple boards.[1]

(See Figure 7.1.)

Materials for trim and mouldings should be constructed from easily shaped stock. Both pine and oak are used when wood trim is desired,

FIGURE 7.1
Wood bases, chair rails, and casings. (Courtesy of Granite Mill)

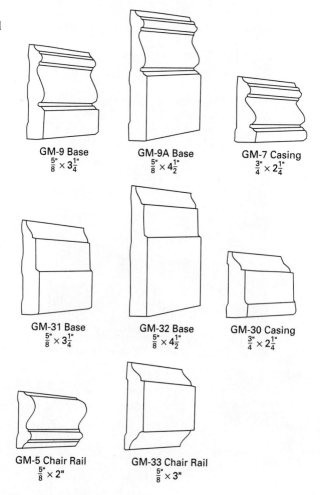

GM-9 Base
$\frac{5"}{8} \times 3\frac{1}{4}"$

GM-9A Base
$\frac{5"}{8} \times 4\frac{1}{2}"$

GM-7 Casing
$\frac{3"}{4} \times 2\frac{1}{4}"$

GM-31 Base
$\frac{5"}{8} \times 3\frac{1}{4}"$

GM-32 Base
$\frac{5"}{8} \times 4\frac{1}{2}"$

GM-30 Casing
$\frac{3"}{4} \times 2\frac{1}{4}"$

GM-5 Chair Rail
$\frac{5"}{8} \times 2"$

GM-33 Chair Rail
$\frac{5"}{8} \times 3"$

and both provide details that are easily discernible and smooth. Trim should always be **mitered** at the corners; that is, the joint should be cut at a 45-degree angle. Also available are medium-density fiberboard (MDF) mouldings for painted interior trims. Other trim materials include solid-surface materials, such as Corian® and Gibraltar®, which are also used for counters. Depending on thickness, these materials are fairly easy to shape.

Bases are a type of moulding universally used to finish the area where the wall and floor meet. There are several reasons for using a base or skirting: It covers any discrepancy or expansion space between the wall and the floor; it forms a protection for the wall from cleaning equipment; and it may also be a decorative feature. The word *base* is used to describe all types of materials, including those mentioned earlier as well as vinyl and rubber.

Baseboard is the term used for wood bases only. When a plain baseboard is used, the wood should be sanded smoothly on the face and particularly on the top edge to facilitate cleaning. The exposed edge should be slightly beveled to prevent breaking or chipping. Traditional baseboards have a shaped top edge with a flat lower part. This design may be achieved with one piece of wood 3½ to 7 inches wide or may consist of separate parts, with a base moulding on top of a square-edged piece of lumber. A **base shoe** may be added to either type. Traditional one-piece baseboards are available as stock mouldings from the better woodworking manufacturers. (See Figure 7.1 for examples.)

For residential use, windows come prefabricated with the **brickmould** or exterior trim attached. The interior casing (the exposed trim) may be flat or moulded and is applied after the window and walls have been installed and the windows **caulked,** a crucial step in these days of energy conservation. The interior casing usually matches the baseboard designs, although the size may vary. (See Figure 7.1.)

Doors, particularly for residential use, often come **prehung.** After installation of the door frame, the space between the jamb and the wall is covered by a casing. This casing matches the profile of the one used around the windows, with the width of the casing determined by the size, scale, and style of the room.

Crown mouldings and **bed mouldings** are used to soften the sharp line where the ceiling and walls meet. Cove mouldings also serve the same purpose—the difference is that crown mouldings are more intricately shaped and cove mouldings have a simple, curved face. Cove mouldings may be painted the same color as the ceiling, thus giving a lowered appearance to the ceiling. Cornice mouldings may be ornate and made up of as many as 10 separate pieces of wood. (See Figure 7.2.)

Chair rails are used in traditional homes to protect the surface of walls from damage caused by the backs of chairs. These rails may be simple strips of wood with rounded edges, or they may have shaped top and bottom edges, depending on the style of the room. (See Figure 7.1.) The installed height of chair rails should be between 30 and 36 inches. When chair rails are painted, they should be made of a hard, close-grained wood. If they are left natural, they should be of the same material and should be finished in the same manner as the rest of the woodwork.

FIGURE 7.2
Ten-piece moulding.
(Drawing courtesy of
Driwood Period Moulding)

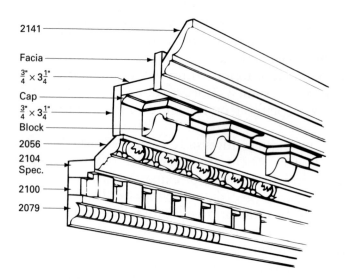

2141
Facia
$\frac{3"}{4} \times 3\frac{1"}{4}$
Cap
$\frac{3"}{4} \times 3\frac{1"}{4}$
Block
2056
2104
Spec.
2100
2079

When plywood panels are used on walls, the edges are sometimes covered with a square-edge batten. In more traditional surroundings, a moulded batten is used.

Picture mouldings, as the name implies, were used to create a continuous projecting support around the walls of a room for picture hooks. Picture moulding has a curved top to receive the picture hook. Of course, when pictures are hung by this method, the wires will be visible, but this method is still used in older homes, museums, and art galleries, where frequent rearranging is required. No damage is done to the walls, as it is with the modern method of hanging pictures. Picture moulding is placed just below or several inches below the ceiling. Wherever the placement, the ceiling color is usually continued down to the top of the moulding.

An infinite variety of patterns may be used for mouldings. They may be stock shapes and sizes or shaped to the designer's specifications by the use of custom-formed shaper blades. This latter method is the most expensive but does achieve a unique moulding.

Wood mouldings may be covered with metal in many finishes (including bright chrome, brass, copper, or simulated metal) for use as picture frame moulding, interior trim, and displays.

All the mouldings discussed thus far have been constructed of wood. When a heavily carved cornice molding is required, the material may be a **polymer.** Focal Point® makes a polymer moulding by direct impression from the original wood, metal, or plaster article. This direct process gives the reproduction all the personality, texture, and spirit of the original, but with several advantages: The mouldings are much less expensive than the hand-carved originals. They are lighter weight and therefore easier to handle; they may be nailed, drilled, or screwed; and they are receptive to sanding. Another feature is that, in many cases, the original moulding consisted of several pieces, but modern technology reproduces multiple mouldings in a one-piece strip, thus saving on installation costs.

Focal Point is authorized to reproduce architectural details for the Victorian Society of America, Colonial Williamsburg® Foundation, National Trust for Historic Preservation, the Frank Lloyd Wright Collection™, and for the Historic Natchez Foundation.

Polymer mouldings are factory primed in white; however, if a stained effect is desired, the mouldings may be primed beige and stained with Mohawk nonpenetrating stain. Careful brush strokes will simulate grain. When stain is skillfully applied, the effect is very convincing.

In Chapter 6, ceiling medallions were mentioned as a form of ceiling decoration. When these medallions were first used as **backplates** for chandeliers, they were made of plaster, but again the polymer reproductions are lightweight and easy to ship. The medallions are primed white at the factory, ready to paint. The use of medallions is not limited to chandeliers. (See Figure 7.3.) They may also be used as a backplate for ceiling fans.

Other materials used in ornate ceiling cornices include gypsum with a polymer agent that is reinforced with glass fibers for added strength. A wood fiber combination may also be used.

Lightweight, QuarryCast®, or glass-reinforced gypsum and cement cast architectural products, including all types of mouldings mentioned previously, are used internationally. Round or tapered column covers, with capitals and base, are also available.

Other reproductions from the past include the dome and the niche cap. When first designed, they were made of plaster or wood, which was then hand carved. Domes and niche caps can provide a touch of authenticity in renovations; in fact, many of Focal Point's designs have been used in restorations of national historical landmarks. Niche caps have a shell design and form the top of a curved recess that usually displays sculpture, vases, flowers, or any other prized possession.

Stair brackets are another form of architectural detail and are placed on the finished **stringer** for a decorative effect. (See Figure 7.3.)

DOORS

An entry door makes a first impression, whether for a private residence or a business. Doors for residential use may be constructed of wood, metal, or fiberglass. In commercial applications, however, doors must be guaranteed not to burn for 1 to 1½ hours because of fire codes. To select a design, look at the exterior of the house to make sure that the design is compatible with the exterior.

WOOD DOORS

Flush doors are perfectly flat and smooth, with no decoration. There are several methods of constructing a flush door. A honeycomb hollow core is used for some interior residential flush doors. (See Figure 7.4.) The core of the door is made of 2- to 3-inch-wide solid wood for the rails and 1 to 2 inches of solid wood for the **stiles,** with an additional 20-inch-long strip of wood, called a lock block, in the approximate hardware location. The area between the solid wood is filled with a honeycomb or ladder core. (See Figure 7.5.) In less expensive doors, this core is covered by the finish veneer. More expensive doors have one or two layers of veneer before the finish veneer is applied. Thus, a flush door may be of three-, five-, or seven-ply construction.

FIGURE 7.3
At the very top, the d'Evereux Rim from Focal Point Architectural Products. Above, the Woodlawn Stair Bracket from Focal Point's National Trust for Historic Preservation Collection. (Photos Courtesy Focal Point Architectural Products, Inc.)

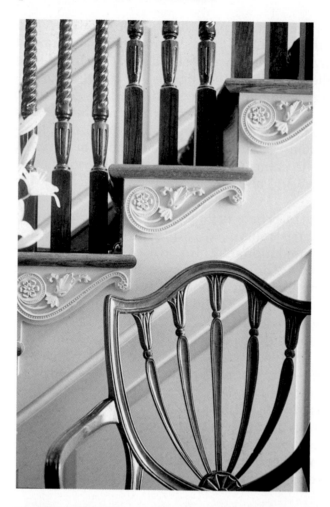

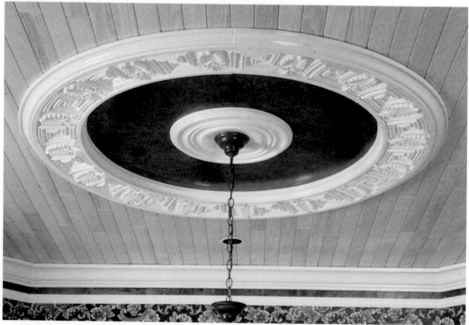

Better-quality flush doors are constructed with a lumber core, also known as staved wood, and wood blocks are used in place of the honeycomb or ladder core of the hollow-core door. The staved or lumber core may or may not have the blocks bonded together. With staved-core

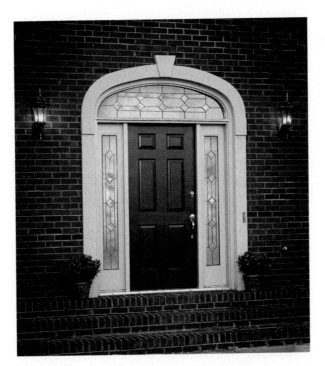

FIGURE 7.4
Avant Steel Door with Regal
Beveled Glass transom and
sidelights makes an
impressive entrance to any
home. (Courtesy of
Peachtree Doors and
Windows Inc.)

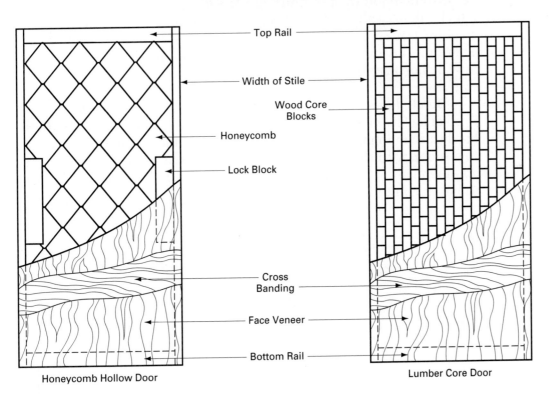

FIGURE 7.5
Door construction.

doors, the inside rails and stiles are narrower than in other flush doors because this type of construction is more rigid. (See Figure 7.5.) Species used for face veneers include hardwoods, such as oak, mahogany, cherry, and maple, and softwoods, such as pine and fir. If the door is to be painted, a "paint-grade" wood door made of softwood should be specified.

Another method of door construction utilizes a particleboard or flakeboard core with a crossband veneer to which the face veneer is attached. A particleboard door core is warp resistant and solid, has no knots or voids, and has good insulation properties and sound resistance (thereby limiting heat loss and transfer of sound waves).

Flush doors for commercial installations may have a high-pressure decorative laminate (HPDL) as the face veneer or, for low maintenance, a photogravure or vinyl covering similar to the paneling discussed in Chapter 5.

Commercial installations of doors do not always require a moulding; the doors are merely set into the wall. In other words, the wall meets the door jamb.

There are three methods of achieving a paneled look in doors. One uses a solid ornate **ogee** sticking; in other words, the stiles and rails are shaped so that the moulding and stile or rails are all one piece of wood. The second method is the same as the first but uses a simpler **ovolo** sticking. The third method uses a **dadoed** stile and rail, and the joining of panel and stile is covered by a separate applied moulding. If the panel is large, it will be made of plywood and a moulding will be used; if the panel is under 10 inches in width, it may be of solid wood (in premium-grade solid lumber is not permitted). Paneled doors reflect different periods, as do paneled walls. When period paneling is used, the doors should be of similar design. (See Figure 7.6.) There are an infinite number of designs for paneled doors. Panels may be horizontal or vertical, small or large, curved or straight, wood or glass.

Dutch doors for residential use consist of an upper and lower part. Special hardware joins the two parts to form a regular door or, with the hardware undone, the top part may be opened to ventilate or give light to a room, with the lower part remaining closed. Dutch doors are used commercially as a service opening. In this case, a shelf is attached to the top of the bottom half. (See Figure 7.7c.)

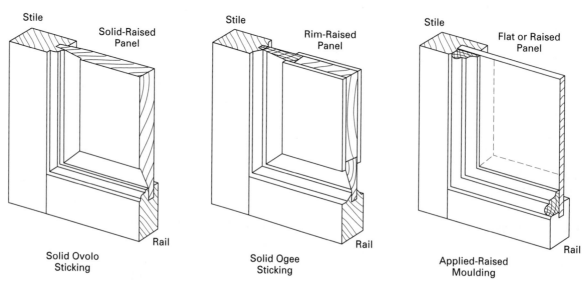

FIGURE 7.6
Paneled doors.

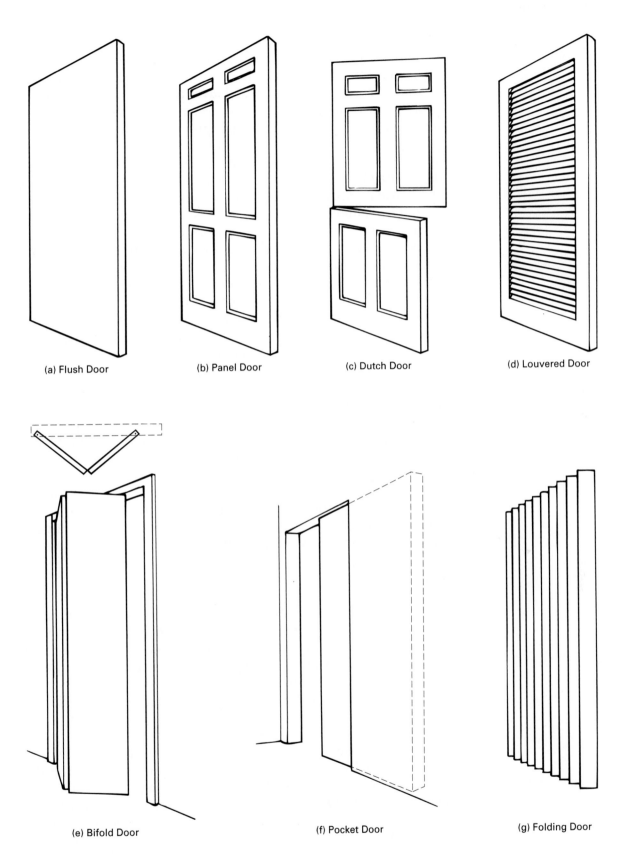

(a) Flush Door   (b) Panel Door   (c) Dutch Door   (d) Louvered Door

(e) Bifold Door   (f) Pocket Door   (g) Folding Door

FIGURE 7.7
Types of doors.

Louvers are used in doors to provide ventilation, such as in cleaning or storage closets, or to aid in air circulation. Louvers are made of horizontal slats contained within stile-and-rail frames. Louvers may be set into wood or metal doors, with the louver at the top and/or bottom, or the center may be all louvered. Some louvers are visionproof, some are adjustable, and others may be lightproof or weatherproof. (See Figure 7.7d.)

One of the most common residential uses for a louvered door is a bifold door for a closet. For a narrow opening, a bifold door consists of two panels; larger openings require a double set of doors opening from the middle. The center panel of each pair is hung from the track, and the outer panels may or may not pivot at the jamb. (See Figure 7.7e.)

A pocket door, or recessed sliding door, requires a special frame and track that is incorporated into the inside of the wall. The finished door is hung from the track before the casing is attached. The bottom of the door is held in place by guides that permit the door to slide sideways while preventing back-and-forth movement. (See Figure 7.7f.)

Folding or accordion doors are used where space needs to be divided temporarily. Folding doors operate and stack compactly within their openings. The panels may be wood-veneered lumber core or particleboard core with a wood-grained vinyl coating. Each panel is 3 5/8 inches or less in width, and folding doors are available in heights up to 16 feet 1 inch. Folding doors operate by means of a track at the top to which the panels are attached by wheels. The handle and locking mechanism is installed on the panel closest to the opening edge. (See Figure 7.7g.)

For an oriental ambience, fixed or sliding **Shoji** panels are available; these are wood framed with synskin inserts, which have an oriental rice paper look. Pinecrest® offers a wide variety of Shoji panels, standard or custom, both fixed and sliding. (See Figure 5.24.)

Glass Doors

Patio doors are similar in construction and appearance to wood-panel entry doors. French doors are often used in residences to open out onto a balcony or patio. They have wood or metal frames and may consist of one sheet of tempered or laminated safety glass, or may have multiple **lights** in each door. Whenever full-length glass is used, by law it must be tempered or laminated. French doors are most often installed in pairs and may open out or in.

When French doors or other styles of doors are installed in pairs, one is used as the primary door. The second one is stationary, with a flush bolt or special lock holding it tight at top and bottom. To cover the joining crack between the pair of doors and to make the doors more weather tight, an **astragal** is attached to the interior edge of the stationary door. Both doors may be used to enlarge the opening. If double doors are used, the astragal is on the exterior edge of the secondary door. Another style of a patio door is the sliding type.

Glass doors for residential use may be comprised of solid wood core, aluminum or vinyl, fiberglass or steel (when sliding and hinged patio doors are considered). Steel and fiberglass doors are foam filled for increased thermal performance. Commercial glass doors must also

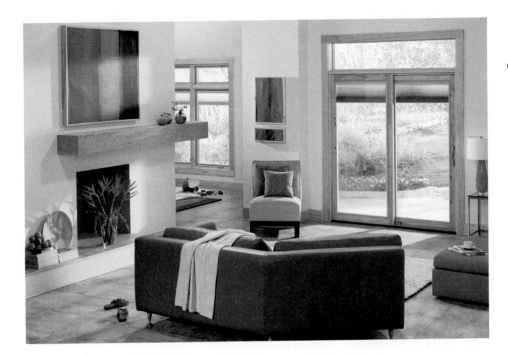

FIGURE 7.8
The Integer Group Image
Pella® Designer Series®
Contemporary Sliding Patio
Door with Between the
Glass Blinds.
(Courtesy of Pella
Windows & Doors)

be made of tempered or laminated glass and are subject to local building codes. The door may be all glass, framed with metal at the top and/or bottom, or framed on all four sides. Because of the nature of an all-glass door, the most visible design feature is the hardware.

Metal Doors

Most metal doors are made of steel, although some are available in aluminum. In the past, metal doors had a commercial or institutional connotation, but today many interior and exterior residential doors and many bifold doors are made of metal. Exterior metal doors were shunned in the past because wood exterior solid-core doors had better insulating qualities. The use of polystyrene and polyurethane as a core has provided residential metal exterior doors with similar insulating qualities, and such doors are not as susceptible to temperature changes and warping as is the wood door.

Surfaces may be factory coated with rust-resistant primer to be painted on-site or vinyl or baked-on polyester finishes embossed with wood grain patterns. Some metal doors are given a wood-fiber coating that can be stained. Higher-end models are actually laminated with a real-wood veneer. Steel doors have a less convincing wood grain than fiberglass doors.

Fiberglass Doors

Fiberglass or fiberglass-composite doors are an alternative to wood. Fiberglass offers six times the energy efficiency as conventional wood doors. Models are available where both the door and sidelite swing open, so large furniture and appliances can pass easily through. An adjustable threshold gives a weather-tight seal, protecting the home from the elements. A **transom** may be added.

Specialty Doors

Special doors must be specified for installations in which X-ray machines will be used. These flush-panel doors have two layers of plywood with lead between the layers; then a face veneer of wood, hardboard, or laminate is applied.

Fire doors have an incombustible material core with fire-retardant rails and stiles covered by a wood veneer or high-pressure decorative laminate. These doors are rated according to the time they take to burn. Depending on materials and construction, this time will vary between 20 minutes and 1½ hours. Local building codes should be consulted before specifying.

For exterior use, a wood door must be of solid construction. Hand-carved doors are available for exterior use, but manufacturer's specifications must be studied carefully because a door that appears to be hand carved may actually be moulded to imitate hand carving at less expense.

Specifications for Doors

Most doors are available prehung (i.e., assembled complete with frames, trim, and sometimes hardware). The bored hole is ready for installation of the lock. This bored hole must have a **backset** that corresponds to the selected hardware. Most prehung doors come predrilled with a 2 3/8-inch hole; however, most designer-type hardware looks better with a 2 3/4-inch backset or even more. The 2 3/8-inch backset, with knob-type hardware, can sometimes result in scraped knuckles.

For prehung doors, door hand is determined by noting the hinge location when the door opens away from the viewer (i.e., if the hinge jamb is on his or her right, it is a right-hand door). In the case of a pair of doors, hand is determined from the active leaf in the same way. If prehung doors are specified, door handing should be included. (See Figure 7.9.)

When standing outside, look at the closed door.

If door swings in:
Handle on right = left-hand door
Handle on left = right-hand door

FIGURE 7.9
Door handing.
(Courtesy of Door and Hardware Institute, "Butts and Hinges," *Tech Talk*, by H. Matt Bouchard, Jr. AHC.)

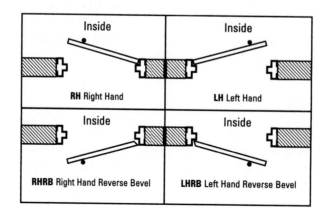

If door swings out:
Handle on right = right-hand door
Handle on left = left-hand door

The following additional information should be provided when specifying doors:

Manufacturer size—including width, height, and thickness.
Face description—species of wood, type of veneer (rotary or sliced). If not veneer, then laminate, photogravure, vinyl coating, or metal.
Construction—cross-banding thickness, edge strips, top and bottom rails, stiles, and core construction.
Finishing—prefinished or unfinished.
Special detailing—includes specifying backset for hardware and any mouldings.
Special service—for example, glazing, fire doors, etc.
Warranty—differs for interior and exterior use.

Reinforced **strike plate** areas are a good security measure, and increasing the distance from the lockset to the deadbolt spreads impact load from potential break-ins, thereby increasing security. Check the frame of the door to be sure it's strong, tight, and well constructed.

DOOR HARDWARE

Most of the following material is adapted, by permission, from the Tech Talk bulletin, "Butts and Hinges," published by the **Door and Hardware Institute (DHI).** This material is technical and has been simplified for ease of understanding.

Hinges

The two parts of a hinge consist of metal plates known as **leaves** and are joined by a **pin** that passes through the **knuckle** joints. **Countersunk** holes are predrilled in the leaves. **Template hardware** has the holes drilled accurately to conform to standard drawings, thus assuring a perfect fit. Template **butt hinges** have the holes drilled in a crescent shape. (See Figure 7.10.)

Door hardware, in general, is not an issue unless it does not work properly. The door unit will not function properly if the proper hinging device is not specified.

There are hinges that will meet all types of applications. The standards developed by the Builders Hardware Manufacturers Association (BHMA) and promulgated through the American National Standards Institute (ANSI) are extremely helpful in making the correct selection of the proper hinge. These standards include ANSI/BHMA A156.1, A156.7, and A156.17.

The following eight points are intended to assist in proper hinge selection.

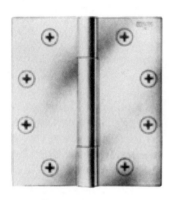

Full Mortise

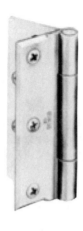

Half Mortise

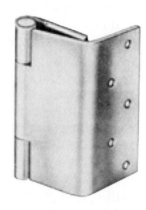

Half Mortise SwingClear

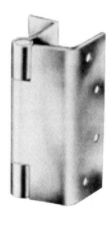

Full-Mortise Swing Clear

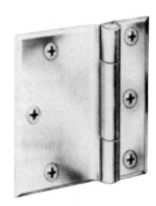

Full Surface

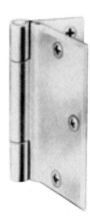

Half Surface

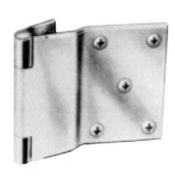

Full-Surface Swing Clear

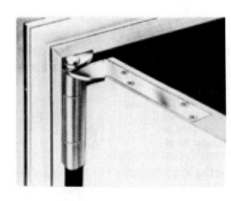

Pivot Reinforced

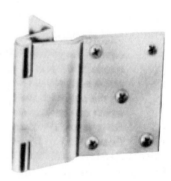

Half-Surface Swing Clear

FIGURE 7.10
Types of hinges.

1. Determine the Type of Hinge

Several pieces of information are needed to select the proper type of hinge. What is the door material (wood or hollow metal)? What is the frame material (wood or hollow metal, channel iron)?

The four classifications of hinges are as follows:

Full mortise—Both leaves are **mortised,** one leaf to the door and one leaf to the frame (WD [wood door] or HM [hollow metal] with WF [wood frame] or HMF [hollow metal frame]).

Half mortise—One leaf is mortised to the door, and the other is surface applied to the frame (HM with CIF).

Full surface—Both leaves are applied to the surface, one to the door and the other to the frame (MCD [metal core door] or HM with CIF [channel iron frame]).

Half surface—One leaf is mortised to the frame and the other is surface applied to the face of the door (WD × WF or MCD × HMF).

There is one easy way to remember what the hinge is called. The full mortise and the full surface really are no problem. However, the half mortise and the half surface are sometimes difficult to keep straight. You need only to remember that *what the hinge is called is what is done to the door.* A half-mortise hinge is *mortised to the door* and surface applied to the frame. A half-surface hinge is *surface applied to the door* and mortised to the frame.

There are several features available for the full-mortise hinge that have to be indicated before going further. One point that must be made when discussing the classification of hinges is the term *swaging.* **Swaging** is a slight offset to the hinge leaf at the barrel. This offset permits the leaves to come closer together when the door is in the closed position. If the hinge were left in the natural state after the knuckle was rolled, the hinge would be referred to as **flatback.** A flatback hinge has a gap between the leaves of approximately 5/32 of an inch. This allows heat and air conditioning to escape, not to mention the unsightly gap between the door and the frame.

The standard swaging on standard-weight and heavyweight full-mortise hinges provides 1/16 of an inch clearance between the leaves when the leaves are in the closed position.

Two additional commonly used features are the nonremovable pin (NRP) and the security safety stud (Sec Std.)

The nonremovable pin has a small set screw in the body of the barrel. This set screw is tightened down against the pin. In most cases the pin has a groove in the position where the set screw makes contact, allowing the set screw to seat. The set screw is positioned so it cannot be reached unless the door is opened. If pin removal is necessary, the set screw merely is removed and the pin is tapped from the bottom in the usual manner.

The security safety stud is another feature that places a stud on one leaf and a locking hole in the other leaf. When the door is closed the stud is anchored into the opposite leaf. Even if the hinge pin is removed, the door is secure because the leaves are locked together. (See Figure 7.11.)

FIGURE 7.11
Nonremovable pin (NRP) and security stud. (Drawings courtesy of Door and Hardware Institute, "Butts and Hinges," *Tech Talk*, by H. Matt Bouchard, Jr. AHC.)

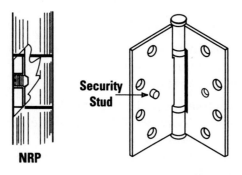

NRP   **Security Stud**

FIGURE 7.12
Raised barrel for square-edged door and raised barrel for beveled-edge door. (Drawings courtesy of Door and Hardware Institute, "Butts and Hinges," *Tech Talk*, by H. Matt Bouchard, Jr. AHC.)

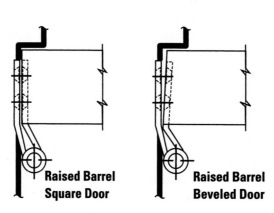

Raised Barrel Square Door   **Raised Barrel Beveled Door**

One important point must be made here. Both these features are intended as *deterrents only*. If someone wants to gain entry through a door badly enough, eventually they will get through!

Another special function available is the *raised barrel* hinge, which is used when the door is set back *into the frame*.

There are three different types of applications: jamb surface mount, raised barrel for square-edged door, and raised barrel for beveled-edge door.

On the jamb-surface-mount application, the door is mounted to accommodate both hinge leaves or what sometimes is referred to as a *double mortised*. The jamb surface mount may be applied to either a square- or a beveled-edge door.

The raised barrel for square-edge door and raised barrel for bevel-edge door are mortised into the frame and door as a standard full-mortise hinge. (See Figure 7.12.)

Depending on the depth of the frame, all three of these applications may restrict the degree of opening.

Another special feature is the *swing-clear* type. This is used mostly in hospitals and institutional buildings when the passage area must be the full width of the opening. One such use would be an 8-foot-wide corridor that requires a full opening for the passage of two beds or carts. With the use of swing-clear hinges, this passage can be accomplished. (See Figure 7.13.)

The hinges are designed to swing the door completely clear of the opening when the door is opened at a 95-degree angle. The standard way to accomplish this degree of opening is to build a

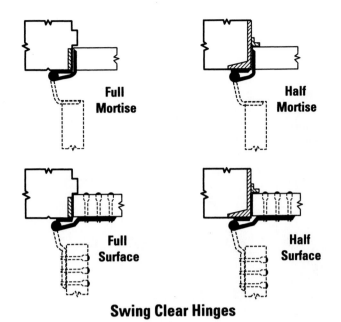

FIGURE 7.13
Swing-clear hinges.
(Drawings Courtesy of
Door and Hardware
Institute, "Butts and
Hinges," *Tech Talk*, by
H. Matt Bouchard, Jr. AHC.)

pocket in the wall to accept the door. This allows the door to be concealed in the wall and not obstruct the flow of traffic.[2]

Soss® Invisible Hinges from Universal Industrial Products are available for light-, medium-, and heavy-duty applications. They are also available for metal cabinet applications. (See Figure 7.14.)

Concealed hinges for cabinets are different in construction from concealed door hinges. They are not visible from the outside of the cabinet but are surface mounted on the inside of the cabinet door. (See Figure 7.14.)

2. Select the Proper Weight and Bearing Structure

Because of the large variety of door sizes and weights, hinges are divided into three groups:
Heavyweight—ball bearing
Standard weight—ball bearing
Standard weight—plain bearing

3. Determine the Size of the Hinge

Two factors determine the weight and structure of the hinge; several bits of information will be necessary:

Door height
Door width
Door thickness
Door weight
Trim dimension required
A general rule of thumb is one hinge for every 30″ of door height or fraction thereof.
Doors up to 60″ in height—two hinges
Doors over 60″ but not over 90″ in height—three hinges
Doors over 90″ but not over 120″ in height—four hinges

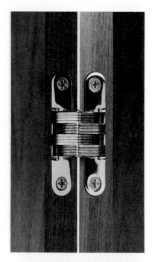

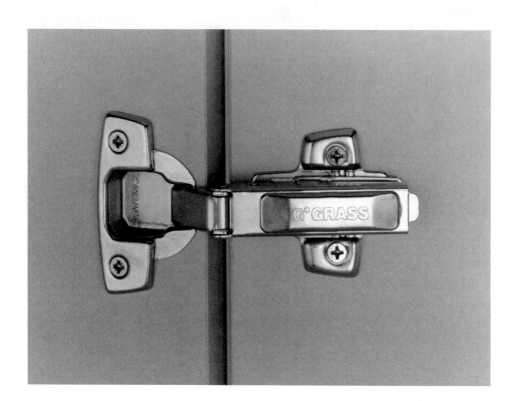

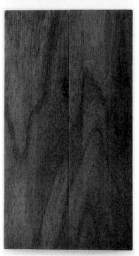

FIGURE 7.14

(a) The G 373 snap-on hinge series offers a low cost solution to a hinge installation. The G 373 offers a 110-degree opening for overlay, half overlay and inset applications. The all-metal hinge has a cup drilling depth of 10.8 mm, allowing for a door thickness from between 13 mm and 22 mm as well as doors with various edge profiles. The G 273 offers adjustment for side, height, and depth. Available in self-closing and free-swinging versions. (Photo courtesy Grass America, Inc.) (b, c) A phrase from Soss Invisible Hinge brochure aptly describes how a Soss hinge appears when the door is open and when it is closed; Now you see it . . . Now you don't. One is open—you see it; the other is closed—you don't see it. (Photo courtesy of Universal Industrial Products)

4. Determine the Type of Material

There are three base materials from which hinges are manufactured: steel, stainless steel, and brass. Each base material has different qualities, as follows:

Steel—This has great strength but is a corrosive material. If the atmosphere in which steel is used is not stable, it will begin to rust. The best application for steel is in a controlled environment, such as inside a building where the temperature and humidity are controlled.

Stainless steel—This also has great strength. It is rust resistant and has decorative value in that it can be polished to a satin or bright finish. Other considerations may be geographical, such as on the seacoast or in industrial areas where acids or atmospheric conditions exist.

Brass—Brass is noncorrosive, rust resistant, and very decorative. However, it has less strength than the steel or stainless-steel material. Brass is often used where appearance is of great concern. Brass may be polished and plated in many various finishes.

Both steel and stainless-steel hinges may be used on listed or labeled door openings (fire rated). Brass material may not be used on fire-rated or labeled openings because of its low melting point.

5. Determine the Type of Finish

All steel and brass material hinges can be plated to match the available finishes that are listed in ANSI/BHMA A156.18, *Materials and Finishes*. Most finishes are lacquered to resist oxidation or tarnishing of the finish. This will be extremely helpful during the specification process.

6. Determine Handing

The hand of a hinge is determined from the outside of the door to which it is applied. Usually, if the locked side of the door opens away (into the area) to the right, it takes a right-hand hinge (also referred to as RH). If it opens to the left, it takes a left-hand hinge (LH). (See Figure 7.15.)

7. Determine Pin and Tip Style

There are a variety of tips from which to choose. The standard in the industry is the flat-bottom tip. These normally are furnished unless something else is specified. The flush/concealed tip is the second most commonly used tip, and this is concealed inside the knuckle. Hospital tips are used primarily for security areas in hospital mental wards and in prison areas. This type of tip prevents hanging any objects on the tip of the hinge. Decorative-type tips are available from most manufacturers, such a *corn, ball, steeple,* and *urn*.

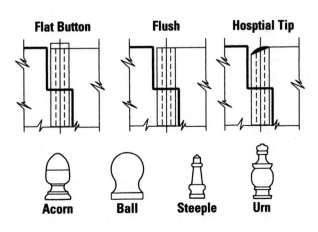

FIGURE 7.15
Pin and tip style.
(Drawings courtesy of
Door and Hardware
Institute, "Butts and
Hinges," *Tech Talk*, by
H. Matt Bouchard, Jr. AHC.)

8. Electric Hinges

Over the past 15 years, hinge manufacturers have made some changes that have revolutionized the hardware industry. With the introduction of electric hinges we now have the ability to monitor the position of the door, transfer power, and incorporate both functions into the same hinge. With this we now have the ability to electrify other hardware items such as locks and exit devices.

Electric hinges can be modified—either exposed on the surface of the hinge or concealed in the hinge. When concealed, the modifications are not visible and normally go undetected by personnel using the openings.

Electrically modified hinges are for low-voltage power transfer only (50 volts or less). Normally modifications are made to full-mortise hinges. Monitoring can be supplied on a half-surface hinge, however, when the need arises.

Most manufacturers require the use of a mortar box or jamb box to protect the wire terminations on the inside of the frame. If this box is not used, the grout that may be poured into the frame will destroy the wiring and usually will void the warranty on the product.

The spring comes in two basic types: *single acting* (full mortise and half surface) and *double acting* (full mortise, half surface).[3] Probably the only time the designer will need this type of hinge is when designing a restaurant, where this type of hinge is used for the entrance and exit doors of the kitchen.

Continuous Hinges

A relatively new concept in hanging doors is the *continuous hinge*. Continuous hinges usually are of a continuous geared type, or the traditional piano hinge . . . . Piano-type hinges are full-length surface applied continuous hinges. They are similar to traditional hinges since their design includes a rolled knuckle and pin. Piano hinges are also designed to distribute the weight of the door along the full height of the door frame. By doing so, localized stress typically found with butt hinges and pivots is eliminated, allowing smooth operation and a longer life for the door opening.[4] (See Figure 7.16.)

Locks

The needs of the client and the expected usage of a lock will determine which lock will be selected. For residential uses, security is probably the foremost criterion, whereas for a commercial installation, heavy usage will necessitate not only a secure lock, but also one built to withstand constant use.

There are three weights or grades of locks: The most expensive is heavy duty; standard duty; and light duty, or builder's grade (the least expensive). The first two types are made of solid metal with a polished, brushed, or antique finish; the light-duty grade has a painted or plated finish that may be removed with wear.

Continuous Hinges

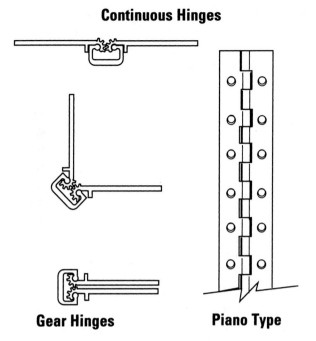

Gear Hinges   **Piano Type**

FIGURE 7.16
Continuous hinges, gear hinges, and piano-type hinges. (Courtesy of Door and Hardware Institute, "Butts and Hinges," *Tech Talk*, by H. Matt Bouchard, Jr. AHC.)

The Door and Hardware Institute describes the four types of locks as follows:

Bored type—These types of locks are installed in a door having two round holes at right angles to one another, one through the face of the door to hold the lock body and the other in the edge of the door to receive the latch mechanism. When the two are joined together in the door, they comprise a complete latching or locking mechanism.

Bored-type locks have the keyway (cylinder) and/or locking device, such as push or turn buttons, in the knobs. They are made in three weights: heavy, standard, and light duty. The assembly must be tight on the door and without excessive play. Knobs should be held securely in place without screws, and a locked knob should not be removable. **Roses** should be threaded or secured firmly to the body mechanism. The trim has an important effect in this type of lock because working parts fit directly into the trim. The regular backset for a bored lock is 2 3/4 inches, but it may vary from 2 3/8 to 42 inches.

Preassembled type—The preassembled lock is installed in a rectangular notch cut into the door edge. This lock has all its parts assembled as a unit at the factory; when installed, little or no disassembly is required. Preassembled type locks have the keyway (cylinder) in the knob. Locking devices may be in the knob or in the inner case. The regular backset is 2 3/4 inches. Preassembled type locks are available only in a heavy-duty weight. [See Figure 7.17.]

Mortise lock—A mortise lock is installed in a prepared recess (mortise) in a door. The working mechanism is contained in a rectangular-shaped case with appropriate holes into which the

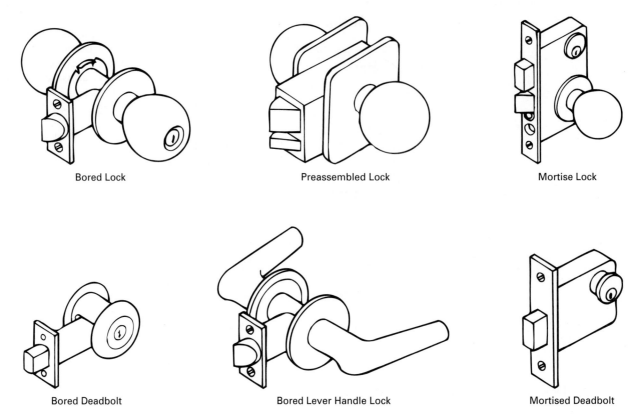

Bored Lock

Preassembled Lock

Mortise Lock

Bored Deadbolt

Bored Lever Handle Lock

Mortised Deadbolt

FIGURE 7.17
Types of locks.

required components (cylinder, knob, and turn-piece spindles) are inserted to complete the working assembly. The regular back-set is 2 3/4 inches. Mortise locks are available in heavy-duty and standard-duty weights. [See Figure 7.17.] **Armored** fronts are also available. To provide a complete working unit, mortise locks, except for those with **deadlock** function only, must be installed with knobs, levers, and other items of trim [emphasis added].[5]

Rim Lock

Rim locks were first used at the beginning of the 18th century and are attached to the inside of the door stile. They are used today in restoration work or in new homes of medieval English, Salt Box, or Cape Cod styles. Because rim locks are exposed to view, the case and other parts are finished brass. The lock achieves its function by means of various types of bolts. The bolt is a bar of metal that projects out of the lock into a strike prepared to receive it.

> The traditional style of surface-mounted rim (or box) locks for doors has been authentically re-created by Baldwin and Designed in cooperation with leading museums and historical foundations.[6]
>
> Powerbolt® provides the convenience of keyless access for today's active lifestyle. The latest in electronic technology operates on just 4 AA batteries and permits access with your personalized code or a key. It is easy to install, easy to program and easy to use. Powerbolt requires no wiring and easily replaces existing door hardware.[7]

The simplest type of door hardware is the passage set, in which both knobs are always free and there is no locking mechanism. An example would be the door between a living room, dining room, and hallway. A **springlatch** holds this type of door closed.

Bathroom doors require a privacy lock. This type locks from the inside in several ways. Some have a push button located on the interior rose, some have a turn or push button in the interior knob, and still others have a turnpiece that activates a bolt. In an emergency, all privacy locks have some means of opening from the outside, either with an emergency release key or a screwdriver.

When the type of use has been decided on, the style of the handle, rose, and finish is selected. There are many shapes of knobs (e.g. ball, round with a semiflat face, or round with a concave face, which may be decorated). Knobs may be made of metal, glass, porcelain, or wood. Grip-handle entrance locks combine the convenience of button-in-the-knob locking with traditional grip-handle elegance. Grip handles should be of cast brass or cast bronze. Interior colonial doors may have a thumb latch installed on the stile surface.

Lever handles are used in private residences and are easier for those with arthritic hands to operate. Levers are also the preferred type for ADA requirements; however, door latch and lockset with door knobs are acceptable. The maximum torque for all door controls (e.g., latch and locksets, door levers, etc.) shall be 8 foot-pounds, with 5 foot-pounds preferred.

When blind persons have access to areas that might be dangerous, such as a doorway leading to stairs, the knob must be knurled or ridged to provide a tactile warning. (See Figure 7.19.) Schlage® manufactures an access bow key with a variety of sizes. The standard bow is 1" across, Hotel bows are 1.5", Access are 1.75", and the Everest® bows are 1.2" across. All Everest key control systems are patented and can only be copied by Schlage locksmiths. For recognition by blind people the larger bow is easily identified. Schlage will also stamp "DO NOT DUPLICATE" on any bow of all versions of its keys at no extra charge, when specified.

Clear finishes take the color of the base metal in the product and may be either high or low luster. Applied finishes result from the addition (by plating) of a second metal, a synthetic enamel, or other material. The most popular of the plated finishes are the chromiums, both polished and satin.

Polished brass and bronze finishes are produced by buffing or polishing the metal to a high gloss before applying a synthetic coating. Satin brass and natural bronze finishes are obtained by dry buffing or scouring, and the resultant finish is then coated. Locks, which include all operating mechanisms, come with numerous finishes, including brass, bronze, chrome, and stainless steel in bright polish, satin, antique, or oil rubbed. Baldwin Hardware Company first produced brass hardware using physical vapor deposition (**PVD**), a process that uses low-voltage ionization to create a stacked finish that is practically indestructible. This finish, when used on brass products from Baldwin, is called the Lifetime® finish.

Roses are used to cover the bored hole in the door and may be round or square, and may also be decorated. Some locks, particularly the mortise type, have **escutcheon** plates instead of roses. These are usually rectangular in shape.

Security, function, and handing are all factors to be considered with regard to mortise locks.

Strictly speaking, the door itself is only right or left hand; the locks and the latches may be reverse bevel. It is necessary, however, to include the term *reverse* and to specify in accordance with the conventions on page 226. This will prevent any confusion regarding which side is the outside, which is especially important when different finishes are desired on opposite sides of the door.

Hardware, in general, may be

1. *Universal.* Used in any position (Example: surface bolt).
2. *Reversible.* Hand can be changed by revolving from left to right, or by turning upside down or by reversing some part of the mechanism. (Example: many types of locks and latches).
3. *Handed (not reversible).* Used only on doors of the hand for which designed. (Example: most rabbeted front door locks and latches).

Although the hardware item specified may be reversible, or even universal, it is good practice to identify the hand completely, in accordance with the convention stated here.[8]

All Schlage locks are reversible. The correct hand, however, should be shown for all pin tumbler locks (small cylindrical pins that form obstacles unless the proper key is used), so that they may be assembled to assure that keyholes are in the upright position. Hand information is also necessary to ensure proper finish of latchbolt and strike for locks that are to be installed on reverse-bevel doors. The assembly must be followed correctly to determine the hand of the door. Some locks must be ordered as right- or left-handed. (See Figure 7.9.)

Security has become an important feature of lockset selection. Most companies manufacture a lockset for which a key must be used on the outside. The lock features simultaneous retraction of both the latch and the deadbolt from the inside, by turning the knob or lever, providing panic-proof (emergency) exiting. Such locks are recommended by police and fire departments to provide compliance with safety and security codes. The distance the belt penetrates the frame is called the **throw**.

Schools, healthcare facilities and commercial offices are becoming more and more aware of the risks associated with easily copied keys. In response to changing security needs, Schlage now offers four primary levels of key control so you can choose the products that match your security needs precisely. You can secure sensitive exterior doors with Primus® key systems without the expense of rekeying the entire facility. Primus keys operate existing Everest® and Classic cylinders. Everest and Classic keys do not operate Primus cylinders.[9]

The patented MacLock® 1500 replaces a deadbolt's single stress point with 28 inches of steel-to-steel surface contact between door and frame. A simple rotation of a key or thumb-turn extends the blade from the door into a strike plate mounted in the door frame. The deadlocked blade distributes stress across 28 inches of hardware, effectively eliminating door and frame tearout, which is common with kick-ins. From the outside, there's no hint that the MacLock is there; all that is visible is a keyed lock that looks like any other deadbolt installation. (See Figure 7.18.)

A door should be controlled at the desired limit of its opening cycle to prevent damage to an adjacent wall or column, to equipment, to the door, or to its hardware. This control is achieved by stops and holders, which may be located on the floor or wall or overhead.

Floor stops are available in varied heights, sizes, shapes, and functions. They may have a mechanism, such as a hook or friction device, to hold the door open at the option of the user. The height of the door from the floor, shape of stops, and location of stops in relation to traffic are important considerations.

Wall stops or bumpers have the advantage of being located where they do not conflict with floor coverings or cleaning equipment. Thus, they do not constitute a traffic hazard.

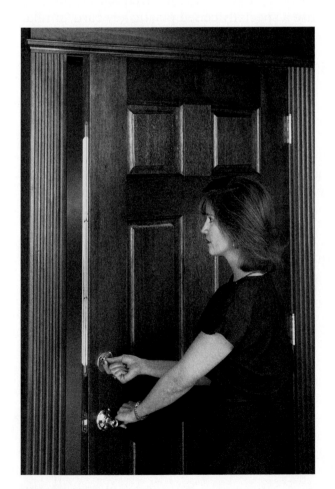

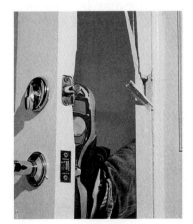

FIGURE 7.18
The large photograph shows the Maclock 1500, with its 28-inch steel blade that fits into the 3H-inch steel strike. The inset photograph shows the contrast with a regular dead bolt in case of a kick-in. (Photographer Winn Fugue; photos courtesy of MacLock Industries LLC.)

For commercial installations, there are two commonly used types of floor holders: the spring-loaded "step-on" type, and the lever or "flip-down" type. Neither type acts as a stop.

Overhead closers used in commercial installations may be either surface mounted or concealed. These devices are a combination of a spring and an oil-cushioned piston that dampens the closing action inside a cylinder. Surface-mounted closers are more accessible for maintenance, but concealed closers are more aesthetically pleasing. An actuator for power operations consists of a round plate with the ADA symbol on it. This actuator provides less than 5.0-lb opening force on a 36" wide door. A three-second delay is required to provide safe passage for a disabled person. (See Figure 7.19.)

In public buildings, all doors must open out for fire safety. A push plate is attached to the door or a fire exit bar or panic bar is used. Slight pressure of the bar releases the rod and latch. For use by disabled individuals, this bar should be able to be operated with a maximum of 8 pounds of pressure.

An electronic eye is not a security measure but provides ease of access. When the beam is broken (i.e., someone steps in its path), the door opens. Locks that open without a key are frequently used for security purposes. Hotels use a specially coded plastic key card, similar to a credit card; the code is changed when the person checks out. Numbered combinations may also be used. The combination may be changed easily, thus eliminating the need to reissue keys. More sophisticated systems can scan and identify the unique pattern of blood cells inside a person's eye, recognize fingerprints or the distinctive profile of a hand, or even respond to a voice whose digitized sound was previously stored in the system.

Plastic key cards and combination codes are often used in restrooms of office buildings and other special areas where access is restricted to certain personnel. In some cases the key cards are used for time-card purposes.

To eliminate having to carry several keys for residential use, all the locksets for exterior doors may be keyed the same. This universal keying may be done when the locks are ordered, or a locksmith can make the changes later (but at a greater expense).

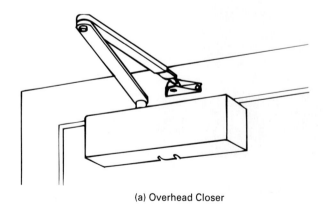

(a) Overhead Closer

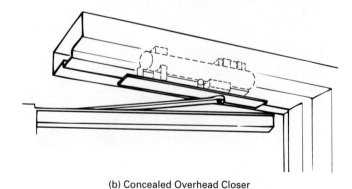

(b) Concealed Overhead Closer

FIGURE 7.19
Overhead door controls.

When specifying locksets, the following information must be provided: manufacturer's name and style number, finish, style of knob and rose, backset, wood or metal door, thickness of door, and door handing.

Lockset installation should be performed by a professional locksmith or carpenter to ensure correct fit (e.g., no door rattles or other fitting problems).

HOSPITAL HARDWARE

Hardware for hospitals and health-related institutions includes items that might not be found in any other type of building. Because the hardware may be used by aged, infirm, sick, or disabled individuals, it must meet all the ADA requirements of safety, security, and protection, and yet be operable with a minimum amount of effort.

Modifications of hinges may include hospital tips for added safety, special length and shape of leaves to swing doors clear of an opening, and hinges of special sizes and gauges to carry the weight of lead-lined doors.

Hospital pulls are designed to be mounted with the open end down, allowing the door to be operated by the wrist, arm, or forearm when the hands are occupied.[10]

BIBLIOGRAPHY

Buchard, Matt, Jr., AHC. "Butts and Hinges," *Tech Talk*. McLean, VA: Door and Hardware Institute, 1998.

Composite Panel Association. *Technical Bulletin, Particleboard and MDF for Shelving*. Gaithersburg, MD: Composite Panel Association, 1998.

GLOSSARY

apron.   Flat piece of trim placed directly under the windowsill.

armored.   Two plates are used to cover the lock mechanism in order to prevent tampering.

astragal.   Vertical strip of wood with weather stripping.

backplate.   An applied decorative moulding used on ceilings above a chandelier or ceiling fan.

backset.   The horizontal distance from the center of the face-bored hole to the edge of the door.

base shoe.   Moulding used next to the floor.

bed moulding.   Cornice moulding.

brickmould.   Exterior wood moulding to cover gap between a door or window and its frame.

butt hinges.   Two metal plates joined with a pin, one being fastened to the door jamb or frame and the other to the door.

casing.   The exposed trim moulding around a door or window.

caulk.   To fill a joint with resilient mastic. Also spelled **calk.**

chair rail.   Strip of wood or moulding that is placed on a wall at the same height as the back of a chair to protect the wall from damage.

cornice.   An ornamental moulding between the ceiling and the top of the wall.

countersunk.   Hole prepared with a bevel to enable the tapered head of a screw to be inserted flush with the surface.

dado. A groove cut in wood to receive and position another member.

deadbolt or deadlock. Hardened steel bolt with a square head operated by a key or turn-piece.

Door and Hardware Institute (DHI). The organization that represents the industry.

escutcheon. Plate that surrounds the keyhole and/or handle.

fascia. The flat, outside member of a cornice placed in a vertical position.

flatback. A hinge that has a gap between the leaves of approximately 5/32 of an inch.

knuckle. Cylindrical area of hinge enclosing the pin.

leaves. Flat plates of a pair of hinges.

lights. Small panes of glass. Usually rectangular in shape.

mitered. Two cuts at a 45-degree angle to form a right angle.

mortised. Set into the surface.

nonremovable. Pins that cannot ride up with use.

ogee. A double-curved shape resembling an S shape.

ovolo. A convex moulding, usually a quarter of a circle.

pins. The bolts of metal holding the leaves together.

polymer. A high-molecular-weight compound from which mouldings are made.

prehung. Frame and door are packaged as one unit.

rails. Cross-members of paneling (walls or doors).

rose. The plate, usually round, that covers the bored hole on the face of the door.

shoe moulding. A small moulding, such as a quarter round, nailed next to the floor on baseboards.

Shoji. Japanese room divider or window consisting of a light wooden frame covered with a translucent material, originally rice paper, but now a less vulnerable manmade material.

soffit. The underside of an overhead surface, such as an arch, cornice, eave, beam, or stairway.

springlatch. Latch with a spring rather than a locking action.

standing trim. Trim that is custom manufactured to a specific length

sticking. The shaping of moulding.

stiles. Vertical members of paneling (walls or doors).

stool. The flat piece on which a window shuts down, corresponding to the sill of a door.

stringer. The diagonal piece of wood that supports that reads of a stairway.

swaging. A slight offset to the hinge at the barrel.

template hardware. Hardware that exactly matches a master template drawing, as to spacing of all holes and dimensions.

throw. The distance a bolt penetrates when fully extended.

transom. The glass area above a door.

NOTES

[1]*Architectural Woodwork Institute Quality Standards Illustrated,* 8th ed. p. 72.

[2]*Basic Architectural Hardware,* (McLean, VA: Door and Hardware Institute, 1985, pp. 8–10.

[3]*Butts and Hinges, Tech Talk,* McLean VA: Door and Hardware Institute, 1998, p. 1.

[4]Ibid.

[5]Ibid.

[6]Baldwin Hardware website, www.baldwinhardware.com.

[7]Weiser Lock website, www.weiserlock.com.

[8]*Basic Architectural Hardware,* p. 10.

[9]*It's Time to Climb Everest,* Schlage brochure, 2000.

[10]*Basic Architectural Hardware,* p. 12.

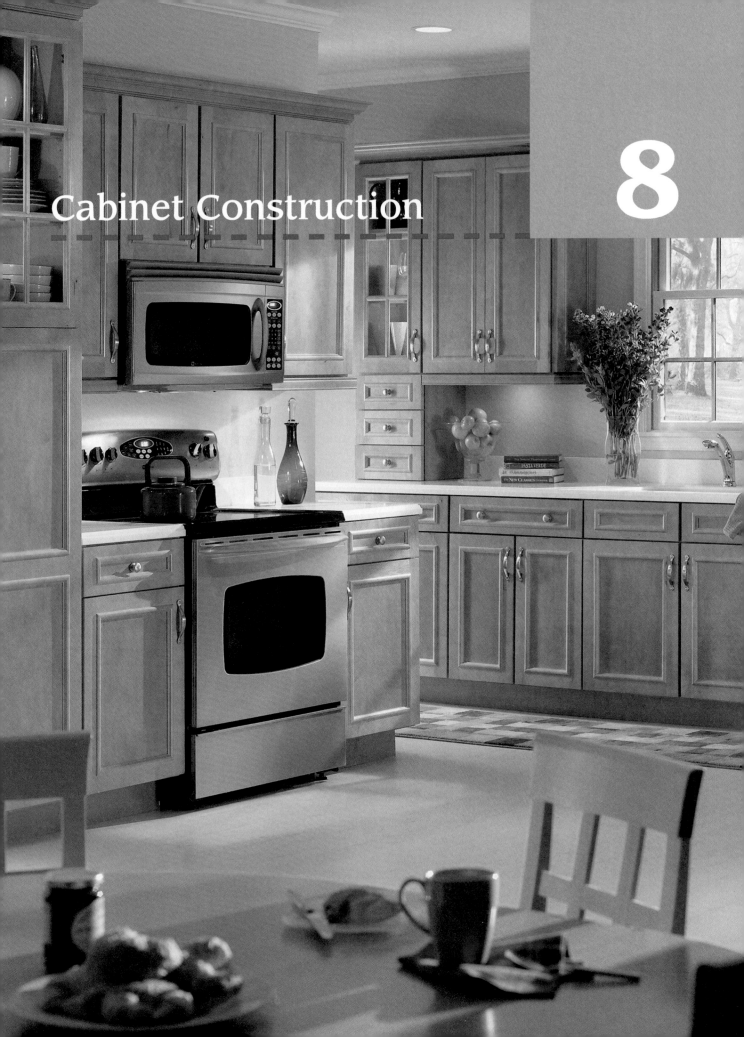

Cabinet Construction

8

To select or design well-made cabinet work, it is necessary to become familiar with furniture construction. By studying casework joints, specifiers will be able to compare and contrast similar items and make an informed decision on which piece of furniture, or which group of cabinets, offers the most value for the money.

Grade must be specified standards provide for three grades: premium, custom, and economy. The following are similar to those for plywood but are repeated here:

Premium grade—The grade specified when the highest degree of control over the quality of workmanship, materials, installation, and execution of the design intent is required. Usually reserved for special projects, or feature areas within a project.

Custom grade—The grade specified for most conventional architectural woodwork. This grade provides a well-defined degree of control over the quality of workmanship, materials, and installation of a project. The vast majority of all work produced is custom grade.

Economy grade—The grade that defines the minimum expectation of quality, workmanship, materials, and installation within the scope of these standards.

Prevailing grade—When the Quality Standards are referenced as a part of the contract documents and no grade is specified, custom-grade standards shall prevail. In the absence of specifications, material shall be mill-option lumber or veneers suitable for opaque finish.

Seismic requirements must be specified—In the absence of specifications, cabinets will not be fabricated to meet any seismic code requirements prevalent in some areas of the world.

Note: Structural lumber (S-DRY) is generally not a suitable casework materials. Rig materials, base frames, kicks, and so on should be made from kiln-dried hardwoods or softwoods with a moisture content of 5 to 10 percent, or a suitable panel product.[1]

When designing casework and specifying materials, several parts need definition. The AWI offers the following "Identification of Parts":

A. Exposed Parts—Surfaces visible when:
1. Drawer fronts and doors are closed;
2. Cabinets and shelving are open-type or behind clear glass doors;
3. Bottoms of cabinets are seen 1219 mm [48″] or more above finished floor;
4. Tops of cabinets are seen below 1829 mm [72″] above finished floor, or are visible from an upper floor or staircase after installation;
5. Portions of cabinets are visible after fixed appliances are installed;
6. Front edges of cabinet body members are visible or seen through a gap of greater than 3.2 mm [1/8″] with doors and drawers closed (sim. Tests 400A-C-1 & 400B-C-1).

Note: For the purpose of factory finishing, both sides of cabinet doors shall be considered *exposed*.

B. Semiexposed Parts—Surfaces visible when:
1. Drawers/doors are in the open position;

2. Bottoms of cabinets are between 762 mm [30"] and up to 1219 mm [48"] above finish floor;

3. All front edges of shelving behind doors.

C. Concealed Surfaces—Surfaces are concealed when:

1. Surfaces are not visible after installation;

2. Bottoms of cabinets are less than 762 mm [30"] above finish floor;

3. Tops of cabinets are 1829 mm [72"] or more above finished floor and are not visible from an upper level;

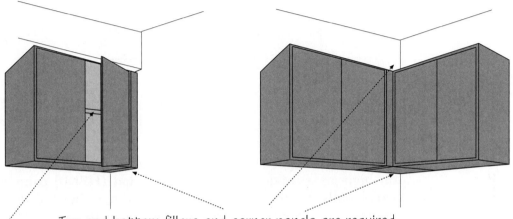

Top and bottom fillers and corner panels are required in Premium Grade, but optional for Custom Grade work.

Contrasting colors may occur (e.g. at door/drawer gaps) unless Exposed and Semi-Exposed finishes are carefully specified by the design professional.

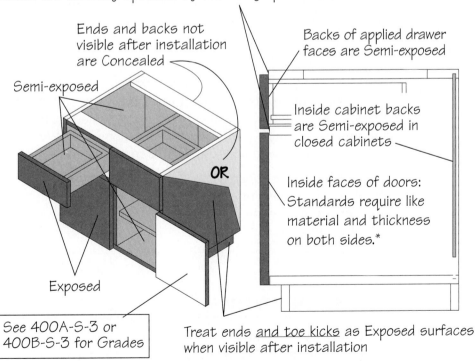

Ends and backs not visible after installation are Concealed

Semi-exposed

Exposed

See 400A-S-3 or 400B-S-3 for Grades

Treat ends and toe kicks as Exposed surfaces when visible after installation

Backs of applied drawer faces are Semi-exposed

Inside cabinet backs are Semi-exposed in closed cabinets

Inside faces of doors: Standards require like material and thickness on both sides.*

OR

FIGURE 8.1
Identification of parts. (Drawing courtesy of the Architectural Woodwork Institute)

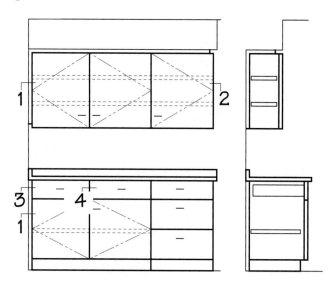

4. Stretchers, blocking, and/or components are concealed by drawers.
5. Corners are created by tall, wall, or base cabinets, and shall be nonaccessible.

Caution: Special consideration should be given to raw wood parts on high-pressure-decorative-laminate-clad (HPDL) cabinets such as wood pulls, wood trims, applied mouldings, banded doors, drawer bodies, and wood cabinet interiors. Specifications regarding the responsibility for finishing (if any) should be clarified by the design professional.[2] Note: A toe kick is required for such items as kitchen cabinets and dressers, to provide a recessed space for toes under doors or drawers. This toe kick is usually 3 inches high and 3 inches deep. For the European kitchen cabinets, the toe space measures 5 7/8 inches high. (See Figures 8.1 and 8.2.)

DRAWERS AND DOORS

Drawer or door fronts may be of one of the five following design categories, and construction will vary with the grade. Custom grade will use glue and finish nail, premium grade will be glued (no nails or other visible fasteners), and economy grade may be nailed.

1. **Flush** overlay construction
2. **Reveal** overlay construction
3. **Reveal** overlay on face frame
4. Flush inset
5. Flush inset with face frame.[3]

A. FLUSH OVERLAY

Doors (1, 2) and drawer faces (3) cover (or nearly cover) the body members (4) of the cabinet, with spaces left between adjacent surfaces sufficient for operating clearance. Flush overlay construction offers a very clean, contemporary look because only the doors and drawer fronts are visible in elevation. When

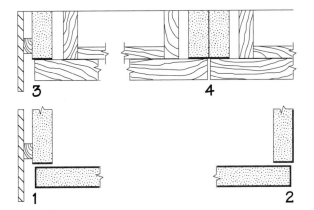

FIGURE 8.3A
Plan section—flush overlay, reveal overlay, reveal overlay (frame), flush inset, and flush inset (frame). (Drawing courtesy of the Architectural Woodwork Institute)

Plan Section - Flush Overlay - Figure 400-03

specified, grain matching between doors and drawer fronts can be achieved by having all pieces cut from the same panel. This style is increasingly popular and lends itself well to the use of plastic laminate for exposed surfaces. Conventional as well as **concealed hinges** are available for a variety of door thicknesses. (See Figure 8.3a.)

B. REVEAL OVERLAY

Doors (1, 2) and drawer faces (3) partially cover the body members or face frames (4) of the cabinet, with spaces between face surfaces sufficient for operating clearance.

In this style, the separation between doors and drawer fronts is accented by the reveal. The style is equally suited to either wood or plastic laminate construction. Although the detail shown here incorporates a reveal at all horizontal and vertical joints, this can be varied by the designer. It should be noted that a reveal over 12.7 mm [1/2"] may, at the woodworker's option, require the addition of a face frame. The addition of a face frame will change the hinge requirements. With or without a face frame, this style allows the use of conventional or concealed hinges. (See Figure 8.3b.)

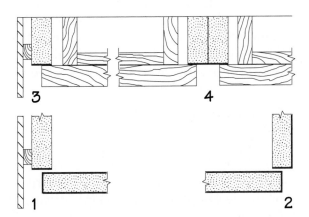

FIGURE 8.3B

Plan Section - Reveal Overlay - Figure 400-04

FIGURE 8.3C

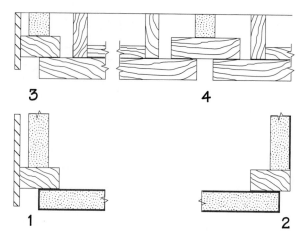

Plan Section - Reveal Overlay (Frame) - Figure 400-05

C. REVEAL OVERLAY ON FACE FRAME

Doors (1,2) and drawer faces (3) are set over face frames or face members (4) on the cabinet. Finished end and scribe details vary with the manufacturer and the QSI Grade specified for the project by the design professional. (See Figure 8.3c.)

D. FLUSH INSET

Doors (1, 2) and drawer faces (3) are inset within members (4) of the cabinet. Gaps between the case and the doors or drawers are often dictated by the operating clearances of the fittings.

With this style of construction, all door and drawer faces are flush with the face of the cabinet. This style is highly functional and allows the use of different thicknesses of door and drawer fronts.

Conventional as well as concealed hinges are available for a variety of door thicknesses. The choice of case and door/drawer material influence the choice of hinges. Conventional butt hinges should be avoided when hinge screws would be attached to the edge-grain of panel products.

This is generally an expensive style due to the increased care necessary in the fitting and aligning of the doors and drawers.

The design features of this casework style are the same as conventional flush with face frame except that the face frame has been eliminated. This style does not lend itself to the economical use of plastic laminate covering finishes. (See Figure 8.3d.)

E. FLUSH INSET WITH FACE FRAME

Doors (1, 2) and drawer faces (3) are inset next to face frames or face members (4) on the cabinet. Finished end and scribe details vary with the manufacturer and the QSI Grade specified for the project by the design professional. Gaps between the case and the doors or drawers are often dictated by the operating clearances of the fittings. With this style of construction, all door and drawer faces are flush

FIGURE 8.3D

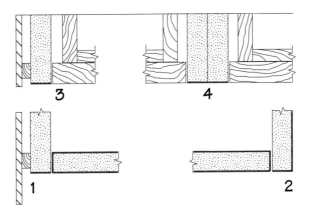

Plan Section - Flush Inset - Figure 400-06

with the face of the cabinet. This style is highly functional and allows the use of different thicknesses of door and drawer fronts.

Conventional as well as concealed hinges are available for a variety of door thicknesses. The choice of case and door/drawer material influence the choice of hinges. Conventional butt hinges should be avoided when hinge screws would be attached to the edge-grain of panel products.

This is generally the most expensive of the four styles shown in this publication due to the increased care necessary in the fitting and aligning of the doors and drawers, in addition to the cost of providing the face frame.

This style does not lend itself to the economical use of plastic laminate covering.

Grain direction (the appearance of the figure) shall run vertically for all doors in every grade, and shall run vertically or horizontally on drawer fronts in custom and economy, with the same direction maintained on any one cabinet or elevations of cabinets. Premium and custom doors shall be set matched. (See Figures 8.3e and 8.4.)[4]

JOINERY OF CASE BODY MEMBERS

The types of joints for drawer construction vary according to grade. Table 8.1, Drawer Construction Techniques, is shown in Section 400B-T-7 of the AWI Standards.

FIGURE 8.3E

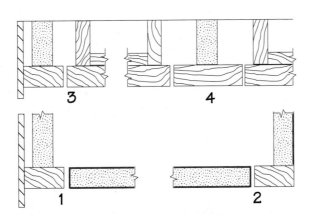

Plan Section - Flush Inset (Frame) - Figure 400-07

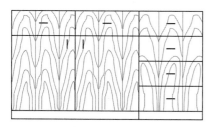

Premium Grade
Doors & Drawer fronts
from sequenced panel sets, well
matched for grain, figure & color

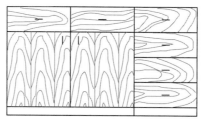

Custom Grade
Drawer fronts no
match required. May be
solid or panel product.

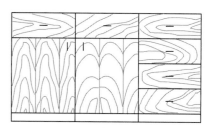

Economy Grade

FIGURE 8.4
Direction and matching. (Drawing courtesy of the Architectural Woodwork Institute)

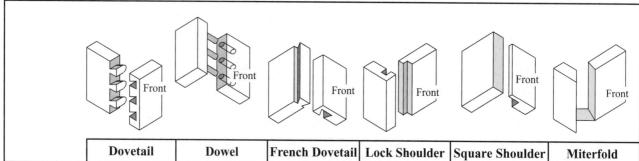

	Dovetail	Dowel	French Dovetail	Lock Shoulder	Square Shoulder	Miterfold
Permitted in Grade	Premium Custom Economy	Premium Custom Economy	Premium Custom Economy	Premium Custom Economy	Economy	Premium Custom Economy
Notes: and Recommended Material Choices [3]		1	2			All four sides and the bottom are machined from one piece
Solid Lumber	√	√	√	√	√	
Veneer Core		√	√	√	√	
Combo. Core		√		√	√	√
Particle Core		√			√	√
Fiber Core		√			√	√

NOTES: In the absence of specifications, the following standards will apply. Where more than one method or material is listed, AWI/AWMAC woodworkers will supply their choice from the alternatives.
1 - The "European" system assembly screw or dowel screw with matching caps is permitted in this configuration when material is 19 mm [3/4"] or thicker
2 - Fully captured bottoms are not feasible when French Dovetail joinery is employed.
3 - While virtually all materials can be painted, stained, finished, or clad with veneers or overlays, solid lumber is usually selected for species and then painted, stained, and/or finished. Panel products may also be painted, stained, and/or finished in their raw state as well as veneered or clad with another product. Thermoset Decorative Overlays are generally limited to particle core panel products.

TABLE 8.1
Drawer Construction Techniques

All drawer bottoms should have a minimum thickness of 1/4 inch and should be captured into **dados** on drawer sides, fronts, and backs.

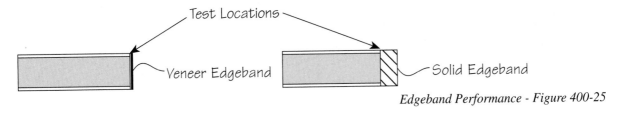

Edgeband Performance - Figure 400-25

FIGURE 8.5
Edgeband performance. (Drawing courtesy of the Architectural Woodwork Institute)

This construction creates a bottom panel that is permanently locked into position.

EDGE TREATMENTS

Edge banding is a method of concealing plies or inner cores of plywood or particleboard when edges are exposed. Thickness or configuration will vary with manufacturers' practices. (See Figure 8.5.)

WOOD CABINETS

For a traditional type of paneling, **stile** and rail construction is used, which consists of a panel that may be flat, raised, or have a beveled edge. The vertical side strips are called stiles, and the horizontal strips at the top and bottom are called rails.

Rails, stiles, and **mullions** may be shaped into an **ovolo** or **ogee** moulding; or, to give a more intricate design, a separate moulding may be added. For raised panels under 10 inches in width, solid lumber may be used in custom grade. For premium grade or wider panels, plywood is used with an attached edge of solid lumber, which is then beveled. (See Figure 8.6.)

Panels are assembled all in one by means of mortise and tenon, or **dowel joints.** At the joining of the panel and the stiles and rails, a small space is left to allow for the natural expansion and contraction of the panel. This type of construction may be called *floating panel construction*, and is advisable where there are great variations in humidity. Panels that are glued have no allowance for this expansion and contraction and may split if movement is excessive. (See Figure 8.7.)

Because the detail and design options in this type of paneling are virtually unlimited, the AWI suggests that the following minimum information be provided for proper estimation and specification:

Panel layout
Grain patterns and relationships
Stile and rail construction
Moulding details
Panel construction
Joinery techniques.

DRAWER GUIDES

Drawer guides are an important feature of well-made casework. They may be constructed of wood or metal. If wood is selected, both male and

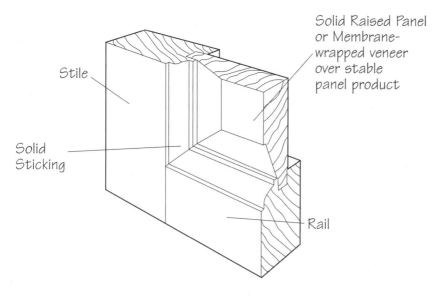

Stile

Solid Raised Panel
or Membrane-
wrapped veneer
over stable
panel product

Solid
Sticking

Rail

Solid Raised Panel - Figure 400-15

Stile

Rim Raised Panel

Solid
Sticking

Rail

Rim Raised Panel - Figure 400-16

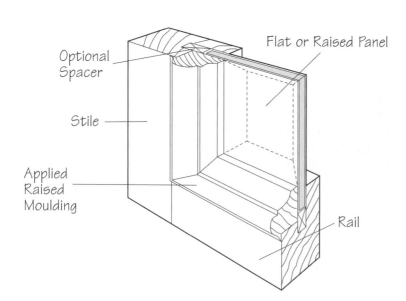

Optional
Spacer

Flat or Raised Panel

Stile

Applied
Raised
Moulding

Rail

Applied Moulding - Figure 400-17

FIGURE 8.6

Panel cabinet doors. These examples illustrate three styles of raised-panel and flat-panel doors. Applied moulding could be used for glass inserts as well. (Drawing courtesy of the Architectural Woodwork Institute)

252

Detail Nomenclature

Familiarity with the labeled details on this page will facilitate communication between architects, designers, specifiers, and woodwork manufacturers by establishing common technical language.

Spline Joint: Used to strengthen and align faces when gluing panels in width or length, including items requiring site assembly.

Stub Tenon: Joinery method for assembling stile- and rail-type frames that are additionally supported, such as web or skeleton case frames.

Haunch Mortise and Tenon Joint: Joinery method for assembling paneled doors or stile- and rail- type paneling.

Conventional Mortise and Tenon Joint: Joinery method for assembling square-edged surfaces such as case face frames.

Dowel Joint: Alternative joinery method serving same function as Conventional Mortise and Tenon.

French Dovetail Joint: Method for joining drawer sides to fronts when fronts conceal metal extension slides or overlay the case faces.

Conventional Dovetail Joint: Traditional method for joining drawer sides to fronts or backs. Usually limited to flush- or lipped-type drawers.

Drawer Lock-Joint: Another joinery method for joining drawer sides to fronts. Usually used for flush-type installation but can be adapted to lip- or overlay- type drawers.

Exposed End Details: Illustrates attachment of finished end of case body to front frame using a butt joint and a lock mitered joint.

Through Dado: Conventional joint used for assembly of case body members. Dado not concealed by application of case face frame.

Blind Dado: Variation of Through Dado with applied edge "stopping" or concealing dado groove.

Stop Dado: Another method of concealing dado exposure. Applicable when veneer edging or solid lumber is used. Exposed End Detail illustrates attachment of finished end of case body to front frame using butt joint.

Dowel Joint: Fast becoming an industry standard assembly method, this versatile joinery technique is often based on 32 mm spacing of dowels.

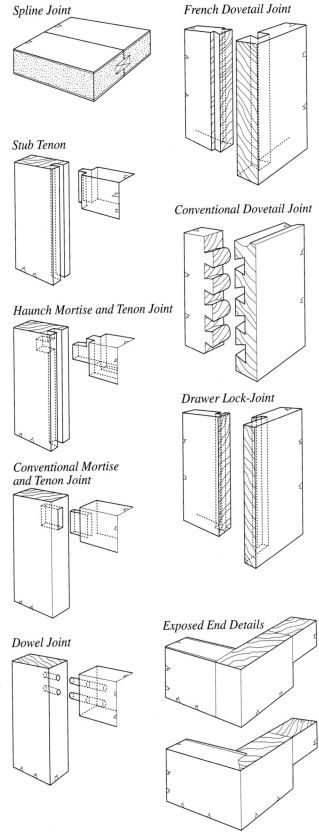

Spline Joint

Stub Tenon

Haunch Mortise and Tenon Joint

Conventional Mortise and Tenon Joint

Dowel Joint

French Dovetail Joint

Conventional Dovetail Joint

Drawer Lock-Joint

Exposed End Details

© 2003 AWI/AWMAC - 8th Edition Quality Standards

FIGURE 8.7
Detail nomenclature. (Drawing courtesy of the Architectural Woodwork Institute)

female parts should be made of wood. Wood drawer guides are found mainly in wood furniture and are usually centered under the drawer, but they may also be attached to the side of the case, with the drawer sides being dadoed to accommodate the wood guide. The reverse procedure may also be used, with the guide attached to the drawer side and the frame dados receiving the guide. Paste wax should be applied to the wood guides to facilitate movement.

Drawer Slide Selection Guide

The type of metal drawer slide selected depends on several factors: travel, width of drawer, action, and load factors.

Table 8.2 serves as both a checklist and a starting point for the discussion of a wide variety of drawer slide systems. Although by no means exhaustive, the characteristics described are often considered the most important by the client, the design professional, and the woodwork manufacturer. The selection of the slide characteristics will affect the usefulness of the cabinets. Careful consideration should be given to avoid "overspecifying" for the purpose intended. The owner and the design professional will be wise to involve an AWI/AWMAC member manufacturer in the design and selection process early in the project. Dimensions use the inch-pound convention.

Knape® and Vogt (KV) provided the following information:

Travel is the maximum extension compared to the closed length. Typically, most slides are either 3/4 or full travel. Special extension

Degree of Extension	☐ STANDARD EXTENSION—All but 4.6" of drawer body extends out of cabinet ☐ FULL EXTENSION—Entire drawer body extends out to face of cabinet ☐ FULL EXTENSION WITH OVERTRAVEL—Entire drawer body extends beyond the face of cabinet
Static Load Capacity	☐ 50 Pounds—Residential/Light Commercial ☐ 75 Pounds—Commercial ☐ 100 Pounds—Heavy Duty ☐ Over 100 Pounds—Special Conditions, Extra Heavy Duty
Dynamic Load Capacity	☐ 30 Pounds; 35,000 cycles—Residential/Light Commercial ☐ 50 Pounds; 50,000 cycles—Commercial ☐ 75 Pounds; 100,000 cycles—Heavy Duty
Removal Stop	☐ INTEGRAL STOP—Requires ten times the normal opening force to remove drawer ☐ POSITIVE STOP—Latch(es) which must be operated/opened to remove drawer
Closing	☐ SELF-CLOSING/STAY CLOSED— Drawer slides will self-close with their related dynamic load when the drawer is 2" from the fully closed position and not bounce open when properly adjusted
	In recent years several hardware manufacturers have developed "drawer systems" of one type or another, nearly all proprietary. In addition to the above criteria, the following should be considered for these system prior to approval for use.
Metal Sided Systems	☐ POSITIVE STOP—Drawer must stop within itself and not rely on the drawer front to stop it ☐ PULLOUT STRENGTH—Systems must demonstrate sufficient strength of attachment of front to sides—design professional should evaluate and approve individually

Source: Table reproduced with permission of the Architectural Woodwork Institute.

TABLE 8.2
Drawer Slide Selection Guide

lengths are available with modified travel. Generally, the longer the travel, the less load a slide can carry and vice versa.

A "3/4 Travel" slide has extension of approximately 75% of its length.

A "Full Travel" slide has extension approximately equal to its length.

An "Over-Travel" slide has travel greater than its length.

Drawer width affects the rigidity of the installation. In wide drawers, the slides will rack from side to side. Excessive racking can degrade performance and shorten life expectancy.

The type of mechanism used to carry the load determines many of the quality aspects of a slide, such as performance, motion, noise, and the "fit and feel." Slides may use rollers, ball bearings, friction fits, or any combination in achieving movement. Generally, better action requires more rollers or ball bearings in supporting and distributing large loads.[5]

Knape & Vogt designates drawer slides in "Pounds Class" categories. KV uses dynamic (rather then static) loading to determine load ratings.

The "Pound Class" categories are used within the slide industry as general guidelines for drawer slide selection. These categories are not the same as actual load ratings. Load ratings vary based on slide length, application, and casegoods construction . . .

Static loads. A static load is a resting load without any motion. Static load capacity is significantly higher than dynamic load capacity.

Dynamic loads. A dynamic load is a load in motion. When a dynamic load gains momentum, it induces more stress and fatigue. Slides must withstand more forces when in motion than when still.

Dynamic loads affect the life and performance of any slide. Other load factors affecting performance are:

1. An evenly or unevenly distributed load.
2. A centered or off-centered load.
3. The load's center-of-gravity relative to the slide's centerline-of-travel.
4. The number of cycles.
5. The speed or frequency of the cycles.
6. The length of cycle stroke.
7. The percent of travel.
8. The stopping force and distance. [emphasis added][6]

Types of mounting include side mount, which requires adequate side clearance and drawer side height; bottom mount, which has limited selection, primarily for pullout shelf applications; and top mount, which also has limited selection, primarily for undercounter drawers.

Other features may include the following: "Stay closed" slides have a built-in feature to prevent unintentional opening. Self-closing drawers will close without assistance from 4 to 6 inches of extension. A positive **stop** with trip latch removal means a trip latch must be activated to affect drawer removal. (This feature prevents drawers from accidentally being pulled completely out of position.) With lift-out removal, a drawer may be lifted from a cabinet when the drawer is fully extended.

CABINET HARDWARE

According to the AWI,

> Architectural cabinet hinges will usually be furnished from the manufacturer's stock unless otherwise specified. The four most common hinge types are show in Table 8.3.

Hinge Type	Butt	Wraparound	Pivot	European Style
Applications	Conventional Flush with Face Frame	Conventional Reveal Overlay	Reveal Overlay Flush Overlay	Conventional Flush without Face Frame Reveal Overlay Flush Overlay
Strength	High	Very High	Moderate	Moderate
Concealed when closed	No	No	Semi	Yes
Requires mortising	Yes	Occasionally	Usually	Yes
Cost of hinge	Low	Moderate	Low	Moderate
Ease of installation	Moderate	Easy	Moderate	Very Easy
Easily adjusted after installation	No	No	No	Yes
Remarks	Door requires hardwood edge	Exposed knuckle and hinge body	Door requires hardwood edge	1. Specify degree of opening 2. No catch required on self-closing styles

© 2003 AWI/AWMAC - 8th Edition Quality Standards

TABLE 8.3
Hinge Selection Guide

Concealed 35-mm Cup Hinge
Installation Requirements

When 35-mm cup hinges are used, plastic insertion dowels to receive the screws of the hinge and 5-mm "Euroscrews" to attach the baseplate are required. The attachment of hinge bodies to particleboard or fiberboard doors with wood screws in the absence of the plastic insertion dowels is not acceptable in premium or custom grade. Manufacturers may use other solutions to assure long-term functionality, as agreed between buyer and seller. At the time of this printing, only hinges showing a small knuckle meet BHMA Grade 1, and no fully concealed 35-mm cup is available tested to BHMA Grade. [See Figure 8.8.] [7]

Grass offers a European-type hinge with a lifetime warranty. There are two different methods of installation: slide-on and snap-on.

Exposed hinges have the knuckle exposed. This type is usually used on traditional-type cabinets. The European-type hinge is completely hidden from view.

A piano hinge or continuous hinge is used on drop-leaf desks and on the doors of some fine furniture. Because piano hinges are installed the whole length of the edge, they support the weight of the door in an efficient manner.

Cabinet doors and drawers may be designed without pull hardware by using a finger pull either as part of the door or drawer construction, or by adding a piece of shaped wood, plastic, or metal to the front of the door. It is necessary to design these finger pulls in such a manner that the doors or drawers open easily (without breaking fingernails).

Cabinet-pull hardware consists of knobs (rounded or square) or handles, ranging from simple metal strips to ornately designed ones. The material from which this hardware is constructed may be wood, porcelain, plastic, or metal. It is necessary to select hardware that is compatible with the design of the cabinets or furniture. For traditional or period cabinets, authentic hardware should be chosen.

Some form of catch is needed to hold cabinet doors shut. There are five different types of catches: **friction,** roller, magnetic, **bullet,** and touch catch. A friction catch, when engaged, is held in place by friction. A roller catch features a roller under tension that engages a recess in the **strike plate.** The magnet is the holding mechanism of a magnetic catch. In a bullet catch, a spring-actuated ball engages a depression in the plate. A touch catch releases automatically when the door is pushed. Many of these catches have elongated screw slots that enable the tension of the catch to be adjusted. Some hinges are spring-loaded, eliminating the need for a catch. (See Figure 8.9.)

SHELVES

For shelves, or when the case body is exposed, the following construction methods are used: Through dado is the conventional joint used for assembly of case body members, and the dado is usually concealed by a case face frame. Blind dado has an applied edge "stopping" or concealing the dado **groove** and is used when the case body edge is exposed. Stop dado is applicable when veneer edging or solid lumber is exposed.

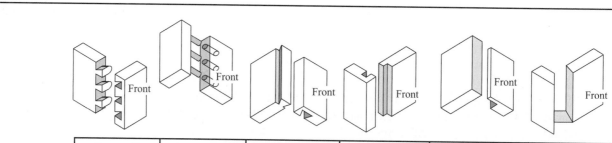

	Dovetail	Dowel	French Dovetail	Lock Shoulder	Square Shoulder	Miterfold
Permitted in Grade	Premium Custom Economy	Premium Custom Economy	Premium Custom Economy	Premium Custom Economy	Economy	Premium Custom Economy
Notes: and Recommended Material Choices [3]		1	2			All four sides and the bottom are machined from one piece
Solid Lumber	√	√	√	√	√	
Veneer Core		√	√	√	√	
Combo. Core		√		√	√	√
Particle Core		√			√	√
Fiber Core		√			√	√

NOTES: In the absence of specifications, the following standards will apply. Where more than one method or material is listed, AWI/AWMAC woodworkers will supply their choice from the alternatives.
1 - The "European" system assembly screw or dowel screw with matching caps is permitted in this configuration when material is 19mm [3/4"] or thicker.
2 - Fully captured bottoms are not feasible when French Dovetail joinery is employed.
3 - While virtually all materials can be painted, stained, finished, or clad with veneers or overlays, solid lumber is usually selected for species and then painted, stained and/or finished. Panel products may also be painted, stained, and/or finished in their raw state as well as veneered or clad with another product. Thermoset Decorative Overlays are generally limited to particle core panel products.

Drawer Joinery - Figure 400-29

400B-T-8

Concealed 35 mm cup Hinge Installation Requirements

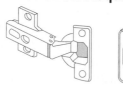

Concealed Hinges Styles - Figure 400-30

When 35 mm cup hinges are used, plastic insertion dowels to receive the screws of the hinge and 5 mm "Euroscrews" to attach the baseplate are required. The attachment of hinge bodies to particleboard or fiberboard doors with wood screws in the absence of the plastic insertion dowels is not acceptable in Premium or Custom Grade. Manufacturers may use other solutions to assure long-term functionality, as agreed between buyer and seller. At the time of this printing, only hinges showing a small knuckle meet BHMA Grade 1, and no fully concealed 35 mm cup is available tested to BHMA Grade 1

FIGURE 8.8
Concealed Hinges Styles. (Courtesy of the Architectural Woodwork Institute)

FIGURE 8.9
Cabinet catches.

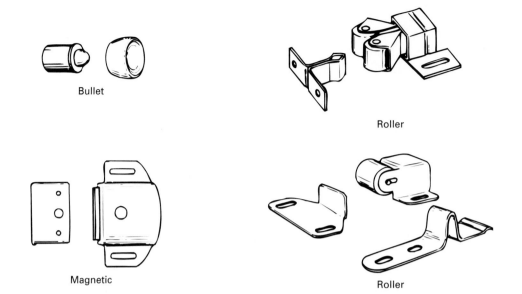

Bullet

Roller

Magnetic

Roller

The span and thickness of shelves varies according to the purpose of the shelves. The AWI provides the following specifications for shelves: "For closet and utility shelving ends and back cleats to receive clothes rods or hooks shall be 3/4 inch × 3$\frac{1}{2}$ inch minimum. Ends and back cleats which do not receive clothes rods or hooks shall be 3/4" × 1$\frac{1}{2}$" minimum. Shelf thickness shall be a minimum of 3/4" if not specified, or shall be as specified by the design professional in relation to anticipated load."[8]

To increase a shelf's visible thickness, a dropped edge or applied piece of wood, called an **apron,** is used.

Particleboard (**PB**) and medium-density fiberboard (**MDF**) are often specified for shelves, and designers should be aware of fairly specific applications. Kitchen cabinets, for example, normally will be designed for a uniform load of 15 pounds per square foot (psf), closets 25 psf, and for books 40 psf. (Table 8.1 lists maximum shelf spans in inches for uniform loading.)

The Technical Bulletin "Particleboard and MDF for Shelving" may be obtained from the Composite Panel Association.

For many common shelving applications, use Table 8.4.

It is designed to quickly determine the amount of load that can be carried on either a **PB** (particleboard) or **MDF** (medium-density fiberboard) shelving system. It is important to understand that the loads shown in the table are in units of pound per square foot (psf). This means that the load is evenly distributed over a one (1)-square-foot (144 inches) area of shelf. The distribution area can be in any shape. For example, it can be 12 inches square, 8 by 18 inches, or any combination of dimensions that equals 144 square inches. Figure 8.11 gives common shelf nomenclature and displays some possible support situations.

To use this table, first determine your estimated shelf loading, then select the desired combination of shelf span, product type, and shelf thickness for your shelf design. The allowable spans are found directly across from the shelf load values. Spans are limited to a maximum of 36 inches.

FIGURE 8.10
Through dado, blind dado,
stop dado, dowel, and Euro
screw methods of shelf
attachment. (Drawing
courtesy of the
Architectural Woodwork
Institute)

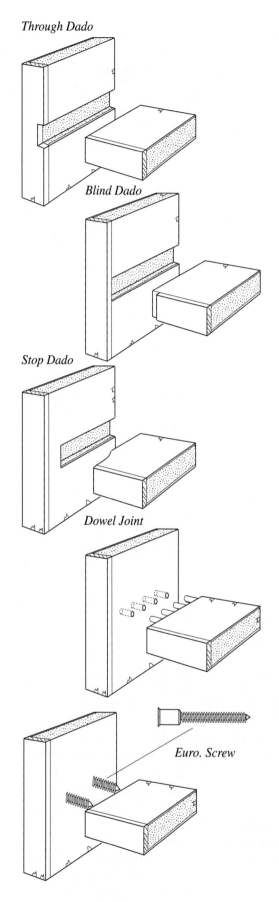

Through Dado

Blind Dado

Stop Dado

Dowel Joint

Euro. Screw

Maximum Shelf Spain (IN.)[1,2]												
Single Span[3]						Multiple Span[4]						
	Particleboard			Medium Density Fiberboard (MDF)			Particleboard			Medium Density Fiberboard (MDF)		
SHELF LOAD	SHELF THICKNESS			SHELF THICKNESS			SHELF THICKNESS			SHELF THICKNESS		
PSF[5]	1/2"	5/8"	3/4"	1/2"	5/8"	3/4"	1/2"	5/8"	3/4"	1/2"	5/8"	3/4"
50	13"	17"	20"	15"	19"	22"	13"	17"	20"	20"	25"	29"
45"	14"	18"	21"	16"	19"	23"	14"	18"	22"	21"	25"	30"
40	15"	18"	21"	16"	20"	24"	15"	19"	23"	21"	26"	31"
35	15"	19"	22"	17"	21"	25"	16"	20"	24"	22"	28"	33"
30	16"	20"	23"	18"	22"	26"	18"	22"	27"	23"	29"	34"
25	17"	21"	25"	19"	23"	28"	19"	24"	29"	25"	31"	36"
20	18"	22"	27"	20"	25"	30"	22"	27"	33"	27"	33"	36"
15	20"	25"	29"	22"	27"	33"	25"	32"	36"	29"	36"	36"
10	23"	28"	34"	25"	31"	36"	30"	36"	36"	34"	36"	36"

[1]For shelves 12 inches or less in depth with continuous support along the back edge of the shelf, the allowable span can be doubled.

[2]A maximum overhang beyond bracket or support not to exceed 6 inches may be added to these spans.

[3]Single Span: shelf simply supported (not fixed or fastened) at its ends only. (see Figure 1)

[4]Multiple Span: shelf simply supported at its ends with a center support. Span lengths refer to the distance from support to support, not the total shelf length. (see Figure 1)

[5]psf. = pounds per square foot

Source: Courtesy of composite Panel Association. Table 1 of Technical Bulletin "Particleboard and MDF for Shelving."

TABLE 8.4
Maximum Shelf Span in Inches for Uniform Loading

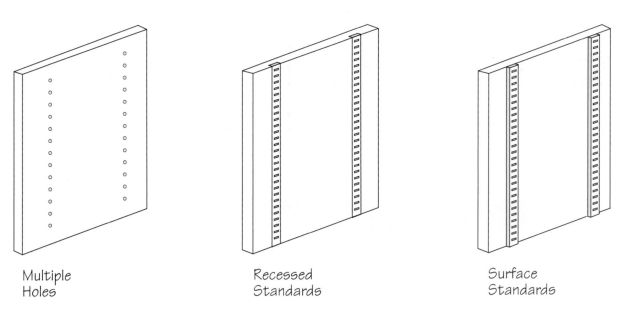

Multiple Holes

Recessed Standards

Surface Standards

FIGURE 8.11
Adjustable shelves. (Drawing courtesy of the Architectural Woodwork Institute)

Shelf loads can vary greatly. For example, kitchen cabinets can reach up to 25 or 30 psf, while bookshelf loads can easily reach 50 psf. It is necessary to know how much weight the shelf will be expected to carry. A single bathroom scale may be used to estimate the anticipated load.

When concentrated (heavy) loads are anticipated, it is important to note that the load acts only on the area where the object makes contact with the shelf. Concentrated loads can produce severe stress on shelves and must be considered carefully. Use the maximum concentrated load as the shelf loading value, rather than the average of all objects to be loaded on the shelf.

The amount of shelf deflects (or bends) depends upon the load, shelf span, and panel thickness. Table 8.4 was designed to limit deflections to a percentage of the shelf span. For example, a shelf with a 24-inch span can be expected to deflect a maximum of 0.10 inches, while a 36-inch span will deflect 0.15 inches (slightly more than 1/8").[9]

When shelves are to be installed permanently, some form of dado may be used for positioning. The type used depends on the frame construction. Another permanent installation uses a wood quarter round on which to rest the shelf. If, however, the shelves are to be adjustable, there are several methods of support. The type used in fine china cabinets is a metal shelf pin. A number of blind holes, usually in groups of three, are drilled 5/8 inch apart in two rows on each interior face of the sides. The metal shelf pins are then inserted at the desired shelf level.

Metal shelf standards have slots every inch, with two standards on each side running from top to bottom of the shelf unit. Four adjustable metal clips are inserted at the same level into these slots. The metal strips may be recessed or surface mounted. This style allows for unlimited adjustment.

For workshop and other informal shelving, metal brackets are attached to the back wall surface instead of to the sides.

BIBLIOGRAPHY

Architectural Woodwork Institute. *Architectural Woodwork Quality Standards Illustrated*, 8th ed. Version 1.0. Reston, VA: Architectural Woodwork Institute, 2003.

Composite Panel Association. Technical Bulletin, *"Particleboard and MDF for Shelving."* Gaithersburg, MD: Composite Panel Association, 1998.

GLOSSARY

apron.   A flat piece of wood attached vertically along the underside of the front edge of a horizontal surface; may be for support (as in bookshelves) or decorative.

bullet catch.   A spring-actuated ball engaging a depression in the plate.

concealed hinge.   All hinge parts are concealed when the door is closed.

dado.   A cross-grained rectangular or square section.

dowel joint.   A joint, usually right angle, using dowels for positioning and strength.

dynamic loads.   A moving load, as opposed to static.

exposed hinge.   All hinge parts are visible when the door is closed.

flush.   The door and frame are level and the frame is completely visible when the door or drawer is closed.

friction catch.   When engaged, the catch is held in place by friction.

groove.   A square or rectangular section cut with the grain.

MDF.   Medium-density fiberboard.

mullion. Vertical member between panels.

ogee. A double-curved shape resembling an S shape.

ovolo. A convex moulding, usually a quarter of a circle.

pivot hinge. Hinge leaves are mortised into the edge of the door panel and set in the frame at the top of both the jamb and door. Some pivot hinges pivot on a single point.

reveal. The small area of the frame that is visible when the door or drawer is closed.

static load. A resting load without any motion. Static load capacity is significantly higher than dynamic load capacity.

stile. Vertical pieces on paneling.

stop. A metal, plastic, or wood block placed to position the flush drawer front to be level with the face frame.

strike plate. Metal plate attached to the door frame, designed to hold the roller catch under tension.

NOTES

[1]Architectural Woodwork Institute, *Quality Standards Illustrated*, 8th ed., Reston, VA: Architectural Woodwork Institute, 2003, p. 122.

[2]Ibid, p. 152.

[3]Ibid, p. 126.

[4]Knape & Vogt, *Full Line Catalog*, p. 4.

[5]Ibid, p. 5.

[6]*Quality Standards Illustrated*, p. 158.

[7]Ibid, p. 271.

[8]Composite Panel Association, Technical Bulletin, "Particleboard and MDF for Shelving," Gaithersburg, MD: Composite Panel Association.

[9]Composite Panel Association, *Technical Bulletin, Particleboard and MDF For Shelving*. Composite Panel Association, Gaithersburg, MD: 20879.

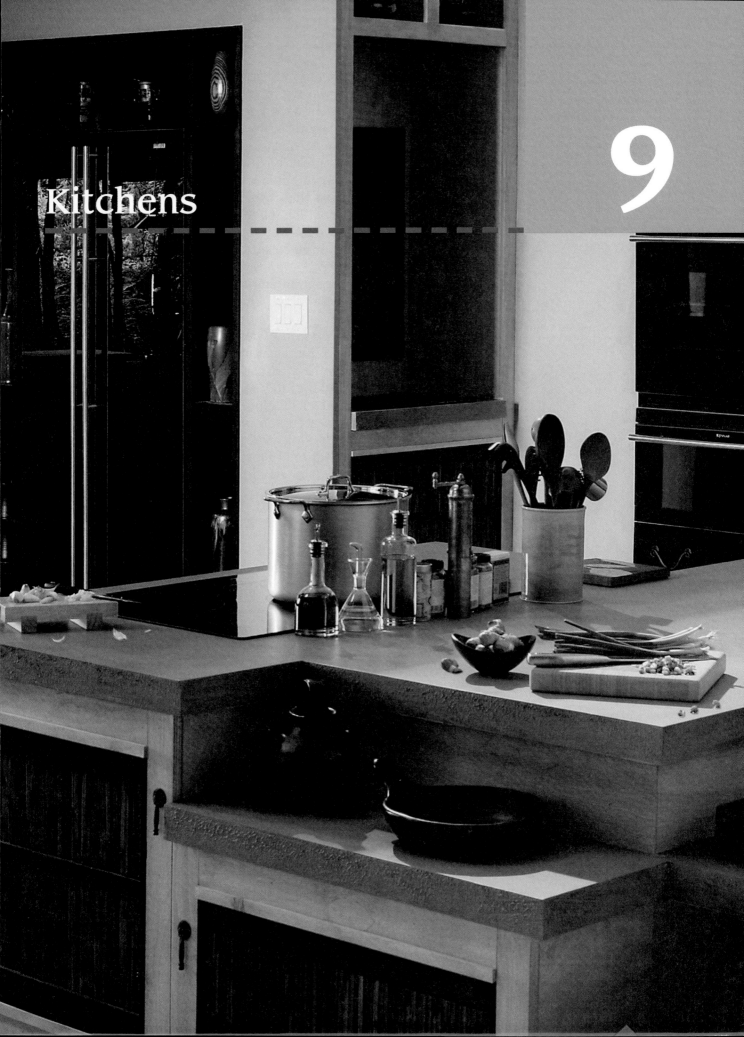

Kitchens

9

The kitchen has undergone many changes over the years. In the Victorian era, the cast iron cookstove was the main source of cooking and heating and, although an improvement over the open fire of the colonial days, much time and labor were required to keep it operating. The coal or wood had to be carried into the house, and the stove required blacking to maintain its shiny appearance. In winter, the heat radiating from the cookstove heated the kitchen and made it a gathering place for the family. In summer, however, to use the stovetop for cooking and the oven for baking, the fire had to be lit, which made the kitchen feel like a furnace. (These traditional wood or wood/coal-burning cookstoves are still available. Some models use gas or electricity but retain the look of a traditional cookstove). (Figure 9.6.)

In the kitchens of the past, in addition to the cookstove, the only other pieces of furniture were tables, chair, and a sink. All food preparation was done on the table or on the draining board next to the sink. There were no counters as we know them today and no upper storage cabinets. All food was stored in the pantry or in a cold cellar. Today, the kitchen has once again become a gathering place for the family. Much family life is centered around the kitchen, not only for food preparation, but also for entertaining and socializing.

The **work triangle,** an area comprised of the distance between your refrigerator, stove, and sink, traces the kitchen's most-traveled areas. Designers from the National Kitchen and Bath Association recommend the following work triangle dimensions and suggestions:

> each leg of the work triangle should measure between 4 and 9 feet in length
> the total length of all 3 legs should be between 12 and 26 feet
> cabinets shouldn't intersect any leg of the triangle by more than 12 inches
> major traffic shouldn't move through the triangle.

Find your floor plan in the work triangle examples shown for ideas about how you can dramatically improve your kitchen's efficiency. You'll save time, energy and miles of extra steps.[1]

In addition to an efficient work triangle, adequate lighting and adequate storage are important. The type of kitchen desired depends on availability of space, lifestyle, and ages and number of family members. Expense and space are the limiting factors in kitchen design. The best utilization of space will create a functional and enjoyable working area. Kitchens are becoming larger and now account for almost 10 percent of the total square footage of a single-family home. They also feature more cabinetry and counter space, and barrier-free products are increasing in importance. GE Appliances publishes a booklet, *Basic Kitchen Planning for the Physically Impaired,* that provides necessary measurements.

Lifestyle involves several factors. One is the manner of entertaining. Formal dinners require a separate formal dining room, whereas informal entertaining may take place just outside the work triangle, with guest and host or hostess communicating while meals are being prepared. If entertaining is done outside the home of a working host or hostess, then the kitchen may be minimal in size. Such things as how the grocery shopping is done also affect the type of cabinets. If grocery shopping is done twice a month, for example, the pantry space should be increased to allow for storage of foodstuffs.

A small kitchen will appear larger with an open plan (that is, without a wall dividing it from the adjacent room). It will also appear larger with a vaulted ceiling. A young couple with small children might require a family room within sight of the kitchen. Teenagers like to be near food preparation areas for easy access to the refrigerator and snacks. All these factors need to be considered when planning a kitchen. Some cooks prefer to work from a pantry and therefore do not need a lot of upper cabinets, whereas others prefer to have a bake center and work from both the upper and lower cabinets.

Gaining in popularity on the west coast is the double island kitchen. One island is for clean up, prep and periodic storage. The other island is the primary workstation, encasing dishwasher, sink and stove top. On a long wall you would have a double oven side by side—versus top and bottom configurations.[2]

According to Linda Trent, "Islands, which may function as eat-in bars, room dividers, and/or work areas, are probably the most sought-after design elements in today's kitchens, because they are attractive and make efficient use of space. Varying island shape can result in interesting angles and efficiencies."[3] One of the links between ergonomics and the new social role of the kitchen is the central island cooktop. (See Figures 9.2 and 9.5.)

Ellen Cheever, Certified Kitchen Designer (**CKD**), ASID, gives the following work simplification techniques for planning a kitchen:

1. Build the cabinets to fit the cook.
2. Build the shelves to fit the supplies.
3. Build the kitchen to fit the family.

FLOOR PLANS

There are infinite variations on basic kitchen floor plans, and this is where customizing comes in. The simplest of all kitchen floor plans is the one-wall design, otherwise known as **pullman, strip,** or **studio.** Here, all appliances and counter space are contained on one wall and, when required, folding doors or screens are used to hide the kitchen completely from view. This is a minimal kitchen not designed for elaborate or family meals.

The **corridor,** or two-wall, plan utilizes two parallel walls and doubles the available space over the one-wall plan. The major problem with this design is through traffic. If possible, for safety's sake, one end should be closed off to avoid this traffic. The width of the corridor kitchen should be between 5 and 8 feet. A narrower width prevents two facing doors from being opened at the same time. For energy conservation, the refrigerator and stove should not face each other directly. (See Figure 9.1.) In an L-shaped kitchen, work areas are arranged on two adjacent walls rather than on two opposite walls; the advantages of this layout are that there are no through traffic and all counters are contiguous. The L-shaped kitchen may also

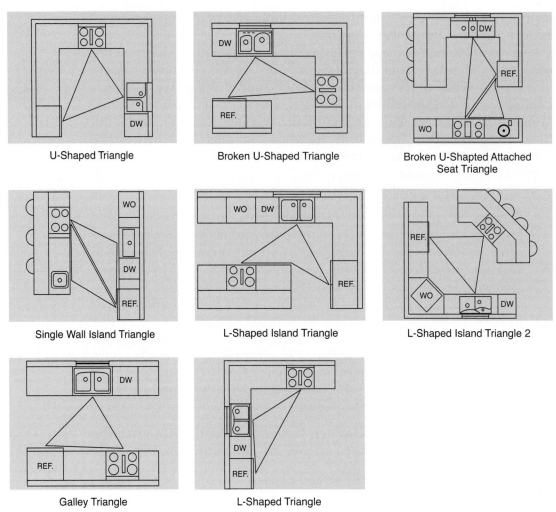

U-Shaped Triangle

Broken U-Shaped Triangle

Broken U-Shapted Attached Seat Triangle

Single Wall Island Triangle

L-Shaped Island Triangle

L-Shaped Island Triangle 2

Galley Triangle

L-Shaped Triangle

FIGURE 9.1
Work triangles. (Drawings courtesy of Kohler)

include an island or a peninsula. This island may simply be an extra work surface, may contain the sink or stove, and may also include an informal eating area. If the island has a raised side facing an eating or seating area, the higher side will hide the clutter in the kitchen.

The U-shaped kitchen is probably the most efficient design. It has three walls of counter space, with no through traffic. Depending on the location of the window, there are at least two walls or more of upper cabinets. The work triangle is easy to arrange in this design, with the sink usually at the top of the U, refrigerator on one side, and range on the other. The refrigerator is always placed at the end of the U to avoid breaking up the counter area and to provide easy accessibility to the eating area. The stove, range, or cooktop is on the opposite side but more centered in the U. Islands also work in a U-shaped kitchen provided that the passageways are more than 4 feet wide.

When planning any kitchen, thought should be given to the activities of each area. The sink area serves a dual purpose. First, it is used for food preparation, such as washing and cleaning fruits and vegetables. Second, after the meal the sink is used for cleanup. In this age of the electric dishwasher, the sink area is generally used only for preliminary cleaning; but in the event of a large number of dishes, sufficient space should be provided next to the sink, 18" on one side and 24" on the other, so a helper can dry the dishes. Counters are generally 36 inches high. They can vary from 42 to 45 inches for those who are standing to 30 to 32 inches for seated cooks and children.

Certain areas of the kitchen require a minimum amount of adjacent counter space. The sink needs 24 to 36 inches of counter space on the dishwasher side and 18 to 36 inches on the other side. For cooktops, 18 to 24 inches should be allowed on either side, and regardless of the type of design, there must be at least 16 inches of counter space on the handle side of the refrigerator, which should be at the end of one side of the counter near the entrance to the kitchen. The refrigerator should not be placed in such a manner that the counter is broken up into small areas.

The refrigerator should be plugged into its own individual 115-volt electrical outlet on a circuit separate from those used for heating and cooking appliances. The refrigerator should be placed in an area that will not receive direct sunlight or direct heat from the home heating system. It should not be placed next to sources of heat, such as next to the range or dishwasher.

The cooking area is considered to be the cooktop area. Many wall ovens are now located in separate areas from the cooktop.

KITCHEN APPLIANCES

Only those appliances that are necessary to a kitchen floor plan will be discussed—in other words, major appliances. Mixers and toasters are outside the scope of this book.

Major appliance manufacturers must comply with Public Law 94–163, enacted by Congress in 1975. This law provides that energy costs for appliances must be calculated as so much per **kilowatt-hour (kwh).** This information must still be supplied on a tag attached to the front of the appliance. Consumers can then calculate their yearly energy cost by finding out their local kilowatt-hour rate. It is important to bear in mind that the higher the local rate, the more important energy conservation features become. It is by using these figures that comparison shopping can be done.

Due to the energy crisis in the winter of 2005, mention is made here of the Energy Star program from the EPA, which is awarded to dishwashers and refrigerators that contribute to savings of both power and water. Significant savings can be realized by minimizing the amount of hot water needed. The water temperature in a dishwasher should be at least 140°F to clean the dishes. All models that are Energy Star–qualified have an internal water heater that boosts the water temperature inside the dishwasher. This allows the thermostat on the household water heater to be turned down to 120 degrees, reducing water heating costs by 20 percent. By federal law, all dishwashers must have a no-heat drying option, resulting in a significant saving of energy. Refrigerators that qualify for the Energy Star program have improved insulation, meaning that the compressor needs to run less often. Heat from the compressor warms the kitchen, resulting in increased air conditioning and higher energy consumption.

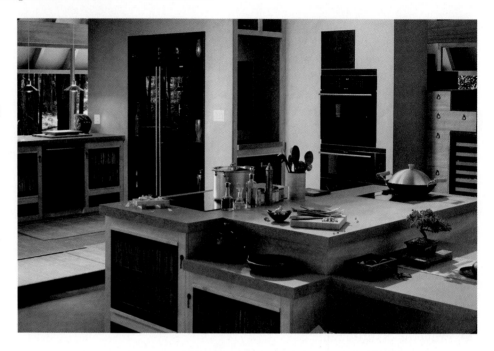

The style of appliances selected may affect the style of cabinetry. Black appliances look better with white or light-colored wood cabinets, whereas freestanding Old World–style stoves may look better with French country cabinetry.

Colored, white, and stainless steel appliances are available. If a change in the decor of the kitchen is planned for the future, white is always a safe choice. All-black appliances are very popular in contemporary kitchens, with black glass fronts on microwaves and ovens. White appliances may have some chrome accents. However, if totally white, they are more expensive than regular black or white appliances.

Jenn-Air® has a full line of floating glass products. The glass fronts are black or white and are available on most of its major appliances. (See Figure 9.2.)

When selecting major appliances, it is important to remember that extra features increase the cost of the appliance. Features selected should be in line with the client's lifestyle.

> Porcelain enamel is most frequently used on surface tops and oven doors because it resists heat, acid, stains, scratches, yellowing, and fading. Baked enamel or electrostatically applied polyester is less durable than porcelain enamel because it is less resistant to stains and scratches; it resists chipping better than porcelain enamel.
>
> Stainless steel is resistant to corrosion, dents and stains and is easy to clean. It may turn dark, however, if it is overheated. Chrome-plated finishes are durable and will not dent easily. Excess heat may cause chrome to discolor over a period of time.[4]

Elmira Stove Works of Ontario, Canada, produces a line of kitchen appliances reminiscent of the old fashioned cast iron cookstove. They are available in white, black, and red with matching panel kits for the

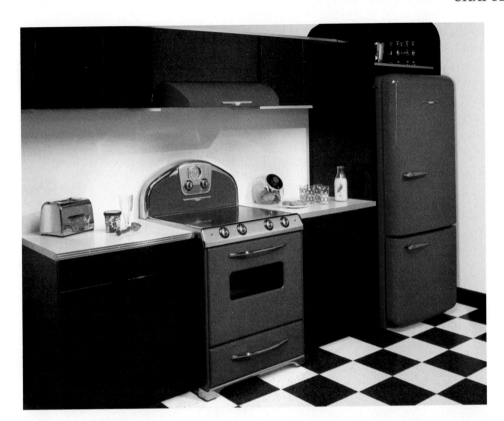

FIGURE 9.3
The fun, funky look of the
"Fab Fifties" is the way
Elmira Stove describes this
1950s retro look. (Photo
courtesy of Elmira Stove
Works)

other kitchen appliances. Their stoves may be all gas or electric or a combination of fuels. Newly introduced by Elmira is the retro look of the 1950s. (See Figure 9.3.)

Refrigerators

The most costly kitchen appliance to purchase and operate is the refrigerator. In fact, the U.S. Department of Energy mandated that 1993 models operate 30 percent more efficiently than 1990 models, and this efficiency has increased. By July 1, 2001, all refrigerators must use 10 percent less energy than previous models. These savings are obtained by better insulation, more efficient compressors, improved heat transfer surfaces, and more precise temperature and defrost mechanisms. The initial increased cost of such methods may be offset by better efficiency over a period of years. As with other appliances, the selection of a refrigerator depends on the client's lifestyle as well as the pocketbook.

For our purposes, the word *refrigerator* will be used instead of *refrigerator/freezer* because we assume that all refrigerators have some form of freezer section. There are a wide variety of features from which to select. These vary from freezers on top, freezers on the bottom, to the Wide-by-Side™ refrigerator from Maytag, where one side is wider than the other, providing an offset appearance of the doors when closed. The freezer section is commonly on top (which is the most energy efficient), but some refrigerators have the freezer section below the regular frozen food storage area.

The refrigerator from the G.E. Profile™ Collection has an Energy Star® rating. This refrigerator has an upper two-door refrigerator and a lower pull-out drawer for the freezer, an internal water dispenser, and electric temperature with digital display.

Sometimes when the doors are the same size on a double-door refrigerator they are called French doors. French Door Bottom-Freezer™ is a trademark of Maytag Corp. For the two different-size doors, the term is *side-by-side* refrigerator. (See Figure 9.4.)

Amana states that "People use their fresh food section almost seven times more than the freezer. That is why they've placed it on top, so

FIGURE 9.4
This kitchen shows the French Door Bottom-Freezer™ refrigerator from Maytag. (Photo courtesy of Maytag Corp.)

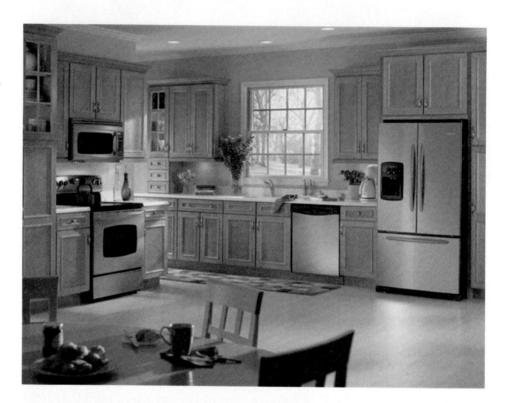

The French Door Bottom-Freezer™ is shown open, displaying the storage capacity.(Photo Courtesy of Maytag)

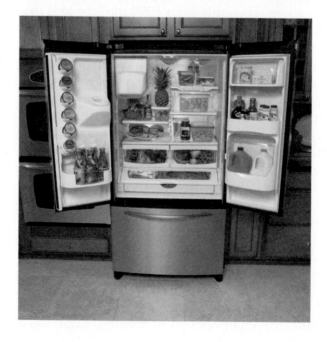

it's easier to get what's in there. Now with the added new Easy Reach Plus™ glide-out freezer drawer, accessing your frozen food has never been easier."[5]

Doors on single-door models that can be reversed are an important feature for those who move frequently. Exterior features include panel adapter kits, which are used on the face of the refrigerator to match other appliances. Stainless steel is the latest finish for appliances.

Side-by-side refrigerators have separate vertical doors for the freezer and refrigerator sections; because the narrower doors have a shorter swing radius, they work well in a galley kitchen or across from appliances with doors. Side-by-side refrigerators are preferred by shorter users and those confined to a wheelchair. Often, this type of refrigerator comes with convenient water and ice dispensers in the door.

Marvel Industries has a new accessible refrigeration that includes a clear ice maker and a refrigerator. Both models install easily into undercounter openings of only 32" high, making them ideal for installations that must comply with the Americans with Disabilities Act (ADA), for areas with limited space, or for universal design projects. This combination is also suitable for executive suites and boardrooms.

Refrigerators are sold by their storage capacity (in other words, by cubic feet of space). It is interesting to note that whereas families and kitchens generally are getting smaller, the size of the refrigerator is staying around 16 to 17 cubic feet. This may be a result of working parents who have less time to food shop, and need to stockpile food, or it may mean that people are entertaining frequently and need to keep food on hand for guests. Sizes of refrigerators vary from 13 cubic feet to 28 cubic feet. The most energy-efficient refrigerator is in the 15- to 20-cubic-foot range.

The average size for refrigerators is 66 1/2 inches high, 35 3/4 inches wide (that is, the refrigerator fits into a 36-inch space), and 30 1/2 inches deep. This depth measurement means that the door of the refrigerator extends beyond the counter by several inches. To design the refrigerator as an integral part of the cabinetry, many manufacturers have recessed the refrigerator coils or placed them above the refrigerator, which makes the refrigerator flush with the edge of the counter; however, this type is usually considerably more expensive than the regular models. The refrigerator door can be covered to match the cabinets, and it can have custom handles. Because this style has no bottom vent, the toe-kick panel can extend from the cabinet across the base of the refrigerator. For new construction, 37 inches of floor space should be allowed for the refrigerator, even if the planned unit is narrower, and accommodations for a water hookup should be made even though the hookup may not be used at the time.

The most common refrigerator features include meat keepers, vegetable storage, unwrapped food sections, adjustable shelves, and humidity-controlled vegetable storage areas. Other interior features might include egg storage, handy cheese and spread storage, and glass shelves that prevent spilled liquids from dripping onto other shelves. The shelves on the doors of both refrigerator and freezer may be fixed or adjustable. The latest feature is a door deep enough to hold gallon containers. Other features include frozen juice can dispensers, ice makers, and ice cream makers within the freezer compartment.

An ice-water dispenser, with cubed and/or crushed ice that is accessible without opening the refrigerator door, may conserve energy and justify the additional expense. Whirlpool's Gold® Kitchen refrigerator comes equipped with an Add-a-Space™ three-position drop-down shelf, In-Door-Ice® ice dispensing system, a triple-action freezer shelf, and three freezer baskets.

One manufacturer offers a third door for access only to the ice cube compartment. Another has a storage unit in the door that can be opened for access to snack items without opening the full-length refrigerator doors. Some companies offer see-through storage bins. U-Line is a manufacturer of Wine Captains, wine storage units that ensure the proper storage temperature for the right wine: red wines are stored in the upper section of the cabinet (approximately 60°F or 15°C); white wines are stored in the middle section (approximately 50–55°F or 10–12°C); and sparkling wines are stored in the bottom cabinet section (about 45°F or 7°C).

The GE Monogram Collection includes a Beverage Center that is large enough for standing containers such as bottles and cans. The door has privacy glass, an innovative liquid-crystal technology that allows you to turn glass from opaque to clear with a simple press of the button. The opaque setting conceals contents from view. This would be a very suitable product for offices, employee lounges, and game rooms. (See Figure 9.5.)

The Wine Chiller holds up to 50 resting bottles of wine. Another appliance in this series is the Icemaker, which produces up to 50 pounds of ice per day.

FIGURE 9.5
This kitchen features rift cut veneer cabinets and stainless steel hardware, a Center island cooking area with an overhead ventilation system. The sink has a goose-neck faucet and there is a double-door refridgerator. Drawers are on both sides of the island and provide plenty of storage. (Photo courtesy of Wood-Mode)

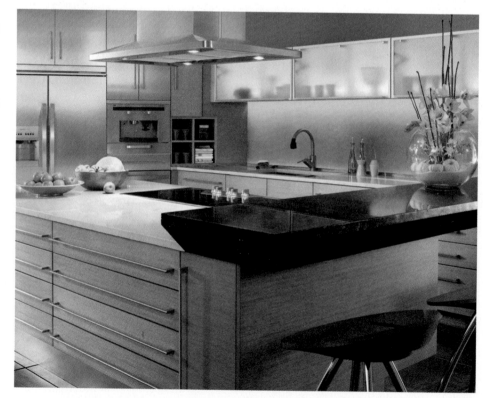

Most manufacturers are interested in energy conservation, and efficiency has greatly improved over the past 15 years. A self-defrosting refrigerator consumes more energy than a manual defrost, but it is much more convenient.

Sub-Zero® refrigerators are designed to be built-in and flush with the adjacent cabinetry. The company offers a complete range of full-size models, from 27 to 48 inches in width and in a variety of configurations. This company's core products, which have the compressors at the top of the units, are 84 inches high and 24 inches deep, the same depth as most cabinets. Sub-Zero's standard units are the only combination units that have two compressors, one for the refrigerator and the other for the freezer, which contributes to fresher food and better energy usage. On the 700 Series units, one unique energy-saving feature is a door/drawer alarm that emits an audible beep after 15 seconds, reminding users that the door or drawer is ajar. Sub-Zero also manufactures two-drawer units, either refrigerators or freezers. These drawers are 34 1/2 inches high, 27 inches wide, and 24 inches deep and can be used in kitchen islands, low peninsulas, or next to a sink. All Sub-Zero's freezer units have an automatic ice maker.

Nylon rollers are provided for moving or rolling the refrigerator from the wall. If the refrigerator is to be moved sideways, a **dolly** should be used to avoid damaging the floor covering.

Ranges

Old-fashioned stoves have been replaced by **freestanding, drop-in,** or **slide-in** range units. Slide-in models can be converted to freestanding by the addition of optional side panels and a backguard. Some ranges contain the cooking units, **microwave/oven,** and/or oven in one appliance, or the oven and cooktop may be in two separate units (often in two separate locations in the kitchen).

Many 30-inch ranges now come with a second oven above the cooktop surface. This may be another **conventional oven** or a microwave. An exhaust fan is incorporated beneath some of the microwave ovens.

Freestanding ranges vary from 20 to 40 inches wide, but most are 30 inches wide. Slide-in ranges usually measure 30 inches wide. A freestanding range has finished sides and is usually slightly deeper than the 24-inch kitchen counter. This type of range may be considered if a change of residence will take place in the near future.

Built-in ranges come in two types: slide-in units or drop-ins, both of which are designed for more permanent installation and are usually placed between two kitchen cabinets. Slide-ins fit into a space between cabinets, and drop-ins fit into cabinets connected below the oven. Drop-ins lack a storage drawer, but both types look alike. The cooking medium may be gas or electricity. Some ranges have the cooking surface flush with the counter, whereas on others the cooking surface is lowered an inch or so. The only difference is that if several large or wide pans are used at the same time, such as during canning or for large parties, the lowered surface is more restrictive. The flush surface permits the centering of the larger pans. The surface of ranges may be white or colored with porcelain-coated steel, stainless steel, tempered glass, or ceramic glass.

FIGURE 9.6
This is the 30" classic gas range with nickel trim from Heartland. Similar models are available for wood burning. (Photo courtesy of Heartland Appliance Inc.)

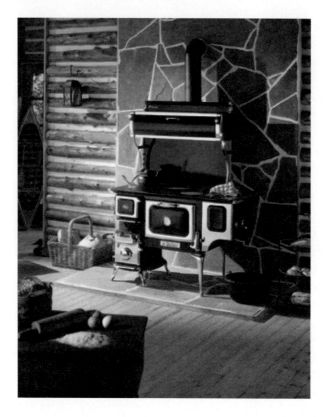

For those who desire state-of-the-art technology combined with authentic 19th-century styling, old-fashioned-type ranges are now available with gas or electricity. These decorative ranges conceal features such as self-cleaning **convection ovens,** digital clock timers, and exhaust vent systems. Several companies manufacture these types of products. Heartland Appliances makes traditional built-in ovens, refrigerators, and wood- or coal-burning cookstoves. (See Figure 9.6.)

Viking Range Corporation, the originator of commercial-type ranges for the home, now has a full line of built-in kitchen appliances in the Designer Series, but not necessarily with a commercial look. The series is available in a variety of colors as well as the classic stainless steel.

Jenn-Air® Pro-Style® cooktops bring commercial style and performance together to make gourmet cooking and gracious entertaining seem effortless. Pro-Style cooktops are stainless steel with details such as oversized knobs and a drop-down control panel to complete the commercial look. The 48" Pro-Style Gas downdraft has two 2-burner modules with an E-ven Heat™ grill assembly with a two-speed downdraft ventilation.

The U.S. Department of Energy estimates that the typical annual cost of operating an efficient gas range is about half the cost of operating an electric range. This only amounts to a dollar or two per month, however, so individual preference is more of a consideration.

Electric Ranges

There are several different types of element choices for electric ranges. The least expensive and most common is the coil element. The most expensive is the European solid disk of cast iron sealed to the cooktop, which some manufacturers refer to as a **hob.** With the solid-electric element, a red dot indicates that the element is thermally protected and will shut down if a pan boils dry. Some elements have a silver dot, a pan sensor that maintains a fairly constant preselected temperature, sometimes with a variance of 20°F. Electric elements heat quickly and can maintain low heat levels.

Another type of element is the radiant **glass-ceramic cooktop,** or smoothtop. When first introduced in 1966 these cooktops were white; now they can be black or patterned grayish-white ceramic glass. The patterned surface shows smudges and fingerprints less than a shiny black surface. All these surfaces are heated primarily by conduction; however, some use halogen. Some smoothtops have quick-heating elements and for safety's sake the indicator lights will stay on as long as the surface is hot. This type of cooktop has a limiter that cycles the burners on and off, restricting the temperature reached by the glass surface. Smoothtops should be cleaned with a special cream, which both cleans and shines the ceramic. These cooktops are usually 30 inches wide. Both radiant and induction methods require flat-bottomed pots of the same diameter.

Two new methods of heating are halogen and induction, both of which are used with glass-ceramic cooktops. The halogen units have vacuum-sealed quartz glass tubes filled with halogen gas that filter out the white light and use infrared as a heating source. The surface becomes a bright red when turned on. Halogen units provide instant on and instant off, and, as with the induction method, the surface unit itself does not get hot. The only heat the glass top may retain is absorbed from a hot pan. Induction elements are the most expensive type.

According to Wolf Appliances,

> How does it work? The electricity flows through a coil to produce a magnetic field under the ceramic cooktop. When an iron or magnetic stainless pan is placed on the ceramic surface, currents are induced in the cooking utensil and instant heat is generated due to the resistance of the pan. Induction only works with cooking vessels made of magnetic materials like stainless steel and cast iron.[6]

When induction-type smoothtops sense overheating, they beep and shut off the power to that burner. Because of the method of heating, induction units turn off the power when a pot is removed. Induction models use electronic touchpads.

For greatest efficiency, all cooking utensils used on an electric range must be flat bottomed to allow full contact with the cooking unit, although induction units will work with slightly warped pans. Usually there are four cooking units, but some of the larger glass cooktops have five or even six units.

Some electric ranges have the controls and clock on a back panel. On separate cooktops, controls are in the front or at the side of the cooktop. On electric ranges, controls may be divided left and right, with the oven controls in between, giving a quick sense of which control works which elements. Controls on the latest cooktops are electronic touchpads.

Cooktops now have concealed or visible hinges that make it easy to clean under the cooktop, where the overflow from drip bowls ends up.

Porcelain drip bowls are much easier to clean than the shiny metal bowls and can be cleaned in the oven during the self-cleaning cycle.

Gas Ranges

Gas cooktops can be made of porcelain-coated steel or stainless steel. One advantage of using gas is that it is easier to moderate temperature changes. Conventional gas burners have grates that hold the pan above the flame. These grates should be heavy enough to support the pan and be easy to clean. Propane burns a little cooler than regular gas. Sealed gas burners are fused to the cooktop, and there are no drip pans; all spills remain on the glass surface, making cleanup easier.

Newer gas ranges have pilotless ignition systems that light the cooking unit automatically from either a spark ignition or a coil ignition. By eliminating the standard, always-burning pilot light, these ranges reduce the gas needed for cooking by 30 percent, keep the kitchen cooler, and prevent pilot outage caused by drafts or other conditions. Electricity must be run to the range to operate the pilotless ignition. In case of electricity failure, the burner may be lit by a match; however, as a safety precaution, the oven cannot be used by lighting a match. If electricity cannot be run to the pilotless range, models with pilot lights are still available. Some gas ranges, such as one from Amana, have a closed-door smokeless broiling option.

One of the trends of the late 1990s was the use of multiburner restaurant-type gas ranges, with six or even eight burners in home kitchens. (Truly commercial ranges are not permitted in a private residence because of the excessive heat generated.) These ranges are freestanding and are very useful when catering for a large crowd or for the gourmet cook.

Gas appliances produce exhaust gases that are better expelled by using a ventilation fan.

Ovens

Electric ovens come in 24-, 27- and 30-inch widths, but some 30-inch ovens require a 33-inch cabinet. Ovens come in two types: self-cleaning (**pyrolytic**) or standard. Self-cleaning ovens have a special cleaning setting that is activated by the timer for the required length of time. This cleaning cycle runs at an extremely high temperature and actually incinerates any oven spills, leaving an ash residue. One of the excellent by-products of a self-cleaning oven is that, because of the high temperatures required to operate the cleaning cycle, the oven is more heavily insulated than is customary and so retains heat longer and uses less energy when baking. Gas ovens are now available that are self-cleaning. At the low end of the price range is the standard oven that requires the use of spray-on oven cleaners. These are becoming hard to find, and most ovens are now self-cleaning.

Ovens cook by one of three methods: radiation, convection, or microwave. Radiant baking is the method used in most ovens. According to Jenn-Air,

While a conventional oven uses radiant heat to warm the food, oven interior and air, convection uses a fan inside the oven cavity to circulate that warm air. The moving air strips away a layer of cooler air that surrounds the food, thus speeding up the baking or roasting process. . . . Jenn-Air's convection ovens have radiant heating elements at the oven's top and bottom, with the fan built into the back for maximum space usage. . . . Meats are juicier, since circulating air seals the outside surface and reduces the evaporation. . . . Because of the way in which the air circulates, cooks can bake three racks of cookies, pizza or other items instead of just one or two.

G.E. offers its Trivection® technology which uses three kinds of heat–thermal heating, convection, and microwave–to cook foods up to five times faster than a traditional oven. A dual loop 2,500 watt wall element surrounds an innovative fan that reverses direction for optimal air and heat circulation, providing even cooking, faster roasting speeds, and multi-rack baking capability. On low heat settings, food can also be dehydrated for long-term storage. The defrosting setting works on the same principle.[7]

However, convection ovens are more expensive than other ovens. Gaggenau offers a combined steam and convection oven.

Exact temperature control and monitoring are extremely important when preparing certain meals. Thanks to the ThermoTest feature, even when lowering the temperature it can be checked to find out when the new required temperature has been reached. In the convection mode, the air, heated by a ring element, is distributed evenly in the oven interior by a fan. With this method different foods can be cooked on several levels evenly without any transfer of taste. The steam oven from Gaggenau is installed completely, which means it is connected directly to the water supply and drainage, thus ensuring an unlimited water supply for all cooking processes. And manual handling of water is now a thing of the past. This is practical, safe, convenient and hygienic—the professional way to add a little moisture during cooking. At the push of a button a burst of steam is added to the food being cooked. This is particularly useful for all yeast mixtures including bread, bread rolls, and sweet yeast pastries.[8]

Built-in ovens are required when using a separate cooktop. These may be single conventional oven units or double oven units with one a conventional type and the other a microwave. Sizes available are 24, 27, and 30 inches. The 24- and 27-inch ovens fit into a standard 27-inch cabinet, but not all 30-inch models fit into a 30-inch cabinet. Some require a 30-inch opening, which only a 33-inch cabinet provides.

Electric ovens may have a solid door, a porcelain enamel door with a window, or a full-black glass window door. Porcelain enamel is available in many colors. Controls may be knobs or electronic touchpads. Electric ovens require the door to be left ajar when the broiling feature is in use, or food will roast. Many new ovens turn off automatically after 12 hours (this is a good safety feature).

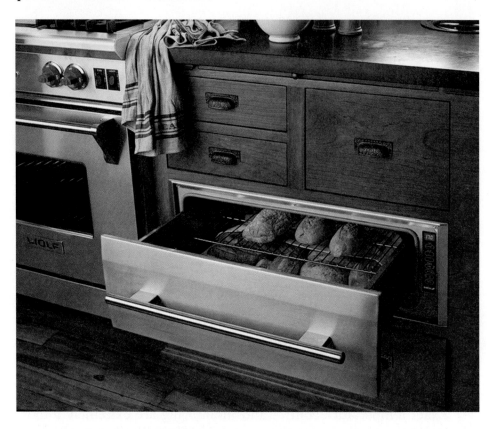

Sometimes double ovens are used, but they do not offer the advantage of waist-level shelves (which are better for disabled individuals). Timers for ovens vary in length from 99 minutes to 10 hours. Warming drawers are becoming more prevalent in upscale kitchens. These thermostatically controlled drawers are designed to keep hot foods hot or crisp prior to serving, and they may also be used for proofing bread. (See Figure 9.7.)

The latest innovative oven is the Advantium™ from General Electric. It is a combination of two technologies, microwave and halogen. The Advantium oven cooks the outside of foods much like conventional radiant heat, while also penetrating the surface so the inside cooks simultaneously. Although halogen light is the primary source of power, a "microwave boost" is added with certain foods. Foods cook evenly and fast, retaining their natural moisture. Halogen has been used before for cooktop cooking, however, this is the first combination in an oven. Two 1500-watt halogen lamps cook from above, where browning is needed most. One 1500-watt bulb cooks from beneath, close to the food for thorough penetration. A turntable ensures that food cooks evenly and consistently every time. The oven converts to a fully functional microwave oven. The Advantium oven can be installed over a warming drawer, above a conventional wall oven, or by itself as its own speed-cooking center. The 120 model plugs into any 120-volt power outlet; the Advantium requires a 240-volt dedicated line to deliver its amazing cooking speed and quality. Some major food companies are now including Advantium speed-cooking instructions on product packaging. The Advantium oven is part of the Monogram Collection. The entire Advantium line received the 2001 American Building Products Award from *Home Magazine*.

Microwave Ovens

Microwave cooking activates the molecules in food about $2\frac{1}{2}$ billion times per second. The friction between molecules produces the heat. Today, most microwave ovens are operated by means of touch controls that electronically monitor the amount of energy from full power to a warming setting or defrost cycle.

Microwave ovens may be programmed to cook whole meals on a delayed-time basis. Some feature recipes that are available at a touch; others use a meat probe to produce meat that is rare, medium, or well done.

Today, most medium-sized models are specifically designed to be mounted over the range (OTR) with built-in recirculating exhaust fans, or under specially sized cabinets (UTC) without a vent.

A microwave's size refers to the cooking cavity. Originally, microwaves were designed to sit on a countertop. Today, most medium-sized models are specifically designed to be mounted over the range (OTR) under specially sized cabinets and have built-in recirculating exhaust fans. Sizes vary from 0.5 cubic foot to 1.3 cubic feet. Microwave ovens are rated by watts, from 600 to 1000 watts. The greater the wattage, the more quickly the oven heats food. The feature used most frequently on a microwave oven is the defrost cycle.

Unlike regular ovens, microwave cooking time varies with the amount of food to be cooked; thus, four potatoes require about 70 percent less energy when microwaved, but 12 potatoes bake more efficiently in a conventional oven.

For safety's sake, some microwaves have child lockouts with keypad releases.

Ventilation Fans

All exhaust systems should move a minimum of 200 cubic feet of air per minute. There are many methods of venting cooking fumes from the kitchen. Ducted fans may be either updraft or downdraft. With updraft, the hood over the cooking surface collects the heat, odors, and fumes and exhausts them to the outside. This method takes up some space in the cabinet over the cooking surface.

There are three types of downdraft fans on the market. The most well-known downdraft is from Jenn-Air, the original manufacturer of cooktops and grill ranges, with a built-in downdraft ventilation and a two-speed fan for flexibility. The higher speed is ideal for grilling and drying, whereas the lower speed provides ventilation for lighter cooking. The lower speed is useful to exhaust heat from the burners during the summer, to avoid overheating the kitchen. Jenn-Air has a vent that goes from the back to the front of the cooking surface. It will also vent the fumes and heat that escape from the oven during the self-cleaning cycle. Downdraft cooking is ideal for peninsulas.

Some manufacturers have a raised vent at the back of the cooktop, which may not always completely exhaust fumes from the front burners, particularly if the pans are very high. A split downdraft consists of two vents on each side of the cooktop surface.

Gaggenau uses the Coanda Effect: An additional fan sends an air-flow towards a cylinder set right at the front of the hood. In an effect known from aerodynamics, the cylinder deflects the air so that it flows back over the cooktop towards the rear of the hood. The backward airflow guides any steam or smoke directly towards the filter area of the hood, ensuring virtually perfect ventilation over the whole of the cooking area.[9]

For cooktops that are in the center of the room, chimney-style island hoods are available that ventilate upwards. For outside walls, an exhaust fan that vents directly outdoors may be used. Ductless or recirculating systems have a **charcoal filter** that filters out odors. (Figure 9.5)

Dishwashers

Dishwashers are 24 inches wide and are usually installed adjacent to the sink so that the plumbing connections are easily made. Dishwashers discharge the dirty water through the sink containing the garbage disposal. Keep sink drain plugs inserted during dishwasher operation to prevent noise transfer through drains.

GE makes a Spacemaker® undersink model for small kitchens. Also available for small families or limited space is the Fisher & Paykel DishDrawer®.

> Since introducing the Dishdrawer to the market, the company has found that clients have used this product in very innovative ways, including recreational vehicles, boats, patio areas and even private corporate jets where space is extremely limited. The DishDrawer is the first certified dishwasher to be used in a Kosher manner. As with most high end appliances the Dishdrawer comes in black, white or stainless steel. It can be fully integrated into a kitchen where it appears to be just another drawer until opened (See Figure 9.8).[10]
>
> The GE Profile® with the SmartDispense™ system is the only dishwasher to automatically dispense just the right amount of detergent based on the home's water hardness into the main wash cycle and every pre-wash to get dishes clean. It's the only dishwasher ever to hold the contents of an entire 45 oz. bottle of liquid or gel dishwasher detergent.[11]

The controls are usually on the front at the top; however, some dishwashers have the controls in the top of the door, so that they are not visible when the dishwasher door is closed.

The EPA's Energy Star program awards manufacturers whose dishwashers can help save money on utility bills through superior designs that require less money and less energy to get the dishes clean. A list of manufacturers who qualify can be found at www.energystar.org/manufacturers.asp. Energy Star does not endorse the manufactured products, companies, or opinions included therein. (See Energy Star logo on page 10, Chapter 1.)

The features most desired in dishwashers are quiet operation, energy and water conservation, and versatile loading. Energy Star–labeled dishwashers save by using both improved technology for the wash cycle and by using less hot water to clean. Construction includes more

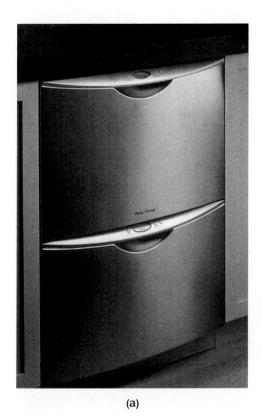

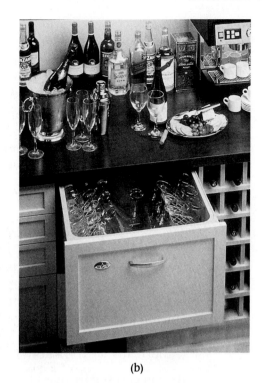

(a)

(b)

FIGURE 9.8
Photo (a) shows a Fisher & Paykel DishDrawer® for the kitchen; (b) shows one used for washing glasses in an entertainment center. (Photos courtesy of Fisher & Paykel)

effective washing action, energy-efficient motors, and other advanced technology such as settings that determine the length of the wash cycle and the temperature of the water necessary to clean the dishes. Available features in dishwashers include a heavy-duty cycle for cleaning heavily soiled pots and pans, a regular cycle for normal soil, rinse and hold for a small number of dishes requiring rinsing, and low-energy wash cycles. Use the sink stopper when the dishwasher is operating.

If the utility company offers lower off-peak rates, a delay-start feature may be desirable. Dishes may be dried by the heated cycle, or for energy efficiency, a no-heat drying cycle may be programmed. To save water and energy, do not rinse dishes before putting them into the dishwasher because a soft food disposer or filtration system is built in. Some foods such as, eggs, rice, pasta, and cooked cereals may need rinsing.

Racks and even dividers are now adjustable, allowing for large-size dishes or wider items that do not fit over the fixed dividers. Some dishwashers have a separate rack on top for silverware, making the silverware easier to get at, easier to clean, and more scratch resistant. A small drop-down rack provides a second rack that enables two rows of cups to be washed in the same space. Water-saver dishwashers are now available that use only 6 gallons per wash.

Frigidaire® has a SpeedClean™ Cycle which provides a 30% increase in washing pressure, powering dishes clean in 50% less time. The Half Load Wash Cycle saves water when washing a small load.[12]

Whirlpool's Gold Kitchen dishwasher loads tall and odd-shaped items in both racks. The LoadLogic™ III feature offers the most flexibility of any of their dishwashers, with a removable upper rack, the AnyWare™ Plus silverware basket, a 3rd cutlery rack for cutlery and utensils, plus much more. The Sani Rinse™ Option helps to eliminate up to 99.999% of food soil bacteria by raising the final rinse temperature to 155 degrees F. The Sani-Rinse option is certified by the National Sanitization Foundation (NSF) to meet household sanitization levels.[13]

The following features are from Asko, an imported dishwasher from Sweden.

The Quiet System™ ensures this is the quietest line of dishwashers—the D3000 series is even 12% quieter than previous models. [It ensures the] lowest water consumption, using under 5 gallons in a Normal program and as little as 2.4 gallons in the Quick Wash program. [The] balanced door remains in whatever position is most convenient, e.g., open just far enough to load/unload the top rack. The height is adjustable from 32-1/4" to 35-1/2", and is ADA (Americans with Disabilities Act) height-compliant.[14]

As you can see from all the features just described, the clients need to choose which are the most important for them. With an open-plan house, sound deadening would be the most important feature; for large parties, capacity would be the best feature.

Raising the dishwasher another 6 inches can save the stress on the back when loading or unloading dishes. This higher counter might be part of a cookbook storage area.

TRASH COMPACTORS

Trash compactors reduce trash volume by 80 percent in less than one minute. Most have some form of odor control and use a compacting ram with the force of approximately 3,000 pounds. In today's society trash disposal has become an expensive service; trash compactors do reduce the volume of trash considerably. They may make trash less biodegradable, however, because of its compacted volume. Trash compactors vary in width from 12 to 18 inches.

In some areas of the United States, as a result of recycling laws, trash compactors may be becoming obsolete. Trash compactors can be used to crush recyclable aluminum cans and plastic bottles, however, making them less bulky. Be aware that some recycling depots require that the cans be in original condition. Where recycling is not required, trash compactors can still be used in the conventional manner.

SINKS

Kitchen sinks are constructed of stainless steel, enameled cast iron, enameled steel, or manufactured materials (usually compression-molded modified acrylic). Each material has its pros and cons.

Stainless steel sinks give a contemporary look to a kitchen and are less likely to cause breakage if dishes are accidentally dropped into them. Finishes may be satin or gloss. Any water spots will leave a spot on the shiny surface, however. In addition, heat from the hot water dissipates more rapidly with a metal sink than with a porcelain enamel model. When selecting a stainless steel sink, the lower the number of the gauge, the thicker the metal will be. Undercoating absorbs sound, protects against condensation, and helps maintain sink water temperature. Like all kitchen sinks there is a great variety of sizes, depths, and number of bowls available in stainless steel. Elkay Manufacturing Company has the following useful hint on selecting a stainless-steel sink: "The deeper the bowl, the straighter the slope, the smaller the radius (the measure of the bowl's corners where the sides and bottom meet), the more useful the sink capacity." Some even come with an integral draining board. KWC offers chromium/nickel stainless-steel sinks with components individually installed under the solid-surface counter. In other words, it may be two round or rectangular sinks separated by a colander. These sinks also have these accessories integrated into one piece.

Porcelain enamel sinks show stains easily, and a scouring powder is usually required to remove such stains. The porcelain may become chipped when hit with a heavy object. Enameled cast-iron sinks provide a colorful touch in the kitchen. However, enameled steel sinks are low cost and lightweight but also less durable than the other types. Sinks made of solid surfaces are easily cleaned, but colors are limited and require an experienced installer, which raises the cost.

Porcelain sinks are highly chip resistant but can break when a heavy object is dropped into them. Porcelain sinks are made from high-fired clay with an enamel finish, a combination that is used more in Europe than in the United States.

Composite or quartz acrylic is the latest material for kitchen sinks. This material produces a color-through sink impervious to stains and scratches. Composite sinks are a combination of natural materials and synthetics.

Some kitchen sinks, such as stainless-steel sinks and those designed to be used with a metal rim, are flush with the counter. Any water spilled on the counter may be swept back into the sink. Self-rimming sinks are raised above the surface of the counter, and any water spilled must be mopped up. Some self-rimming sinks have predrilled holes, which must be ordered to suit the type of faucet to be used. The old standard had three holes, or four holes if a spray or soap dispenser was to be used. With the increasing use of single-lever faucets with self-contained pullout sprays, however, only one hole may be needed. (See Figure 9.9.) Some models of stainless-steel sinks have knockout holes started in their undersides for extra accessories. An extra hole may be needed for a water purifier, hot water dispenser, cold water dispenser, and soap/lotion dispenser. Under-mounted, flush-mounted, and integral or molded sinks have the faucets on the counter. Very contemporary kitchens have sinks with wall-mounted faucets. When the faucet is pointed down it is called a **bib** (like an outside hose faucet). (See Figure 9.9.)

FIGURE 9.9
Amarilis/heritage bar pantry faucet. (Photo courtesy of American Standard)

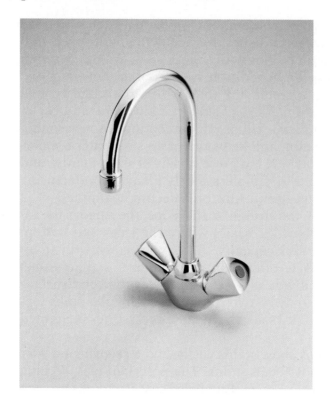

Single-compartment sink models should be installed only where there is minimum space. One-bowl models do not provide a second liquid disposal area if the bowl is in use. For corner installations L-shaped double model are available. A single-bowl sink, called a bar sink or hospitality sink, is often placed in a separate area of the kitchen, usually in an island. These sinks typically have a high arc bar faucet (See Figure 9.9.)

In triple sinks one of the bowls is usually shallower and smaller than the other two and may contain the garbage disposal unit. Some sinks have small colanders for draining pastas or cleaning vegetables, or fitted wooden cutting boards. Other sinks have a ribbed area for draining dishes. Instead of the normal square or rectangular sinks, they may be D-shaped, have lower divides between sinks, different depths, and so on. (See Figure 9.8.)

Aristech Acrylics LLC is pleased to announce a new and exciting line of sink and vanity bowl products. The new sinks and bowls are manufactured by Schock in Germany, a long-time respected name in solid surface sink production. Our new sink line includes seven unique models; two double-bowl kitchen sinks, three modular kitchen sinks, and two vanity bowls in today's most popular sizes. All sinks and bowls are available in White, Ivory, and Crème and feature a ten-year limited warranty. Our selection of extra large, extra deep acrylic kitchen sinks and food preparation basins are designed to meet the demands of today's active lifestyles.[15]

Corian, when used as a material for kitchen sinks, may or may not be an integral part of the counter.

The width of a kitchen sink varies between 25 and 43 inches. Some sinks with attached drain boards are almost 50 inches wide. New sinks have the drain at the rear, which means there is a flat area for food preparation and more accessible storage space under the sink.

Accessories for sinks may include a fitted cutting board, where waste material may be pushed off one corner into the sink. Wire or plastic colanders are another feature and are useful for holding food or vegetables that require rinsing.

GE's booklet "Real Life Design Kitchens" deals with special-needs users. One of the comments of GE is that we are all different—different heights, ages, abilities, strengths, weaknesses, and preferences. Yet our homes are designed for a "standard" person. The universal design is a natural, logical, people-first approach to design. This kitchen illustrates living space that is simply beautiful and one that can be easily used and enjoyed by everyone. For example, a rolling table placed beneath the GE Profile Built-in Convection Microwave Oven gives a seated cook or child plenty of workspace. "A mechanized adjustable height sink is so innovative that one might easily overlook its other outstanding features, like the high contrast faucet with single control and a pull-out nozzle, the soap dispenser and the pop-up drain control."[16] (See Figure 9.9.)

Accessible Designs Adjustable Systems, Inc. offers an a adjustable sink, as well as adjustable ranges and adjustable storage cabinets.

The oversized, ADA-compliant Assure kitchen sink allows the cook to sit or stand while working. Featuring a large, comfortably deep work basin and a small disposal/prep basin, Assure offers a barrier-free workspace in a modified apron-front design. Made of KOHLER® Cast Iron, Assure is a pleasing blend of function and design. This model features a tile-in or undercounter installation and a three-hole faucet drilling.[17]

Maintenance

Kitchen sinks should only be cleaned with mild powders or paste cleaners. Steel wool or heavy-duty abrasive powders should not be used. A mirrored-finish stainless sink can be cleaned with a special automotive polishing compound to maintain its sheen.

Kitchen Faucets

Faucets do not come with the kitchen sink and can sometimes be as expensive as the sink itself. Faucets constructed of chrome-plated steel should be all chrome-plated steel, with no parts chrome-plated plastic, because plating over plastic will gradually peel off with use. In the past, the order of durability was chrome, colors, and then brass. This is because colored and brass faucets had a transparent coating applied over the finish. Brass and copper are the latest finishes for kitchen faucets. Delta, a Masco company, has a brass faucet with Brilliance® (as described in Chapter 7, page 237). Due to this finishing method, brass faucet sales for kitchens and bathrooms have dramatically

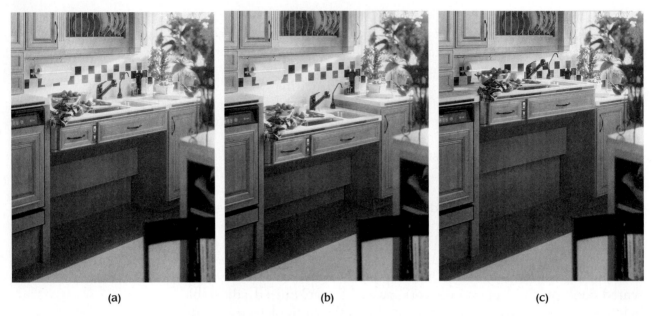

(a)   (b)   (c)

FIGURE 9.10
These three photos show how adaptable the sink from GE "Real Life Design Kitchen"s can be: (a) is counter level, (b) is below, and (c) is above. (Photo courtesy of GE Corp.)

increased in the past few years; however, the brass color varies with each manufacturer.

Moen developed a new copper finish in response to the growing use of copper cookware and accessories by gourmet chefs and today's style-conscious homeowner. Moen's brass finish and brushed stainless finish come with a Moen-patented, titanium-strengthened LifeShine® technology guaranteed not to tarnish, corrode, or discolor.

A mixing type of valve, with which hot and cold may be blended with one handle, allows one-handed operation. Single-handle faucets meet ADA requirements. Another type of ADA-approved handle is the wristblade handle. One problem is that the handle may be accidentally turned on when in the hot position, and a burn can result. To prevent burns, the water heater should be set at 120°F. Most kitchen faucets have a hose attached for spraying the sink and washing vegetables. Several manufacturers provide lifetime warranties on their valves. Price Pfister offers the Pforever Warranty™, which covers material and workmanship for the life of the product on all noncommercial products. Price Pfister's commercial products carry a 10-year warranty. Moen® warrants to the original purchaser that its faucets will be leak and drip free during normal domestic use for as long as the purchaser owns them. If the faucet should ever develop a leak or drip during this time, Moen will provide, free of charge, the parts necessary to put the faucet back in good working condition. These warranties are important because the cost of replacing a faucet can be very expensive.

A gooseneck faucet is higher than normal and may be used for the kitchen but is more frequently used in a bar sink. Moen has designed its new kitchen faucet longer than the customary length. Delta's new Innovations® line also has an extended 9 1/4-inch spout, for greater convenience. This faucet comes with a half-ball handle, whereas the veggie

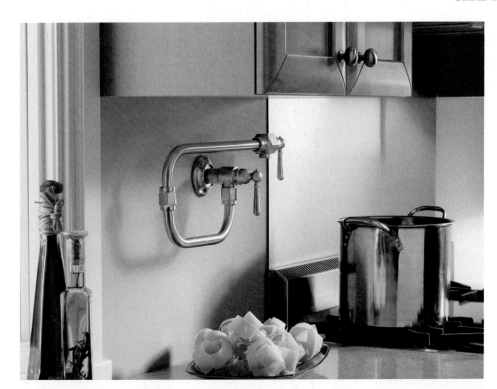

FIGURE 9.11
HiRise kitchen pot filler.
(Photo courtesy of Kohler)

sprayer makes washing quick and easy. Delta's Signature® line also has a 9 1/4-inch spout, with the escutcheon plate (the base) sloped toward the sink area for easy runoff of water.

For the home chef, Kohler has a HiRise kitchen pot filler with a 24" reach. This is available in deck-mount or wall-mount version. This means that cook pots filled with water do not have to be carried from sink to stove, but can be filled at the stove (See Figure 9.11.)

Kohler Co. is a world leader in products for the kitchen and bath as well as home furnishings. It markets such products under the brand names of Kohler plumbing, Sterling plumbing, Kallista, Ann Sacks, Robern mirrored cabinetry, Canac cabinetry, Baker and McGuire furniture, and, in Europe, under the brand names of Jacob Delafon and Neomediam in plumbing products and Sanijura in bath cabinetry.

Several hot water dispensers on the market provide very hot water (about 190°F), for use in making hot drinks and instant soups. Franke and In-Sink-Erator have introduced models that dispense both hot and cold water through one faucet. The extra hole in the sink may be used for these dispensers as well as for purified water.

Because of increasing awareness of water conservation, plumbing manufacturers are now making 2.5- to 2.7-gallons-per-minute-flow kitchen faucets.

European faucets are often called **taps.**

KITCHEN CABINETS

Stock kitchen cabinets usually start at 15 inches wide and come in 3-inch increments up to 48 inches. The depth of lower cabinets is 24 inches and the depth of upper cabinets is 12 inches. Filler strips

FIGURE 9.12
Wood Mode kitchen city
lights. Wood Mode was
named the number-one
choice for kitchen cabinets
by designers in a *House &
Garden* poll. (Photo courtesy
of Wood-Mode)

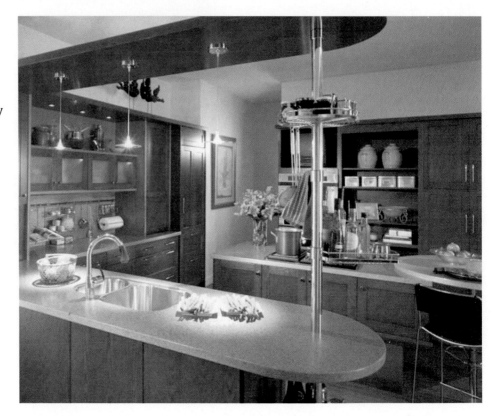

are used between individual cabinets to make up any difference in measurements.

Kitchen cabinets are usually made of all wood or wood with decorative laminate doors. Solid wood is required for raised-panel designs. For dimensional stability, a medium-density or multidensity fiberboard (MDF) is used for the case and shelves, and the edges are banded with a wood veneer that matches the door and drawer fronts. The interior of the cabinets is often coated with a PVC plastic material that reflects light, making it easier to find items inside and easier to clean. Undercabinet appliances are also popular and free the counter of clutter.

When looking at the construction of kitchen cabinets, it would be wise to reread Chapter 7's information on cabinet construction. All better-quality cabinets will meet the criteria set forth in that chapter. (See Figure 9.12.)

The kitchen is a very personal room, and the style of cabinets selected should reflect the client's lifestyle. At one extreme are kitchens in which everything is hidden from sight (behind solid doors) and counters are empty. The other extreme is the kitchen with raised panel doors, shaped at the top, often with glass inserts, and shelves on which personal collections and/or kitchen utensils are displayed. Glass doors should be used with glass shelves for displaying decorative items, or the impact on the viewer is lost. (It is also important to consider what will be visible through the glass doors.). Another style of kitchen uses open shelves for the storage of dishes and glasses; a pantry is used for food storage. Most kitchens fall somewhere between these extremes, but kitchens should be personalized for the client.

Wood cabinets may use flush overlay, reveal overlay, or, for more traditional styles, an exposed frame with a lipped door. The face surface of the door may be **plane,** have a flat or raised panel, or have mouldings applied for a traditional approach. Contemporary kitchens may have not only flush overlay doors, but flush overlay in combination with linear metal or wood decorative strips, which also function as drawer and door pulls. Perma-Edge® from Wilsonart International has matching mouldings for doors and drawers.

The traditional front-frame cabinet construction and the European-style frameless construction (sometimes referred to as 32-mm cabinets) are both popular. Thirty-two millimeters is the spacing of predrilled holes in the cabinet sides for shelf spacing. Shelves in all cabinets should be fully adjustable to accommodate the needs of the user. A well-stocked kitchen requires a minimum of 50 square feet of shelf space and a minimum of 11 square feet of drawer space. Pots and pans are more readily accessible if drawers, rather than base cabinet shelves, are used for storage.

When the frameless type of construction is used, it will have an opening 1 1/2 inches wider than that in conventionally constructed cabinets. A quality frameless cabinet is as strong as a face-frame cabinet, with 1/2-inch-thick sides and a 1/4-inch-thick back. There is very little cost difference between framed and frameless construction. (See Figure 8.4.)

Many special features may be ordered for the custom-designed kitchen, which will add to the cost of the installation. However, these may be ordered to fit the personal and budgetary needs of the client. Following is a list of some of the available features.

1. Base sliding shelves make all items visible, which eliminates the need to get down on hands and knees to see what is at the bottom of a base unit.

2. A bread box may be contained within a drawer with a lid to help maintain freshness.

3. A cutting board, usually made of maple, that slides out from the upper part of a base unit is convenient and will help protect the surface of the counter from damage. A cutting board should not be placed directly over a drawer that might be needed in conjunction with the cutting board.

4. Lazy susans in corner units or doors with attached swing-out shelves utilize the storage area of a corner unit. Another use for the corner unit is the installation of a 20-gallon water heater, which provides instant hot water for the kitchen sink and the electric dishwasher and prevents waste of water. A second water heater can be installed close to the bathroom to conserve energy and avoid having to wait for the hot water to reach the bathroom.

5. Dividers in drawers aid in drawer organization, and vertical dividers in upper or base units utilize space by arranging larger and flat items in easily visible slots (thus avoiding nesting).

6. Bottle storage units have frames to contain bottles.

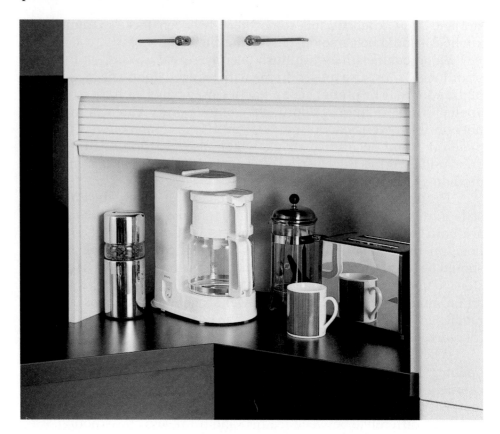

7. Spice racks may be attached to the back of an upper door or built into a double-door unit. A special spice drawer insert allows for easy visibility of seasonings.

8. Hot pads may be stored in a narrow drawer under a built-in cooktop.

9. A tilt-down sink front may hold sponges, scouring pads, and other cleaning materials.

10. Wire or plastic-coated baskets for fruit and vegetable storage provide easily visible storage.

11. A wastebasket attached to either a swing-out door, a tilt-down door, or sliding out from under the sink provides a neat and out-of-sight trash container.

12. Appliance garages are built into the back of the counter and enclose mixers, blenders, and other small appliances. The garage may have tambour doors or may match the cabinets. (See Figure 9.13.)

13. Portable recycling units have been on the market for some time. Some states and cities have comprehensive recycling laws, and both custom and stock cabinets offer multibasket recycling units (the four-unit model is most popular). Manufacturers recommend putting one single recycling unit near the sink for compostables, and then two away from the food preparation area, one for aluminum cans and the other for bottles. Local building codes should be checked to see whether some type of venting is necessary for the cabinet under the sink. (See Figure 9.14.)

14. A mixer can be placed in a base unit and gas cylinders raise or lower in and out of the cabinet. (See Figure 9.15.)

Several kitchen cabinet companies publish brochures that will assist in kitchen planning. These brochures include questionnaires that cover such issues as height of primary user, type of cooking to be performed, and what the client may or may not like about the current kitchen plan.

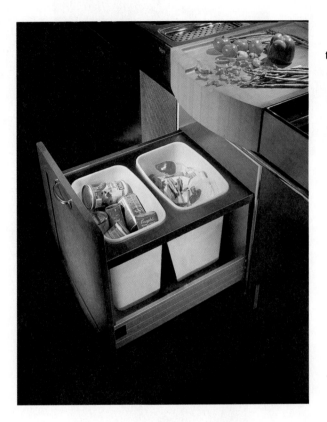

FIGURE 9.14
A recycling drawer under the cutting board. Leftovers from the cutting board can conveniently be scraped into the pull-out waste bin. The second bin is for cans. (Photo Courtesy of Neff Kitchens)

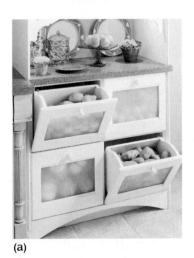

(a)

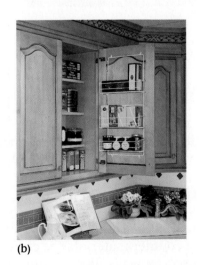

(b)

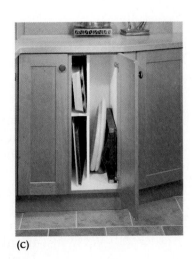

(c)

FIGURE 9.15
(a) Tip-out bins for potatoes, etc. (b) Spice cabinet. (c) Tray and cookie sheet dividers. (d) Corner turntable. (e) Tip-out drawer and undersink unit. (f) Pantry unit. (g) Pull-out pantry unit. (h) Knife drawer. (i) Pot drawer. (Photos [a] to [f] courtesy of Wood Mode® Inc. Photos [g] to [i] courtesy of Neff® Kitchens)

(Continued)

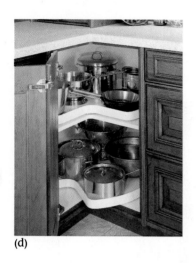

(d)

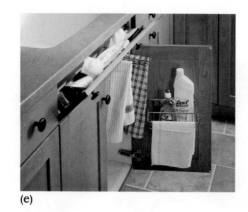

(e)

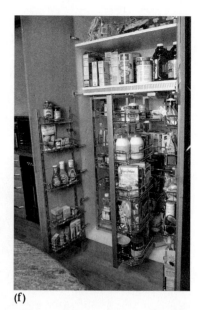

(f)

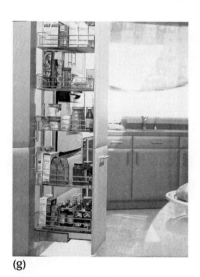

(g)

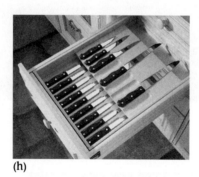

(h)

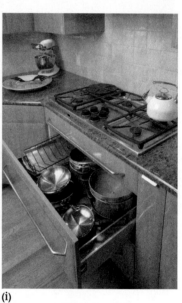

(i)

FIGURE 9.15
(Continued)

COUNTER MATERIALS

Counters may be of the following materials: decorative laminate, ceramic tile, wood, marble, travertine, solid-surface materials, solid-surfacing veneer (SSV), stainless steel, granite, or slate.

Decorative Laminate

In some areas of the United States, decorative laminate is the most commonly used counter material. The construction is exactly the same as for laminate used on walls. For countertop use, two thicknesses are available; a choice of one or the other depends on the type of counter construction. For square-edged counters, the general-purpose grade is used. If it is necessary to roll the laminate on a simple radius over the edges of the substrate, a **postforming** type is specified. The postforming method eliminates the seam or brown line at the edge of the counter.

For counters that require a chemical-resistant laminate, Wilsonart Chemsurf® is a good solution. It is used in laboratory counters, hospitals, beauty salons, photographers' darkrooms, and similar areas where chemicals are used.

Wilsonart International now has the capability of producing digital graphics, as shown on the company's website, www.wilsonart.com/design. These include children's drawings, an epicurean series featuring such things as hot peppers, and many other exciting patterns. The epicurean series would make a fun backsplash, perhaps in a family room or kitchen.

Installation

Postformed countertops must be constructed at the plant rather than at the job site, because heat and special forming fixtures are used to create the curved edge. The counter may be manufactured as a single unit, or each postformed side may be manufactured separately. By manufacturing each side separately, any discrepancy in the alignment of the walls can be adjusted at the corner joints.

For square-edged counters, the edge is applied first and then routed smooth with the substrate. The flat surface is then applied, and the overlapping edges are routed flush with the counter surface.

Another method is to apply the flat surface first and rout the apron to accommodate such edge treatments as Wilsonart's custom edges.

Wilsonart® Custom Edges add a rich, luxurious look to a countertop, transforming the ordinary into the extraordinary. Laminate edges are available in two bevel-edge profiles and offer an affordable way to enhance your countertop and eliminate the brown line of traditional laminate countertops. Wood moldings in red oak or hard maple are available in square, half round and bevel edge designs.[18] [See Figure 9.16.]

Bevel Edge Style - FE, SE

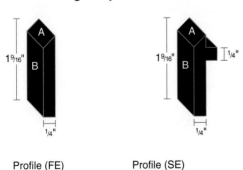

Available Patterns/Finishes: All Wilsonart Laminate

Laminate Bevel Edge Style - FE, SE
Select any combination of laminates for A and B planes, or create a sculpted look by using the same pattern on your top and edge.

Wood Style - HT-1, HT-11, KT-1

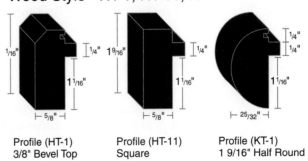

Available Species: Red Oak, Hard Maple

Wood Style -
Available in Red Oak and White Maple solid wood.
Can be stained to match cabinetry or other wood finishes.

FIGURE 9.16
Wilsonart decorative edges. (Drawings courtesy of Wilsonart International)

A decorative laminate surface is durable, but it is not a cutting surface and will chip if heavy objects are dropped onto it.

For high-use and heavy-wear areas such as fast-food countertops, supermarket check-out stands, and bank service areas, a 0.125-inch thickness of decorative laminate is available.

Maintenance

Decorative laminate may be cleaned with warm water and mild dish soaps. Use of abrasives or special cleansers should be avoided because they may contain abrasives, acids, or alkalines. Stubborn stains may be removed with organic solvents or two minutes of exposure to a hypochlorite bleach, such as Clorox®, followed by a clean-water rinse. The manufacturer's specific instructions and recommendations for cleaning should be followed.

Ceramic Tile

Ceramic tile is a popular material with which to cover kitchen counters. To facilitate cleaning, the **backsplash** may also be covered with tile.

> Crossville has a new product for use on a backsplash, Questech® Metals. These polished, embossed, patterned tiles are sold in sets of three and are available in copper, nickel silver and bronze, and are combined with ceramic tile for a custom kitchen backsplash.[19]

Ceramic tile is a durable surface; however, the most vulnerable part is the grout, which can absorb stains unless a stain-proof grout is specified. A grout sealer or lemon furniture oil will also seal the surface of the grout so that stains will not penetrate.

Around the sink area, the ceramic tile counter may be carried down the front to the top of the doors below. This is reminiscent of old farmhouse kitchens and protects wood cabinets from water.

Because of the hard surface of the tile, fragile items that are dropped on the counter will break, and if heavy objects are dropped, the tile may be cracked or broken. Sufficient tile for replacements should be ordered.

Installation

When installing a ceramic tile counter, it is recommended that an exterior-grade plywood be used as the substrate. The remaining installation procedure is the same as for floors and walls.

Maintenance

Maintenance of ceramic tile counters is the same as that for ceramic tile floors.

Wood

Wood counters are usually made of a hard wood, such as birch or maple, and are constructed of glued strips of wood that are then sealed and coated with a varnish. Unsealed wood will permanently absorb stains. Wood counters should not be used as a cutting surface because the finish will become marred. A special area may be set aside for cutting purposes or a slide-out bread board can be installed. Any water accumulating around the sink should be mopped up immediately, as a wood surface can become damaged from prolonged contact with moisture. Wood counters may be installed in a curved shape by successively adding a strip of wood, gluing, and clamping it. When dry, another piece is added.

Marble

Marble has often been used as a material for portions of the countertop. Today, in some expensive installations, marble may be used for the entire counter area. Some people like to use a marble surface for rolling out pastry or making hand-dipped chocolates. As mentioned in the section on marble floors, marble may absorb stains. This tendency may cause unsightly blemishes on marble countertops. Heavy items dropped on a marble surface will crack it.

Maintenance

Stain removal from marble countertops is the same as for marble floors.

Quartz

> The only producer of quartz in the United States is Cambria. The beauty of quartz is reminiscent of granite, but is available in a color range that expands the design options. . . . It is twice as strong as granite, and resists staining and abrasion. . . . This product may be used in commercial kitchen Splash Zones and Food Zones. It has the same certification as stainless steel.[20]

Maintenance

Wipe with warm water. Unlike other countertops, there is no sealing, buffing, or reconditioning needed.

Concrete

A concrete counter may be poured on-site or at the factory. It is poured with reinforcements added and then allowed to cure. It is usually ground with diamond cutters and then sealed with several coats of epoxy. Maintenance is to apply a high-quality water-based liquid wax every nine months to a year.

Travertine

When travertine is used as a counter material, it must be filled. Maintenance of travertine countertops is the same as for marble floors.

Granite and Slate

Granite has become a very popular material for kitchen counters in up-scale houses. However, granite will absorb stains, and therefore should be sealed. Construction of the cabinets must be strong enough to support the extra weight of stone.

Slate may be used as a counter material but it also needs to be sealed.

Maintenance

Maintenance of granite and slate countertops is the same as that for granite walls and slate floors.

Solid-Surface Materials

Corian, a product invented by DuPont, is an advanced blend of natural materials and pure acrylic polymer, and combines the smoothness of marble with the solid feel of granite and the workability of wood. Corian is manufactured as a continuous cast-sheet product. The sheets are precut into specific lengths at the plant. It is available in sheets of 1/4, 1/2, and 3/4 inch thicknesses and in a wide variety of double- and single-bowl kitchen sinks and lavatory styles. Corian is nonporous and highly resistant to abuse; even cigarette burns, stains, and scratches can be removed with household cleanser or a Scotch-Brite® pad. Because Corian is acrylic, it can be formed to a very tight radius before the inside of the curve becomes too compressed and the outside too stretched. Other brands of solid-surface materials are made of polyester, which resists tight radii. Dark colors may perform differently from light colors.

Solid-surface materials may have thicker, built-up edges, made by using joint adhesive, and can be routed into a variety of decorative treatments, including bullnose edges and "sandwich" inserts. (See Figure 9.17.) Solid-surface manufacturers may be able to supply custom colors for large projects.

Wilsonart SSV (solid-surfacing veneer) is 1/8 inch thick and Gibraltar®, also from Wilsonart International, is ¹/₂ inch thick, and both materials match their laminates exactly, so a coordinated look can be obtained although different materials are being used. To add to this coordinated look, Wilsonart now has decorative accessories and countertop accessories available in matching Gibraltar.

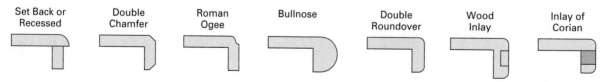

| Set Back or Recessed | Double Chamfer | Roman Ogee | Bullnose | Double Roundover | Wood Inlay | Inlay of Corian |

FIGURE 9.17
Edge treatments for counters.

Surell® is a solid-surface material from Formica®, and Swanstone® is a reinforced solid-surface material that is compression molded under extreme heat and costs less than other solid-surface materials.

Maintenance

Most stains on solid-surface materials wipe off with a regular household detergent. Because of the solid composition of these materials, most stains stay on the surface and may be removed with any household abrasive cleanser or Scotch-Brite pad gently rubbed in a circular motion. Cigarette burns and cuts may be removed with very fine sandpaper, 120 to 140 grit, and then rubbed with a Scotch-Brite pad. If the surface is highly polished, repolishing may be required to blend the damaged area.

Stainless Steel

All commercial kitchens have stainless-steel counters because these counters can withstand scouring, boiling water, and hot pans. Stainless-steel counters can be installed in private residences, if desired, providing a high-tech look.

Maintenance

One of the problems with stainless steel is that the surface may show scratches, and with hard water the surface shows water spots. Water spots may be removed, however, by rubbing the damp surface with a towel, and scratches gradually blend into a patina. Apart from possible scratches and spots, stainless steel is extremely easy to maintain.

FLOORS

Kitchen floors may be ceramic tile, quarry tile, wood, laminate, or any type of resilient flooring. The choice of flooring will depend on the client's needs and personal wishes. Some people find a hard-surfaced floor to be tiring to the feet, whereas others are not bothered by the hard surface. Wood floors need to be finished with a durable finish that will withstand any moisture that may be spilled accidentally. Resilient flooring may be vinyl, cushioned or not, or the new rubber-sheet flooring.

WALLS

Kitchen walls should be painted with an enamel paint that is easily cleansed of grease residue. The backsplash may be covered with the same decorative laminate as used on the counter, applied either with a cove or a square joint. Ceramic tile may be used in conjunction with a ceramic tile counter or with a decorative laminate counter. Mirror may also be selected for kitchen walls; it provides reflected light and visually enlarges the appearance of the counter space. A completely scrubbable wallcovering is another alternative material for the backsplash.

CERTIFIED KITCHEN DESIGNERS

A Certified Kitchen Designer (CKD) is a professional who has proven his or her knowledge and technical understanding through a stringent examination process conducted by the Society of Certified Kitchen Designers, the licensing and certification agency of the American Institute of Kitchen Dealers. A CKD has technical knowledge of construction techniques and systems used in new construction and light exterior and interior remodeling, including plumbing, heating, and electrical.

A CKD will provide a functional and aesthetically pleasing arrangement of space depicted in floor plans and interpretive renderings and drawings. In addition to designing and planning the kitchen, the CKD supervises installations of residential-style kitchens. An interior designer would be well advised to work with a CKD.

BIBLIOGRAPHY

American Gas Association. *Buyer's Guide, Efficient Gas Ranges*. 1991.

Consumer Reports. "Cooktops, a Remodeler's Dream?" July 1994.

Consumer Reports. "Wall Ovens, a Cooktop's Complement," July 1994.

Jenn-Air Company. *Solid Element Cooktops*. Indianapolis, IN: Author, 1985.

Whiteley, Peter O. "Choosing a Kitchen Sink," *Sunset Magazine*, January 1993.

GLOSSARY

backsplash.   A protective area behind a counter

bib.   A downward-facing faucet.

charcoal filter.   A frame that contains charcoal particles, which filter the grease from the moving air.

CKD.   Certified Kitchen Designer.

convection oven.   Heated air flows around the food.

conventional oven.   Food is cooked by radiation.

corridor kitchen.   Two parallel walls with no contiguous area.

dolly.   Two- or four-wheeled cart used for moving heavy appliances.

drop-in range.   Ranges designed to be built into base units.

freestanding range.   Ranges having finished sides.

glass-ceramic cooktop.   A smooth ceramic top used as a cooking surface in electric ranges.

hob.   Sealed solid element providing a larger contact area with the bottom of the pan and better control at low-heat settings.

kilowatt-hour (kwh).   A unit of energy equal to 1,000 watt hours.

microwave/oven.   Heat is generated by the activation of the molecules within the food by the microwaves.

plane.   A flat surface.

postforming.   Heating a laminate to take the shape of a form.

pullman kitchen.   A one-wall kitchen plan.

pyrolytic action.   An oven that cleans by extremely high heat, incinerating any residue to an ash.

slide-in range.   Similar in construction to a drop-in range, except that the top edges may overhang the side; therefore, this type must be slid in rather than dropped in.

strip kitchen.   One-wall kitchen plan.

studio kitchen.   One-wall kitchen plan.

tap.   European word for faucet.

work triangle.   An imaginary triangle drawn between the sink, refrigerator, and cooking area.

NOTES

[1]Kohler website, "Work Triangles," www.kohler.com.

[2]Kevin Henry, "The Evolution of the Modern Kitchen," *Pure Contemporary Magazine,* March 2005.

[3]Linda Trent, "Combining Kitchen and Bath Elements," *Interiors & Sources,* April 1994.

[4]*Buyer's Guide to Energy-Efficient Gas Furnaces & Appliances,* Arlington, VA: American Gas Association.

[5]Amana website, www.amana.com.

[6]Wolf Appliances website, www.subzero.com.

[7]GE Appliance website, www.geappliances.com.

[8]Gaggenau website, www.gaggenau.com.

[9]Ibid.

[10]Fisher & Paykel website, www.fisherpaykel.com.

[11]GE Appliances website, www.geappliances.com.

[12]Frigidaire website, www.frigidaire.com.

[13]Whirlpool website, www.whirlpool.com.

[14]Asko website, www.askousa.com.

[15]Avonite website, www.avonite.com.

[16]GE Appliances website, www.geappliances.com/shop/dsgn_cntr/universaldesign.htm.

[17]Kohler website, www.kohler.com.

[18]Wilsonart International website, www.wilsonart.com.

[19]Crossville website, www.crossvilleinc.com.

[20]Cambria website, www.cambriausa.com.

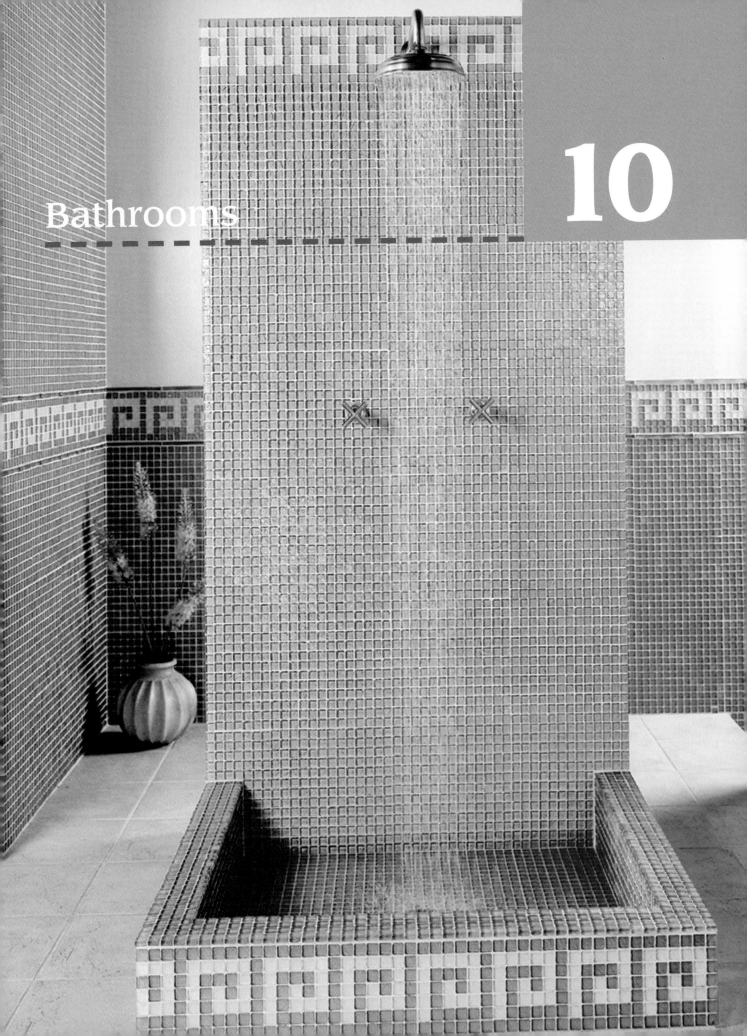

Ancient Greek cities featured large public baths where one could take a hot and cold bath and then get a rubdown with olive oil. Public bathing was also practiced by the Romans, who used aqueducts to bring water to the people of Rome. Their bathing facilities consisted of dressing rooms, warm rooms, hot baths, steam rooms, recreation rooms (where the bather exercised), and cold baths, as well as a swimming pool. These bathing facilities were an early version of present-day spas. After the fall of the Roman Empire, during the Dark Ages, bathing became much less frequent. In the 1800s and early 1900s, one often reads, the Saturday-night bath was a ritual. A metal tub was brought into the heated kitchen, and hot water was poured in by hand. Almost 90 percent of the modernization of bathrooms has occurred in the past 25 years.

American hotels originated the idea of bathing rooms, and the first one was built at the Tremont House in Boston in 1829. The idea proved very popular and spread to other hotels and private homes throughout the United States. As a nation, Americans take more baths and showers than any other people in the world. The realities of the 2000s, however, include both energy and water conservation. According to Linda Trent, "The graying of America combined with new awareness of the needs of the physically challenged have increased demand for both safety features and barrier-free or accessible products that are attractive and functional, particularly in hospitality, commercial and multi-housing construction and renovation."[1]

Because all bathrooms have the same three basic fixtures, it is the designer's challenge to create a bathroom that is not only unique but functional. A knowledge of the different materials used in these fixtures and the variety of shapes, sizes, and colors will help designers meet this challenge.

PLANNING A BATHROOM

Eljer offers the following suggestions for planning a better bathroom: The size of the family needs to be considered. The more people who will use a bathroom, the larger it should be. There should also be more storage, more electrical outlets, and perhaps more fixtures. If the bathroom is to be used by several people at the same time, compartmenting can often add to utility.

The family schedule should also be considered. Where several people depart for work or school at the same time, multiple or **compartmented** bathrooms should be considered. Two lavatories will allow a working couple to get ready for work at the same time.

The most economical arrangement of fixtures is against a single **wet wall.** Economy, however, is not the only factor to be considered. Plumbing codes, human comfort, and convenient use require a minimum separation between and space around fixtures. The minimum size for a bathroom is approximately 5 feet by 7 feet, although, if absolutely necessary, a few inches may be shaved off these measurements. Deluxe bathrooms may be very large and incorporate a seating area or an exercise room and/or a **spa.**

In a corridor-type bathroom, there should be 30 inches of aisle space between the bathtub and the edge of the counter or the fixture opposite. The bathtub should only be placed under the window if there is privacy and the walls and window frames are tiled to retain watertight integrity. This window location is often used in the master bathroom. There should be a minimum of 24 inches in front of a toilet to provide knee room. When walls are on either side of the toilet, they should be 36 inches apart. If the **lavatory** or bathtub is adjacent to the toilet, then 30 inches will be sufficient.

The lavatory requires elbow space. Five feet is the recommended minimum length of a countertop with two lavatories. The lavatories should be centered in the respective halves of the countertop. For a sit-down **vanity,** the counter should be 7 feet long, with 24 inches between the edges of the lavatories for greatest comfort. Six inches minimum should be allowed between the edge of a lavatory and any side wall.

The location of the bathroom door is extremely important. The door should be located so it will not hit a fixture, because such poor placement would eventually cause damage both to the door and the fixture. A sliding pocket door may have to be used to prevent this.

All bathroom fixtures, whether tubs, lavatories, toilets, or **bidets,** come in white and in standard colors that are more expensive than white fixtures. High-fashion colors—even black—cost 40 percent or more than white fixtures. Care should be taken not to select fad colors that will become dated, because bathroom fixtures are both difficult and expensive to replace when remodeling. To obtain a perfect match, all fixtures should be ordered from the same manufacturer. Colors, even white, vary from one manufacturer to another.

FLOORS

Bathroom floors should be of a type that can be cleaned easily, particularly in the area of the bathtub, shower, and toilet. Ceramic tile may be used, but it should not be highly glazed because glazed tiles, when used on a floor, can be slippery when wet. Other types of flooring material that can be used for the tub area include wood with a good finish, laminate, or any of the resilient flooring materials.

Carpeting may be used in the master bath but is not suggested for a family bath because of a likelihood of excessive moisture, causing possible mold and mildew.

WALLS

Wallcoverings are often used in bathrooms. Vinyls or vinyl-coated wallcoverings are recommended because they are easy to wipe dry and maintain. Bathroom walls should be treated (before applying wallcovering) to prevent possible mildew (see Chapter 2, page 34). Most of the manufactured materials used for counters can be used to cover vertical surfaces, either on the wall or as a shower enclosure (e.g., Syndecrete®, discussed in Chapter 1). If an acrylic shower and tub **surround** is not used, ceramic tile is installed because of its vitreous quality.

Only semigloss paint or enamels that can withstand moisture should be used on bathroom walls.

BATHTUBS

The typical tract-home bathtub is 5 feet long, 30 inches wide, and, in less expensive styles, only 14 inches deep. Tubs that are 6 feet long are available, however, for those who like to soak. Tub height, measured from the floor, may vary (15, 16, or even 22 inches). Tub heights of 14 inches are convenient for bathing children. The depth figures represent the outside tub measurements, however, and allowing for the **overflow** pipe, a 14-inch tub height does not permit the drawing of a very deep bath.

Many semicustom homes feature 5' × 42" or 6' × 42" oval tubs in master baths. There are so many sizes and shapes of tubs, however, that there is no longer an "average" size.

Most state laws require that all bathtubs installed today have a **slip-resistant** bottom. Many tubs also come with a handle on one or both sides, which is extremely useful for the elderly or infirm.

The straight end of the bathtub contains the drain and the plumbing, such as faucets or **fittings,** and the overflow pipe; therefore, the location of the bathtub must be decided before the order is placed. Bathtubs may be ordered with a left or right drain, all four sides enclosed, the front and two sides enclosed, or the front and one side enclosed. For a completely built-in look, a drop-in model may be specified.

The drop-in model is sometimes installed as a sunken tub. Although a sunken tub may present a luxurious appearance, it can be difficult to get in and out of such tubs. In addition, sunken tubs can be difficult to clean. Cleaning a sunken tub means lying flat on the floor to reach the interior. Sunken or recessed tubs can present a safety hazard in that small children may crawl into the bathtub and hurt themselves or, at worst, drown.

Bathtubs are manufactured of several materials. The old standby is the porcelain enameled cast-iron tub, which was originally a high-sided bathtub raised from the floor on ball-and-claw feet with the underside exposed. This style is still available today in a modernized version from Kohler. Both the modernized version, Tellieur Suite, and the Historic™ bathtub are shown in Figure 10.1.

The porcelain enamel gives better color than other materials and is approximately 1/16 of an inch thick, but this finish can be chipped if a heavy object is dropped on it. Therefore, bathtubs should be kept covered with a blanket or a special plastic liner until construction has been completed.

A cast-iron bathtub is the most durable bathtub available, but it is expensive and heavy; it may weigh as much as 500 pounds. Therefore, the floor should be strong enough to bear the combined weight of the tub, the tub full of water, and the bather. Formed steel tubs with a porcelain enamel finish were developed to provide a lightweight (about 100 pounds) tub that would be less expensive than cast iron. Formed steel tubs are ideally suited for upper-story installations or for remodeling because they are easier to move into place than cast-iron tubs. A formed steel tub is noisier than a cast-iron tub, but a sound-deadening coating may be applied to the underside at an extra cost. If the bathtub does not come with an insulated coating on the outside, a roll of fiberglass insulation can be wrapped around the tub. This insulation not only helps the tub retain heat longer, but it also helps reduce noise. Because of the

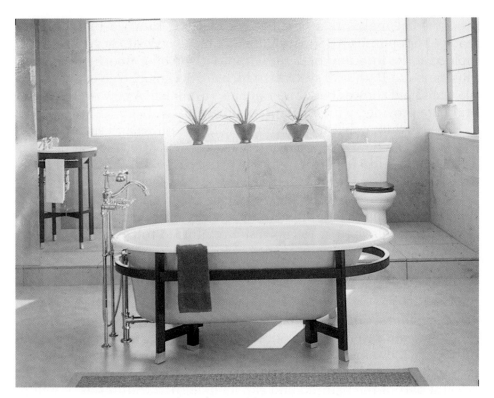

(a)

FIGURE 10.1
Tellieur Suite is shown in the large photo. A modernized version of the claw-foot bathtub is shown in the small photo. (Photo courtesy of Kohler Company)

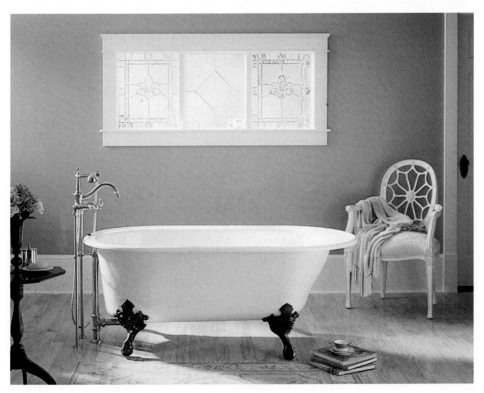

(b)

properties of steel, formed steel bathtubs may flex; therefore, they do not have as thick a layer of porcelain enamel as do cast-iron tubs.

If a cast-iron or steel bathtub is badly stained or chipped, it can be "replaced" without tearing out the walls to get access to the old tub. The product that makes this possible is called Re-Bath®, a bathtub liner made of nonporous ABS (acrylonic butadiene styrene) acrylic, custom molded to fit into any bathtub without disturbing flooring, walls, or plumbing. Re-Bath wall systems, which are designed to go over existing tile walls, and shower base liners are also available. A new overflow and drain are provided with Re-Bath tub liners.

Heavy-duty polyester reinforced with fiberglass and surfaced with a **gel coat** can be used for bathtubs. In specifying this type of tub, it is important to select a name brand. There are currently many poor-quality units on the market produced by a process that does not require a large investment. Consequently, the tubs can crack easily and lose their surface rapidly. Good maintenance practices and avoidance of abrasive cleansers are mandatory for polyester-reinforced tubs. Some manufacturers recommend using a coat of marine wax or a good automotive wax to restore the shine to dulled surfaces of gel-coat tubs.

Another type of lightweight bathtub is acrylic reinforced with fiberglass. This type of bathtub does not have such as a high gloss as the gel-coated ones, but maintenance is easier.

There are several advantages to acrylic-reinforced fiberglass bathtubs. First, they are much lighter weight than steel or cast iron, although they may not be as durable. Second, the tub surround can be cast as an integral part of the bathtub and can include such features as a built-in seat, soap ledges, and grab bars. The latter type of tub can be installed only in new construction, because the tub and surround are too large to be placed in a remodeled bathroom. For remodeling, molded tub units are available with wall surrounds in two, three, or four pieces that pass easily through doorways and join in the recessed bathtub area to form a one-piece unit.

Soaking tubs are also made from reinforced fiberglass. Instead of sitting or laying in the tub, one sits on a molded, built-in seat, and the tub is filled to the requisite depth. Some soaking tubs are recessed into the floor, and the bather steps over the edge and down into the tub; others are placed at floor level and require several steps to reach the top. Soaking tubs should not be installed in every bathroom in the house, because it is impossible to bathe small children in such tubs and the elderly or infirm will find it too dangerous to enter and leave a soaking tub. A regular bathtub should be installed in at least one bathroom in the house.

Jacuzzi was the inventor of the whirlpool bath, and his name is contained in both the Webster's and Oxford dictionaries. The name Jacuzzi® has become synonymous with whirlpool baths, but it is a registered trade name only to be used with Jacuzzi products. Whirlpool baths are generally bathroom fixtures; they must be drained after each use. The Jacuzzi uses continuous cast acrylic, reinforced with fiberglass for added strength. Quiet jets are placed low in the bath for the best results in hydrotherapy. These whirlpool jets create a circular pattern of bubbles as the air/water mixture flows into the tub, providing a deeply penetrating massage.

Jacuzzi's newest bath combines two exquisite hydrotherapy experiences. When operated as a whirlpool bath, patented Jacuzzi® Therapro™ jets create an extra wide, circular flow of air and water that deliver a powerful full-body massage, while Accupro™ jets ease tension with targeted deep tissue massage. When operated as a Pure Air® bath, Jacuzzi's patented 360 degree balanced airflow system produces thousands of warm effervescent bubbles.[2]

MORPHOSIS® ALPHA is the beginning of a new hydromassage concept conceived by renowned design house Pininfarina and inspired by nature that envelops, charms, and amazes. The arch that runs above the whirlpool bath represents a lovingly protective gesture, an abstract concept of a seashell, of a sail or of contemporary architecture. The perfection of double whirlpool baths: a unique idea to be shared between the two of you.[3]

Most companies manufacture a corner bath, which can be either a plain bath or, more often, a whirlpool. The corner location gives a feeling of openness because the tub does not have walls surrounding it and is only used for bathing, not for showering.

Spas or hot tubs are similar to whirlpool baths but need not be drained after each use. They are equipped with heat and filtration systems. Because the same water is recirculated, daily testing and maintenance of the proper water chemistry are required. Spas may be installed outside in warmer climates or in an area other than the bathroom. They have many of the same features as the whirlpool baths but are larger (64 to 84 inches long, 66 to 84 inches wide, and 28 to 37 inches high). Spas come with factory-installed redwood skirts and rigid covers.

Tub surrounds and shower enclosures may also be reinforced fiberglass, as mentioned previously, or they may be decorative laminate, ceramic tile, solid ABS, or solid acrylic. Many of these surrounds and enclosures have integrated tubs with built-in whirlpool systems. The all-in-one type eliminates the need to caulk around the area where the tub and surround meet. Failure to install and caulk the tub surround properly is the major cause of leaks in the tub area. When designing a bathroom, the bathtub should be placed where an access panel can be installed to simplify future plumbing repairs. Access *must* be provided to any whirlpool equipment to facilitate future maintenance. (See Figure 10.2.)

Ceramic tile is installed as described in Chapter 3. The substrate must be exterior-grade plywood or a special water-resistant grade of gypsum board. The backer board, mentioned in Chapter 4, also makes a suitable substrate. Particular attention must be paid to the application of the grout, because it is the grout that makes ceramic tile a waterproof material. When a cast-iron tub is used, the extra weight may cause a slight sagging of the floor. Any space caused by this settling should be caulked immediately.

SHOWERS

Showers may be installed for use in a bathtub or they may be in a separate shower stall. There should always be at least one bathtub in a house, but stall showers may be used in the remaining bathrooms. When used with a bathtub, the tub spout contains a **diverter** that closes off the spout and diverts the water to the shower head. A bathroom with

FIGURE 10.2
The Premier Stratford. This full-depth walk-in bathtub has a door that closes securely and is available with a hydrotherapy system, choice of showers, seat boosters, hand grips, and many other options. (Photo courtesy of Premier Bathtubs)

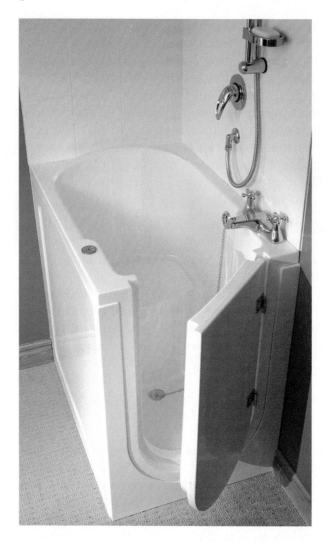

a shower instead of a tub is designated as a three-quarter bath. (See Figure 10.3.)

Stall showers are 34 inches square; a slightly larger 36-inch square is recommended if space is available. These are minimum requirements; deluxe showers may be 48 inches square or even 60 × 36 inches wide. The larger ones usually include a seat.

Stall showers may be constructed entirely of ceramic tile; in other words, the sloping base and walls are all made of tile. When installing a ceramic tile shower area, particular attention should be paid to the waterproof base and to the installation procedures supplied by the manufacturer or the Tile Council of North America. Other stall showers have a **preformed base,** with the surround touching the top of the 5- to 6-inch deep base. This preformed base is less slippery than a base of a tile but not quite as aesthetically pleasing. Shower walls may be constructed of any of the solid-surface materials. (See Chapter 9, p. 298.)

The standard height of a shower head is 66 inches for men and 60 inches for women, which puts the spray below the hairline. These measurements mean that the plumbing for the shower head must break through the tub or shower surround. Therefore, it is recommended that

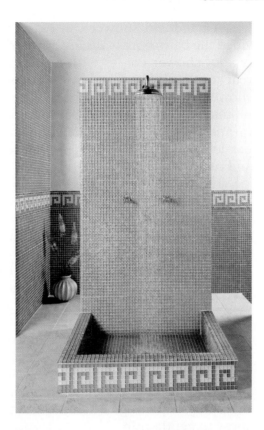

FIGURE 10.3A
This freestanding shower uses illuminessence glass mosaic tile, which won first place in the Ceramic and Tile category of *Flooring Magazine's* Innovation Award in 2004.The shower uses various 1″ × 1″ illuminessence glass water crystal mosaics in a combination of clear and frosted. (Photo courtesy of Crossville Inc.)

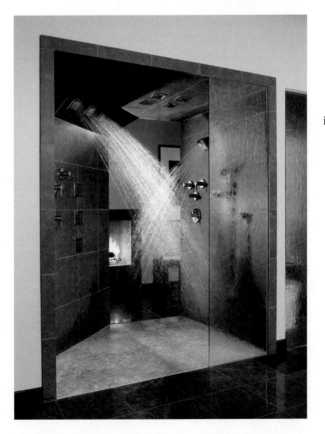

FIGURE 10.3B
Kohler elevates the act of showering to a luxurious experience that can be customized to accommodate individual preferences. With innovative products that are inspired by the evocative power of water, including single-function and multifunction showerheads with large diameters, as well as bodysprays and handshowers that offer unique water delivery, it's easy to create an experiential showering environment. (Photo courtesy of Kohler)

the shower **feed-in** be 74 inches above the floor. When placed at this height, the shower head should be adjustable so it can be used to wash hair or to hit below the hairline.

A handheld shower can easily be installed in any bathtub, provided the bathroom walls are covered with a waterproof material. This type of shower comes with a special diversion spout, and the water reaches the shower head by means of a flexible metal line. One type of shower head is hung on a hook at the required height. Another type is mounted on a 5-foot vertical rod and attached to the water outlet by means of a flexible hose. This full-range sliding-spray holder or grab bar locks at any desired height. The spray holder is both adjustable and removable.

Handheld showers have several advantages. Such showers can be hung at a lower level for use by children and can be used to rinse the hair of young children without the complaint of "the soap is getting in my eyes." In addition, handheld units may be used to clean and rinse the interior of the bathtub.

Shower heads more than 5 to 10 years old use between 3 and 8 gallons of water per minute. Replacing one of these with a model achieving a flow of 2.4 gallons per minute or less will save the average household almost 12,000 gallons of water annually. Water is a limited resource and should be conserved. Some cities have mandated 2.4-gallon shower heads. Water conservation does not mean a skimpy shower. Speakman Anystream® shower heads will automatically adjust water flow to compensate for available pressure. By means of the spray-adjusting T-handle, output ranges from bracing needle spray to gentle rain.

> Every aspect of the new GROHE Movario shower products line is geared toward individualizing showering choices. The line includes shower heads, hand showers and accessories all designed from top to bottom to satisfy ergonomic needs as well as meet market demand for multiple spray options and large spray faces for wide whole-body water coverage. At the heart of GROHE's Movario line, however, is the new RotaHead-System that enables Movario hand showers to convert from shower head to body spray functionality with the simple twist of a wrist.[4]

There are several ways to keep water within the shower area. One way is to hang a shower curtain from rings at the front of the shower. A shower curtain is a decorative feature, but unless care is taken to ensure placement of the shower curtain inside the base when using the shower, water may spill over onto the floor, causing a hazard. Glass shower doors are also used (the type depends on local building codes). All shower doors are made of tempered glass, but some codes require the addition of a wire mesh. These glass doors may pivot, hinge, slide, or fold. The major maintenance problem with glass doors involves removing soap and hard-water residue from the glass surface and cleaning the water channel at the base of the door. A water softener greatly reduces or even eliminates this residue. Some shower units are designed with close-fitting doors that completely enclose the front of the unit and become steam systems with a **sauna** effect

> The Allegro™ line from Sussman Lifestyle Group of contemporary saunas is a luxurious addition to almost any bathroom, master bedroom, exercise area or spare room in the home. Their

winding curves accentuate sleek shapes, while wide glass walls create a sense of bright spaciousness. Quality construction, high-grade woods, and abundant accessories qualify these enclosures as exceptional quality furniture.

Each Allegro sauna is modular in construction and self-contained. All large sections such as ceiling panels, benches, supports, trimming and lighting are ready for assembly, allowing installation in less than one afternoon. . . for a Lifetime of Pleasure®.[5]

Master bathroom showers are often designed so that no door or curtain is required. These shower stalls have walls so placed that the water is contained within the wet area.

Pittsburgh Corning Glass Block Shower systems supply the custom-built glass block shower—without the "custom" hassle. These systems are pre-designed to include, Premiere series glass block, customized acrylic bases in two standards colors, and five designer colors. The walk-in style is 72" × 51" and features a curved wall at the entrance. A door 28" × 69" in clear or hammered glass and gold or silver frames is included for the Classic and Neo Angle models. (See Figure 10.4.)

Wheelchair-accessible stall showers are available and vary in size from 42 by 36 inches to 65 by 36 inches, all with an interior threshold height of only 1/2 an inch. Units with integral seats have the seat placed toward the front of the enclosure for easier access. Hewi, Inc., manufactures a wide variety of accessories that will make for an accessible shower. These accessories include a fold-up seat, hanging seats, and grab bars, all available in 12 colors.

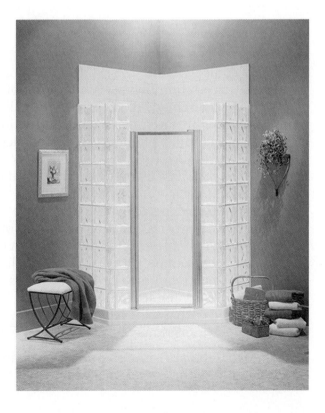

FIGURE 10.4
The Neo Angle shower from Pittsburgh Corning. (Photo courtesy of Pittsburgh Corning)

TUB AND SHOWER FAUCETS

Tub/shower combinations may be of two different types: deck mounted or wall mounted. Deck mounted are used only for tubs. Both types are available in single or dual control (hot and cold water are controlled together or separately). A shower-only unit has wall-mounted controls, which may be single or dual control. Single controls regulate the temperature of the water more easily. Two choices are available with a tub/shower combination: two sets (one for the tub and the other for the shower) or one set, with a diverter. The diverter in tub/shower combinations is most commonly a diverter-on-spout. After the water temperature is balanced, the diverter is pulled up to start the shower. To stop the flow of water to the shower head, the diverter is pushed down. The handle diverter design has three handles and, by twisting the middle handle, the water is diverted to the shower head. The two other handles control the hot and cold water. This handle diverter has 8-inch **centers.**

Most shower heads are adjustable and change the flow of water to drenching, normal, or fine spray. Some shower heads have a pulsating flow that provides a massaging action. Conventional shower heads use from 6 to 8 gallons of water per minute. Plumbing codes are being amended to make 2.7 gallons of water per minute at 60 psi the maximum amount of water that can be used. Antiscald controls are required by law on all shower heads. Many manufacturers have similar multijet showers.

Fast-flowing Roman tub valves feature high-flow 3/4-inch valves. This type of valve enables whirlpool baths to be filled rapidly, provided a large-capacity water tank is used. Like all other types of faucets, shower heads may come in white, brass, or a combination of brass and chrome.

LAVATORIES

Lavatories come in many sizes, shapes, and materials according to personal and space requirements. Many types of materials are used, but most lavatories are made of vitreous china. All of the following materials may be used, however: glass, cast iron, stainless steel, sculpted marble, china or ceramic, enameled steel, polished brass, or solid-surface materials. (See Figure 10.5a-d.)

Lavatories are usually round or oval, but they may also be rectangular, or even triangular for corner installations. Sizes range from 11 × 11 inches for powder rooms to 38 × 28 inches.

Pedestal lavatories are a newer style of lavatory, but they are probably more suitable in a master bathroom because they do not provide the adjacent counter area usually needed in family bathrooms. They may be as streamlined or decorative as desired. To compensate for the lack of counter space, some pedestal lavatories are as large as 44 × 22 inches, with a wide ledge surrounding the bowl area.

Built-in lavatories may be one of six types:

1. They may be self-rimming (where a hole is cut into the counter smaller than the size of the lavatory and the bowl is placed so that

the edge is raised above the level of the counter). With a self-rimming sink, water cannot be swept back into the bowl and must be mopped up.

2. For a flush counter and bowl installation, the lavatory may be installed with a flush metal rim. This is a popular and inexpensive style but can cause a cleaning problem at the juncture of the rim and the countertop.

3. The integral bowl and counter, such as those made of solid-surface materials, is another option. With this type, which may be placed virtually anywhere on the vanity top, the countertop and bowl are seamed for a one-piece look, with the faucets usually mounted on the counter.

4. An old-fashioned wall-hung installation is quite often used in powder rooms or for wheelchair users.

5. The lavatory is installed under the counter. This type of installation is generally used with a tile, marble, or synthetic countertop. Under-the-counter installations are becoming very popular and require that the fittings be deck mounted.

6. The lavatory can be installed above the counter; this is a modern version of the pitcher and bowl set of the Victorian era.

Glass lavatories are available in clear glass, cobalt, and aquamarine. Another specialty lavatory is a solid brass self-rimming bowl, which adds an elegant look to a bathroom. For a unique lavatory, a self-rimming painted ceramic washbasin may be used. These specialized sinks have wall- or counter-mounted faucets.

Porcher, from American Standard, has 20 custom colors and 11 special finishes, including polished copper, polished gold, and polished platinum. Porcher also offers embellishments of these same metals in a wide variety of patterns.

Lavatories come punched with one hole or three holes. The single hole is for European-style single-hole faucets. With single-control fittings and 4-inch centerset fittings, the third hole is for the **pop-up** rod. In wide-spread fittings, however, the third hole is used for the mixture of hot and cold water.

Some lavatories are punched with one or two extra holes. These holes are used as a shampoo lavatory and have a retractable spray unit. The second extra hole is for a soap or shampoo dispenser. Shampoo lavatories are extremely useful for a family with children because the bowl is usually installed in a 32-inch-high vanity (in contrast to the 36-inch height of a kitchen sink). Some styles of shampoo lavatories feature spouts that swing away.

In imported brochures, lavatories are often referred to as **basins.**

LAVATORY FAUCETS

Many types of lavatory faucets are currently available. The single-handle faucet was the invention of Alfred M. Moen, who invented it after being burned by the sudden flow of hot water. **Center-fit** faucet fittings have been used ever since the 1980s. With these units, the two handles and spout are in one piece, with a 4-inch spread. The

FIGURE 10.5A
Porcher Rock Ice.
(Photo courtesy of
American Standard)

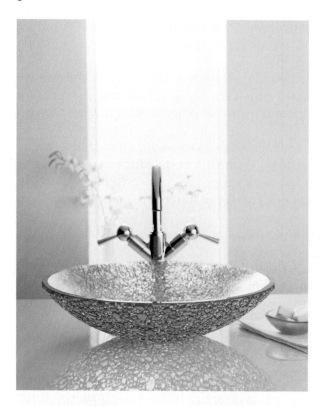

FIGURE 10.5B
Glass sink and counter with
wall-mounted faucet.
(Photos b, c, and d courtesy
of Kohler)

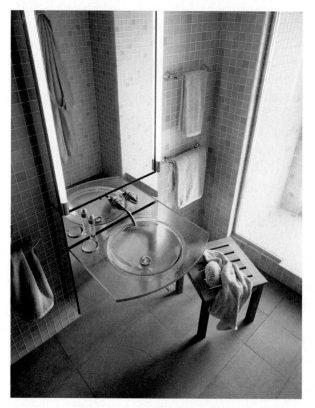

single-control unit with a 4-inch spread has a central control that
regulates both temperature and rate of flow. This single-control unit
may also work by means of a lever that, when pulled up, increases the
flow of water and, when pushed down, decreases the flow. Temperature

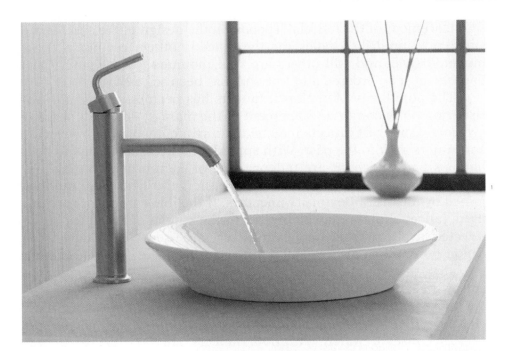

FIGURE 10.5C
Basin mounted on the counter with single-handle faucet.

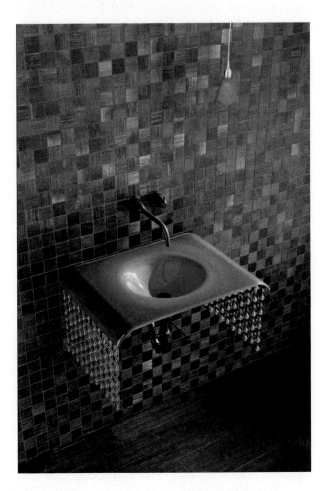

FIGURE 10.5D
Wall-hung all-in-one sink and counter with wall-mounted faucet.

is controlled by moving the lever to the right for cold and to the left for warm or hot water. For arthritis sufferers, the lever faucet is easier to operate than a knob type.

Placement of the faucets depends on the design of the sink. Some sinks have predrilled holes for the faucets, others require a deck-mounted style, and still others are wall mounted. (See Figure 9.11.) Faucets must be ordered after the sink has been selected.

The popularity of center-fit faucets has been declining; spread-fit fittings now comprise 80 percent of the market, and their share is growing. Center-fit faucets may be making a comeback, however, as consumers look to the past. With spread-fit faucets, the hot and cold handles and the spout are independent of each other. To make installation and choice of faucet sets easier, the fittings should be joined by means of flexible connectors. If flexible connectors are not used, faucet choices may be limited to the spread of the holes in the selected lavatory. When center-fit fittings are used, a plate covers the center hole. When a spread-fit fitting is used, the center hole accommodates the spout. Mini-wide faucets offer the appearance of spread-fit faucets and fit the common 4-inch center fit. Mini-wides are more difficult to clean, however, because the faucets are very close together.

To conserve water, bathroom faucets are now set to a flow of 2 gallons per minute. Most manufacturers are using a ceramic disc cartridge inside the faucet; ceramic disc cartridges are considered the most durable, especially with problem water. The cartridge helps prevent dripping, which can waste gallons of water each year.

Several companies are now manufacturing faucets designed as barrier-free products with water conservation in mind. When the faucet's electronic sensor beam is broken by the hands, water flows at the preset temperature. Savings of up to 85 percent over normal water usage are typical. Additional energy savings are realized because hot water is conserved.

Faucets may be polished chrome, black chrome, polished brass, or even gold plated. A current trend is to use two different finishes on the same faucet, such as black chrome with polished chrome and/or polished brass, or wood and brass. Brushed nickel with brass is often used. Two finishes are often used on what is known as the ring handle (circular handles with no extended part). Delta Faucet Company manufactures ring handles suitable for retrofit, so the bathroom can be given a new appearance without great cost.

Usually chrome is the most durable finish, followed by colors and then brass. With the introduction of the PVD process, brass is now a viable choice. Delta, a Masco company, uses Brilliance® on its brass bathroom fittings, with the pop-up drain (usually the first part of the faucet assembly to show wear) also being coated.

Translucent and metal handles have slight indentations to provide a nonslip surface. The handles may also be of a lever type. The traditional shape for spouts is being replaced by a more delicately curved shape, which is popular in Europe. The Roman-style faucets previously used for bathtubs are now being used for lavatories.

The new Europlus II® faucet from GROHE has a user-friendly "loop style" handle, making one-finger control of both water temperature and volume effortless. This is a particularly important consideration for people with physical limitations. (See Figure 10.6.)

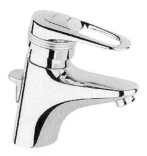

FIGURE 10.6A
The Grohe Europlus II Faucet with loop handle.
(Courtesy of Grohe, America, Inc.)

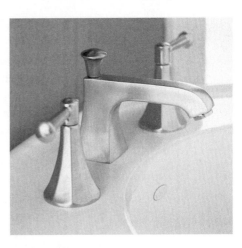

FIGURE 10.6C
The Bol™ Ceramic Faucet. (Photo
Courtesy of Kohler)

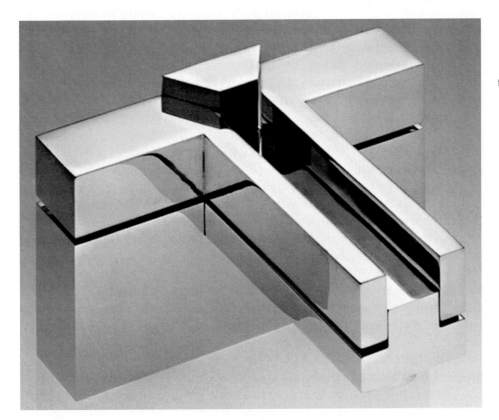

FIGURE 10.6B
The Phoenix Lav Set. The
handles of this unique 4″
center faucet turn outward
to operate. (Photo Courtesy
of Paul Decorative)

Pull-out spouts, which have previously been a feature of kitchen
faucets, are now used for lavatories.

Wrist-control handles, which meet the standards of the Americans
with Disability Act, do not require turning or pulling but are activated
by a push or pull with the wrist rather than the fingers.

TOILETS

In Europe, a toilet is often called a *water closet*. The plumbing trade frequently uses that term, or *closet*, when referring to what the layperson calls a toilet. In some areas of the United States, the toilet may also be called a commode. We will use the word *toilet* in the text because this is the more common word, but when talking to a plumber, *closet* is more correct.

Toilet bowls and tanks are constructed of vitreous china. Only vitreous china can withstand the acids to which a toilet is subjected. Most toilets are designed with water-saving devices that are important both economically and environmentally.

There are two basic shapes to a toilet: regular or round bowl and the elongated bowl. Most toilets do not come with a toilet seat; therefore, it is important to know the shape of the toilet before ordering a seat. Some special-shape expensive toilets come with a seat. More space, (usually 2 inches) is required for installing an elongated-bowl toilet. Local building codes will provide space requirements.

Toilets may be wall hung, which leaves the floor unobstructed for easy cleaning, or floor mounted. Wall-hung toilets have a wall outlet; in other words, they flush through a drain in the wall. To support the weight of a wall-hung toilet, 6-inch studs must be used and an L-shaped unit called a chair carrier must be installed.

Floor-mounted toilets flush through the floor or the wall. For concrete floor construction, wall outlets are suggested to eliminate the extra cost of slab piercing.

Another choice in the design of toilets is whether tank and bowl should be a **low-profile,** one-piece integral unit, or whether the tank and bowl should be in two pieces. For space saving in powder rooms or bathrooms, a corner toilet, an Eljer exclusive, is available. An old-fashioned ambience can be created by using an overhead wall-hung tank with a traditional pull chain. In areas where condensation on the toilet tank is a problem, an insulated tank may be ordered.

All toilets are required to have a visible water turn-off near the bowl on the back wall in case of a faulty valve in the tank.

Toilets have different flushing actions: gravity flush and pressure assisted. Gravity flush uses nothing more than water weight to generate flushing pressure and will work with very low **water pressure** from the water supply system. The pressure-assisted type is described next.

The 1992 National Energy Policy Act limited water use for new toilets to 1.6 gallons per flush, compared with the typical 3.5-gallon models. For a family of four, that amounts to a savings of more than 11,000 gallons of water per year. A European import even has double-handed flushers to vary how much water is used in each flush. However, when this new law went into effect, the new toilets were not very efficient and often resulted in double flushes, which defeated the purpose of the law. All the major plumbing manufacturers now use the *FLUSHMATE*® vessel from the Sloan Valve company.

The toilet actually contains a tank inside a tank. That is, the pressure-assist vessel resides within the tank of the toilet. When you lift the lid, you see the pressure-assist vessel. This vessel holds all of the water used by the toilet.

As water enters the vessel . . . the air inside is trapped and compressed. A built-in regulator limits incoming water pressure to 35 pounds per square inch, or about the same as a garden hose.

When the vessel's internal pressure reaches 35 psi the toilet is ready to flush. When flushed air pressure pushes water through the toilet at almost three times the rate of a traditional gravity system. The whole flush cycle takes less than a minute. (The pushing action of the pressure-assist vessel requires the bowl to be designed differently, which means a gravity toilet cannot be retrofitted with a pressure-assist vessel.) [See Figure 10.7.][6]

Flushmate-equipped water closets have **trapways** specifically designed to allow waste to be extracted earlier in the flush. Water is contained in the Flushmate vessel, resulting in a nonsweating

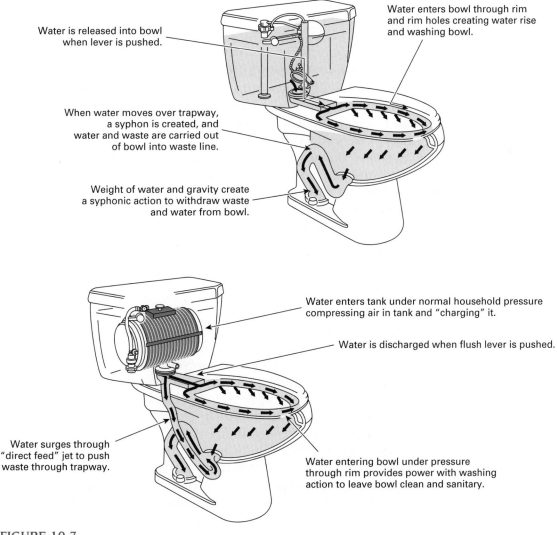

FIGURE 10.7
Flushing action. (Courtesy of American Standard Inc., *The Bathroom Book***)**

toilet—so the floor around the toilet remains dry and there is no need for an insuliner tank.

Toto®'s Dual-Max (Flushing system allows you to choose appropriate level of water usage-without comprising flushing performance. Select either 1.6 gallons per flush or .09 gallons per flush, and Dual-Max delivers optimum flushing performance while offering maximum water conservation.)[7]

Kohler produces the Ingenium™ flushing system, which results in a quiet, controlled flush that minimizes noise and splash while the sustained swirling motion of water rinses the bowl clean. Another of Kohler's innovations is the Purist Hatbox toilet. (See Figure 10.8.)

Allow 36 × 36 inches of clearance space in front of the toilet or bidet, 16 inches from the center of the fixture to an adjacent wall or fixture.

Toilets for elderly and disabled individuals have an 18-inch-high seat, whereas regular toilet seats are 15 1/2 inches high. Higher toilets may also have a set of metal rails or armrests for extra support. The height of the seat on one-piece toilets may be less than 18 inches. (See Figure 10.9.)

BIDETS

Although bidets are common in Europe, they are only now becoming an accepted fixture in American bathrooms, and only in more sophisticated types of installations. A bidet is generally installed as a companion and adjacent to the water closet or toilet and is used for cleansing the perineal area. Bidets do not have seats. The user sits astride the bowl, facing the controls that regulate water temperature and operate the pop-up drain and transfer valve. Water enters the bidet via the spray rinse in the bottom of the bowl. A bidet may also be used as a foot bath when the pop-up drain is closed.

When the fresh water supply is below or directly involved with piping, a **vacuum breaker** must be installed.

COUNTERTOPS

The term *vanity cabinet* is not technically used in the architectural profession. Ready-made bathroom cabinets containing the lavatory are so often called and sold by this name, however, that this term is used to refer to the prefinished cabinet with doors underneath the countertop. Vanity cabinets may be ordered with or without a finished countertop. The lavatory is purchased separately. Other types of vanities come with the countertop and bowl molded in one.

A ready-made vanity is between 29 and 30 inches in height. For a master bathroom in a custom-designed house, the counter can be raised to suit personal requirements; however, some building codes state that at least one vanity in the house must be at the lower height.

Most custom-designed bathrooms have specially designed cabinets containing the lavatory with a storage area beneath. A bathroom countertop may be made of the same materials as a kitchen counter,

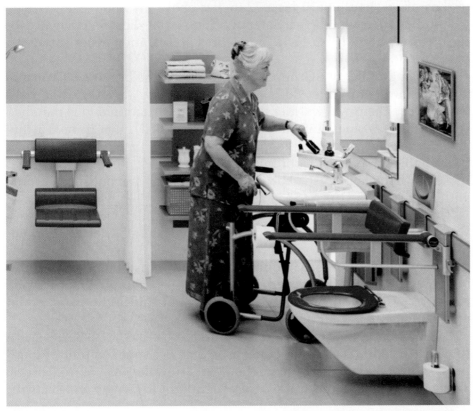

FIGURE 10.8
Purist Hatbox toilet. (Photo
courtesy of Kohler)

FIGURE 10.9
Barrier Free Bathroom.
(Photo courtesy of Pressalit
Care, Inc.)

although marble is more frequently used in bathrooms than in kitchens.

Solid-surface materials for countertops, vanities, lavatory bowls, showers, and bathtubs are becoming increasingly popular because they are versatile and attractive.

ACCESSORIES

There should be 22 inches of towel storage for each person. Towels should be within convenient reach of the bath, shower, and lavatory. Soap containers may be recessed into the wall, such as those used in the tub area. For the lavatory with a counter, a soap dish can be a colorful accessory. A toilet tissue dispenser should be conveniently placed next to the toilet. Many faucet manufacturers that make designer model faucets also make bath accessories to match.

Ergonomic design is a fundamental element of HEWI products for universal design. These include either fixed or stationary support bars—which may also be used as towel bars—grab bars, and an adjustable mirror, with nylon frame and lever-handle turn control.

Ground fault interrupter (**GFI**) electrical outlets must also be provided for the myriad of electrical gadgets used in the bathroom. All switches should be located so they cannot be reached from a tub or shower area. (This is usually stated in local building codes.) All electrical switches should be at least 60 inches away from water sources.

Mirrors may be on the door of a built-in medicine cabinet, or they may be installed to cover the entire wall over the counter area. When used in the latter manner, mirrors visibly enlarge the bathroom. The top of the mirror should be at least 72 inches above the floor.

Robern manufactures a Safety Lock box that slides into a wall cabinet, as shown in Figure 10.10, and stores prescription drugs safely out of reach.

Sussman Lifestyle Groups has introduced the brand new Warma-Towel®, an amenity that adds comfort and cozy warmth to the bath experience. The towel warmer is all-brass construction and is matched with a stainless-steel built-in heater for controlled, quiet heat. Warma-Towel comes in a variety of floor, pivoting, and wall models. Each model is available in polished chrome, polished brass, Regal gold, bright nickel, satin nickel, brushed black nickel (pewter), and polished chrome with Regal gold accents. (See Figure 10.11.)

Special cabinets may contain pull-out laundry hampers, tilt-out waste baskets, drawer organizers for cosmetics and toiletries, and appliance garages for personal appliances.

Ventilating fans are required in bathrooms that do not have windows that can be opened. Broan-Nutone manufactures a wide range of ventilation products for residential and light commercial applications.

Broan has a new exhaust fan, Solitaire® Ultra Silent® Series, with the industry's lowest sound levels, as low as 0.3 sones (a unit of loudness), which is silent to the ear and measurable only by machines. These fan units incorporate a 7-watt nightlight for safety and security.

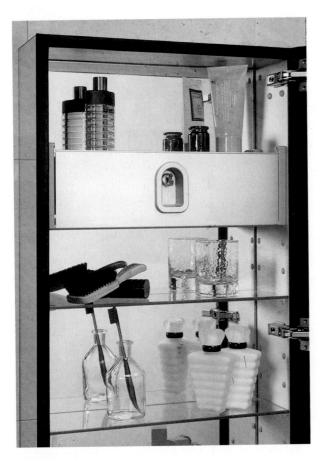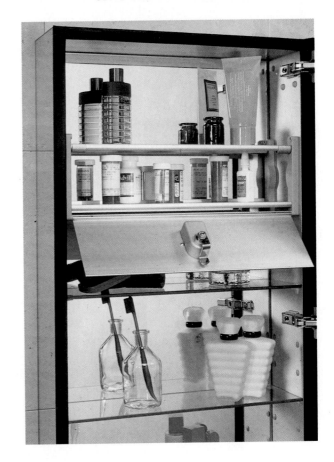

FIGURE 10.10
The Safety Lock medicine cabinet from Robern is shown open and closed. This Safety Lock box offers a safe place to store prescription drugs out of reach of children. (Photos courtesy of Robern Inc.)

Ventilating fans for bathrooms often incorporate a light and sometimes a heater.

Certified Bathroom Designers (**CBDs**) perform the same services for bathroom design as CKDs do for kitchen design.

PUBLIC RESTROOMS

The bathrooms previously discussed were designed to accommodate one or two people at a time. In public restrooms, however, conditions and location may mean that the bathroom will be used by many people at the same time. (This includes not only people who can walk, but those who use wheelchairs and those who walk with impaired mobility.)

Title III of the ADA requires all new construction of public accommodations and commercial facilities meet or exceed ADA Accessibility Guidelines for Buildings and Facilities (ADAAG) specifications.

According to Bobrick Washroom Equipment Inc.,

Public washrooms are one of the most critical building amenities with regard to accessibility and function for people with disabilities. With one in four persons becoming disabled sometime during

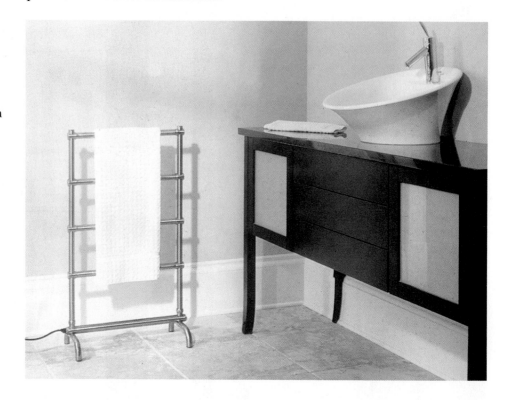

their life, washrooms need to be responsive to a wide range of human needs and abilities: including people without disabilities and those using wheelchairs and walking aids, people with sight or hearing disabilities, impaired coordination, cardiac or pulmonary disorders, and even people affected by temporary illness, pregnancy, or advanced age. The ADA requires that all washrooms, whether newly constructed or remodeled, be usable by people with disabilities. This means that some of each type of fixture or feature must meet barrier-free requirements. . . . **All building plans, however, should be confirmed with local jurisdictions to ensure job compliance.**[8]

Bobrick publishes a brochure, *Barrier-Free Washroom Planning Guide*, that includes diagrams to aid in making public restrooms accessible for wheelchair-bound individuals. (See Figure 10.12.) This planning guide also has specifications for water closets serving children ages 3 through 12, and also the forward and side reach of various ages of children.

Universal design can be accomplished in some instances by simply using the same item for everyone; sometimes positioning an item differently; at other times by modifying or replacing a single manufactured feature of an item; and in some circumstances by replacing an item with one that is more adjustable or adaptable. Universal design eliminates radically different looking items and special labels (e.g., handicapped), and the stigma associated with them, while providing choices for all users.[9]

Elkay offers a wide selection of items that are ADA compliant, such as water coolers, drinking fountains, sinks, and faucets. Elkay's drinking fountains have the WaterSentry Filter System, which removes lead,

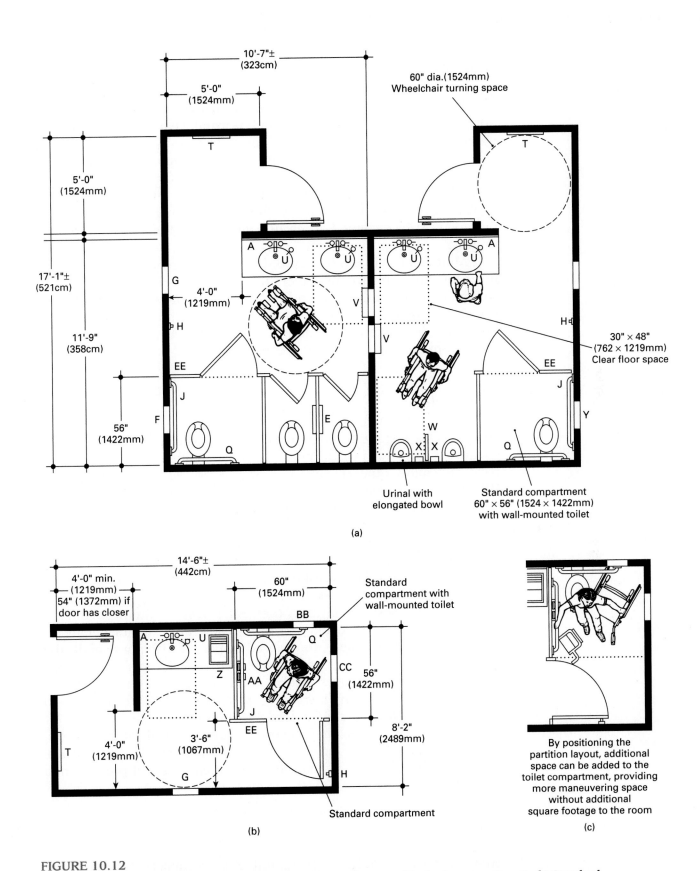

FIGURE 10.12

Small barrier-free public washrooms. (a) Small public washroom with single compartment. (b) Standard compartment meeting minimum ADAAG requirements. (c) Standard alcove compartment provides greater accessibility. By positioning the partition layout, space can be added to the toilet compartment, providing more maneuvering space without adding square footage to the room. (Courtesy of Bobrick Washroom Equipment Inc.)

Labels within figure (a):
- 10'-7"± (323cm)
- 5'-0" (1524mm)
- 60" dia.(1524mm) Wheelchair turning space
- 5'-0" (1524mm)
- 17'-1"± (521cm)
- 11'-9" (358cm)
- 4'-0" (1219mm)
- 30" × 48" (762 × 1219mm) Clear floor space
- 56" (1422mm)
- Urinal with elongated bowl
- Standard compartment 60" × 56" (1524 × 1422mm) with wall-mounted toilet
- (a)

Labels within figure (b):
- 14'-6"± (442cm)
- 4'-0" min. (1219mm) 54" (1372mm) if door has closer
- 60" (1524mm)
- Standard compartment with wall-mounted toilet
- 56" (1422mm)
- 8'-2" (2489mm)
- 4'-0" (1219mm)
- 3'-6" (1067mm)
- Standard compartment
- (b)

Labels within figure (c):
- By positioning the partition layout, additional space can be added to the toilet compartment, providing more maneuvering space without additional square footage to the room
- (c)

chlorine, and sediment from the water. It also provides an extra level of protection by removing cysts, such as cryptosporidium and giardia, from the water.[10]

Public restrooms receive much physical abuse, most of which is not premeditated but occurs through normal wear and tear. Unfortunately, vandalism is a major problem; therefore, fixtures and materials must be selected for durability. Bobrick manufactures a line of Maximum-Security Accessories™ that are mostly secured from the rear. Mirrors are bright, polished stainless steel. A two-stall restroom in a small restaurant and a multistall restroom in a huge recreational facility must be designed differently with this potential for vandalism in mind.

Maintenance is another factor in the selection of materials and fixtures for public restrooms. Floors are usually made of ceramic tile or similar material and require a floor drain, not only for an emergency flooding situation, but also to simplify cleaning and disinfecting of the floor. For the hospitality buildings, such as hotels, durable and functional commercial accessories are available.

Lavatories

To aid in cleaning the counter areas of public restrooms, vitreous china lavatories with flush metal rims are most frequently specified. Such lavatories allow quick cleaning of any excess water on the counter. White sinks are usually selected in restrooms for two reasons: They are cheaper and cleanliness is more easily visible.

Lavatories come with three holes punched in the top, but soft or liquid soap dispensers may be installed in a four-hole sink. Or, the soap dispenser may be attached to the wall above each lavatory or between two adjacent ones. For freestanding applications, wall-hung vitreous china lavatories may be specified.

A specially designed lavatory that meets ADA requirements must be installed to enable the seated person to reach faucet handles. Faucets, toilets, and washroom accessories used by people with physical disabilities must meet ADA specifications for controls and operating mechanisms (push buttons, valves, knobs, and levers): *They must be operable with one hand, without tight grasping, pinching, or twisting of the wrist, and with a force that does not exceed 5 pounds of force.*

Because some wheelchair occupants are paraplegic, it is important to turn down the temperature of hot water to 110°F and wrap the waste pipe with some form of insulation. These measures will prevent inadvertent burns.

Faucets

Some companies specialize in manufacturing faucets designed to be used in public restrooms. These faucets are available with **metering devices,** usually of the push-button type, that can be adjusted to flow for 5 to 15 seconds. This metering conserves energy and water and prevents accidental flooding. Other faucets have an electronic eye; when the beam is broken, the faucet turns on and stays on as long as there is continuous motion (such as hands being washed) in the sensor field. By reacting to motion and not to beam obstructions, they can help conserve water, minimize vandalism, and reduce maintenance time. Common obstructions, such as soap and water, will not disrupt normal operation. If the sensor is covered completely, the faucet will shut off in 12 seconds. Most electronic faucets have temperature controls to eliminate the chance of scalding.

Faucets manufactured for commercial use can be fitted with anti-vandal devices, which require special tools to dismantle.

Toilets

Wall-hung toilets are often used in public restrooms to facilitate cleaning. The toilet seats do not have lids and must have an open front. To aid in quicker maintenance and to avoid vandalism, toilets in public restrooms do not usually use a conventional tank, but instead have a **flush valve.** This valve requires greater water pressure than residential toilets, but uses less water and is easier to maintain. This type of valve is not used in private residences because it is too noisy. It may be operated by hand or sometimes by a foot pedal.

Installation of the Sloan OPTIMA®-equipped Flushometer provides the ultimate in sanitary protection and automatic operation plus the water economy that makes it the most advanced flushing system ever. There are no handles to trip or buttons to push. The Flushometer uses adaptive infrared technology to sense the user's presence and initiates the flushing cycle once the user steps away.

Another electronic method of flushing is that when there is no longer pressure on the seat, the toilet will flush automatically.

There is a great need for more stalls in ladies' rooms than in the men's restrooms. Some architects are beginning to realize this need after seeing long lines outside the ladies' rooms at sporting events and other public affairs.

Several different types of **urinals** may be used in the men's room. All are constructed of vitreous china, and all have integral flushing rims. One type is a stall urinal mounted on the floor. Others may be wall hung. A wall-hung unit with an elongated front is designed for use by the physically disabled, and meets ADA requirements. Urinals also have automatic flushing similar to the toilets mentioned earlier.

Stall Partitions

There are many different styles of stall dividers and many different materials from which to select. The **pilasters** may be floor anchored, ceiling hung, overhead braced, or floor-to-ceiling anchored. Ceiling types minimize maintenance but require structural steel support in the ceiling. Stalls are 32 to 36 inches wide and 56 to 60 inches high. However, doors are 22 to 29 inches wide for in-swinging doors and 32 to 36 inches wide for out-swinging doors. The difference in the width measurement is made up by stiles, which vary between 3 to 24 inches, depending on requirements. Doors of regular stalls open into the stall, whereas some wheelchair-accessible stalls have out-swinging doors that are 34" wide with an overall size of 60" wide by 59" deep.

Bobrick, in its *Barrier-Free Washroom Planning Guide,* offers complete instructions regarding size and location of stalls, toilets, lavatories, and all accessories.

The material used for partitions may be galvanized steel primed and finished with two coats of baked enamel, stainless steel, seamless high-pressure decorative laminate, or even marble. All of these finishes come in a variety of colors and may be coordinated with the colors used for washroom accessories, vanity centers, shelves, and countertops.

When the design of restrooms dictates, entrance screens for privacy should be used. It is important to consider the direction the door opens and placement of mirrors to ensure privacy.

Urinal screens are used in men's restrooms. These screens may be wall hung, floor anchored, ceiling hung, or supported by a narrow stile going from floor to ceiling, in a similar manner to the stall partitions. Urinal screens are placed between each urinal or between the urinal area and other parts of the restroom.

Accessories

Washroom accessories must not project more than 4 inches into a clear access aisle if their leading edge is between 27 and 80 inches above the finish floor; if their leading edge is at or below 27 inches, then they may project any amount as long as the required minimum width of an adjacent clear access aisle is maintained. This standard is specifically designed to ensure detection by visually impaired people. It is recommended that all floor-standing and surface-mounted units projecting more than 4 inches be located in corners, alcoves, or between other structural elements so as not to be a hazard to visually impaired people or interfere with access aisles or wheelchair turning areas. Fully recessed accessories are the preferred choice throughout universally designed washrooms.

As mentioned previously, soap dispensers may be installed on the lavatory rim itself. This type is preferable because any droppings from the dispenser are washed away in the bowl; the dry-powder type usually leaves a mess on the counter area. To meet ADA standards, soap dispensers installed over lavatories must be mounted so that their push buttons are no higher than 54 inches above the finish floor. Paper towel dispensers should be within easy reach of the lavatory, along with towel disposal containers. Sometimes both these accessories come in one wall-hung or wall-recessed unit. Another method of hand drying is the heated air blower. At the push of a button, heated air is blown out and the hands are rubbed briskly until dry. This type of hand dryer eliminates the mess of paper towel disposal, but if the dryer breaks down there is no way to dry the hands. Newer hand dryers operate electronically, similar to automatic faucets; in other words, they start when the hands are positioned under the blower and turn off when the hands are removed. There are also automatic motion-controlled paper towel dispensers, which spew out a sheet of paper towels.

Each toilet compartment requires a toilet tissue dispenser; an optional accessory is the toilet seat cover dispenser. A feminine product disposal container is necessary in each stall in a ladies' room. A napkin and tampon vending machine should be placed outside, near the toilet stalls. A hook for hanging pocketbooks and jackets is optional in toilet stalls. The preferred location for a hook is on the handle side of the door so no personal items are left behind. Another optional accessory in ladies' toilet stalls is a flip-down shelf that holds packages off the floor area.

In stalls for use by individuals with disabilities, stainless steel grab bars are required by law to be mounted on the wall nearest the toilet. They are 1 1/2 inch in diameter and 1 1/2 inches from the wall and 33 inches from the floor. Local building codes vary, so it is important to consult the codes for exact measurements.

There are two methods of transfer for wheelchair-bound people, depending on their abilities. Those who are able to stand with support can pull themselves upright by means of the grab bars. Others have to use the side transfer method, in which the arm of the wheelchair is removed and the individuals lean across the toilet and pull themselves onto the seat. The side transfer method requires a larger stall, because the chair must be placed alongside the toilet; front transfer requires only the depth of the chair plus standing room in front of the toilet.

BIBLIOGRAPHY

Bobrick Washroom Equipment Inc. *Barrier-Free Washroom Planning Guide*. Los Angeles, CA: Author, 2005.

Mazzurco, Philip. *Bath Design*. New York: Whitney Library of Design, an imprint of Watson-Guptil Publications, 1986.

GLOSSARY

basin.   A European term for a lavatory.

bidet.   A sanitary fixture for cleansing the genitourinary area of the body.

CBD.   Certified Bathroom Designer.

center fit.   Two handles and one spout mounted on a single plate.

centers.   Another way of saying "on centers"; in other words, the measurement is from the center of one hole to the center of the second hole.

compartmented.   Bathroom divided into separate areas according to function and fixtures.

diverter.   Changes flow of water from one area to another.

feed-in.   Where the rough plumbing is attached to the fittings.

fitting.   Another word for the faucet assembly; a term used by the plumbing industry.

flush valve.   Designed to supply a fixed quantity of water for flushing purposes.

gel coat.   A thin outer layer of resin, sometimes containing pigment, applied to a reinforced plastic moulding to improve its appearance.

GFI.   Ground fault interrupter. A special electrical outlet for areas where water is present.

lavatory.   The plumbing industry's name for a bathroom sink.

low profile.   A one-piece toilet with almost-silent flushing action. There are almost no dry surfaces on the bowl interior.

metering device.   A preset, measured amount of water is released when the metering device is activated.

overflow.   A pipe in bathtubs and lavatories used to prevent flooding. The pipe is located just below the rim or top edge of these fixtures.

pedestal.   A lavatory on a base attached to the floor rather than set into a counter surface. The base hides all the waste pipes that are usually visible.

pilaster.   Vertical support member, varying in width.

pop-up rod.   The rod that controls the raising and lowering of the drain in the bottom of the lavatory.

preformed base.   Shower pan or base of terrazzo or acrylic.

sauna.   A steam bath of Finnish origin.

slip-resistant.   Special material on the bottom of the tub to prevent falls.

spa.   Whirlpool-type bath for more than one person, with a heating and filtration system. Frequently installed outside in warmer climates.

spread.   Distance between holes of a bathtub or lavatory faucet.

surround.   The walls encircling a bathtub or shower area.

trapway.   The snake-like tubing at the back of the toilet that water flushes through. The better designed and larger the trapway, the less chance there is for clogs.

urinals.   Wall-hung vitreous plumbing fixtures used in men's rooms, with flushing devices for cleaning purposes.

vacuum breaker.   A device that prevents water from being siphoned into the potable water system.

vanity.   Laypersons' term for a prefabricated lavatory and base cabinet.

water pressure.   Measured as so many pounds per square inch, usually 30 to 50 psi.

wet wall.   The wall in which the water and waste pipes are located.

wrist control.   Long lever handles operated by pressure of the wrist rather than with fingers.

NOTES

[1]Linda Trent, "Combining Kitchen and Bath Elements," *Interiors & Sources*, April 1994.

[2]Jacuzzi website, www.jacuzzi.com.

[3]Ibid.

[4]Grohe America website, www.grohe.com.

[5]Sussman Lifestyle Group website, www.sussmanlifestylegroup.com.

[6]Flushmate website, www.flushmate.com.

[7]Website www.totousa.com.

[8]Bobrick Washroom Equipment Inc., *Barrier-Free Washroom Planning Guide*, Los Angeles, CA: Author, 2005, p. 2.

[9]Ibid.

[10]Elkay ADA Compliant Products, Elkay, Oak Brook, IL 60523.

Measurements

METRIC CONVERSION TABLE

This simple metric conversion chart contains equivalents only for the linear measurements taken from the textbook.

Some other quantities such as gallons, pounds, square yards, and temperatures may be converted from the following figures:

To convert square yards to square meters multiply square yards by .80

To convert gallons to liters, multiply gallons by 3.8

To convert pounds to kilograms, multiply pounds by 0.45

To convert Fahrenheit to Celsius, subtract 32 from the Fahrenheit amount and multiply by 5/9

IN.	CM	IN.	CM	IN.	CM	FT	M
1/000	0.003	4	10.16	36	91.44	1	3.05
1/16	0.16	4 1/4	10.80	37	93.98	2	6.10
3/32	0.24	5	12.70	39	99.06	3	9.14
1/8	0.32	6	15.24	40	101.60	4	12.19
5/32	0.40	7	17.78	42	106.68	5	15.24
3/16	0.48	8	20.32	44	111.76	6	18.29
1/4	0.64	9	22.86	46 1/2	118.11	7	21.34
5/16	0.79	10	25.40	48	121.92	8	24.38
3/8	0.95	11	27.94	52	132.08	9	27.43
7/16	1.11	12	30.48	54	137.16	10	30.48
1/2	1.27	14	35.56	55	139.70	12	2.7
5/8	1.59	15	38.10	59	149.86	15	4.5
3/4	1.91	18	45.72	60	152.40	22	6.6
7/8	2.22	19 1/2	49.53	64	162.56	25	7.5
1	2.54	20	50.80	66 1/2	168.91	28	8.4
1 1/16	2.70	22	55.88	72	182.88	37	11.1
1 1/4	3.18	23	58.42	78	198.12	64	19.2
1 1/2	3.81	24	60.96	82	208.28	66	19.8
2	5.08	27	68.58	84	213.36	100	30.0
2 1/4	5.72	29	73.66	90	228.60		
2 3/8	6.03	30	76.20	91	231.14		
2 3/4	6.99	30 1/2	77.47	96	243.84		
3	7.62	32	81.28				
3 1/8	7.94	33	83.82				
3 5/8	9.21	34	86.36				
3 7/8	9.84	35 3/4	90.81				

Index